Muscles, Nerves and Movement
KINESIOLOGY IN DAILY LIVING

D0745342

Muscles, Nerves
KINESIOLOGY

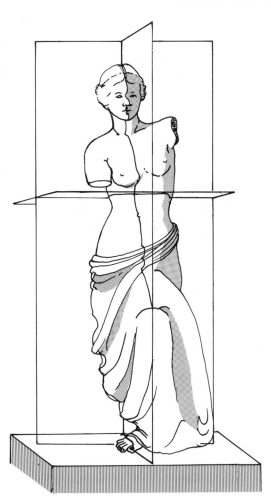

and Movement
IN DAILY LIVING

SECOND EDITION

BARBARA TYLDESLEY TDipCOT MEd
Department of Occupational Therapy,
School of Health Sciences,
University of Liverpool,
PO Box 147,
Liverpool L69 3BX

JUNE I GRIEVE BSc MSc
Formerly Department of Occupational Therapy,
School of Health and Paramedical Studies,
Brunel University College,
Osterley Campus,
Borough Road,
Isleworth,
Middlesex TW7 5DU

Blackwell Science

© 1996 by
Blackwell Science Ltd
Editorial Offices:
Osney Mead, Oxford OX2 0EL
25 John Street, London WC1N 2BL
23 Ainslie Place, Edinburgh EH3 6AJ
238 Main Street, Cambridge
  Massachusetts 02142, USA
54 University Street, Carlton
  Victoria 3053, Australia

Other Editorial Offices:
Arnette Blackwell SA
  224, Boulevard Saint Germain
  75007 Paris, France

Blackwell Wissenschafts-Verlag
GmbH
  Kurfürstendamm 57
  10707 Berlin, Germany

  Zehetnergasse 6
  A-1140 Wien
  Austria

All rights reserved. No part of
this publication may be reproduced,
stored in a retrieval system, or
transmitted, in any form or by any
means, electronic, mechanical,
photocopying, recording or
otherwise, except as permitted by the
UK Copyright, Designs and Patents
Act 1988, without the prior
permission of the publisher.

First edition published by
Blackwell Scientific Publications 1989
Reprinted 1991, 1993, 1995
Second edition published by
Blackwell Science Ltd 1996

Set in 10 on 13 pt Palatino
by Best-set Typesetter Ltd., Hong
Kong
Printed and bound in Great Britain by
The Alden Press, Oxford and
Northampton

The Blackwell Science logo is a
trade mark of Blackwell Science Ltd,
registered at the United Kingdom
Trade Marks Registry

DISTRIBUTORS

Marston Book Services Ltd
PO Box 269
Abingdon
Oxon OX14 4YN
(*Orders:* Tel: 01235 465500
        Fax: 01235 465555)

USA
Blackwell Science, Inc.
238 Main Street
Cambridge, MA 02142
(*Orders:* Tel: 800 215-1000
        617 876-7000
        Fax: 617 492-5263)

Canada
Copp Clark, Ltd
2775 Matheson Blvd East
Mississauga, Ontario
Canada, L4W 4P7
(*Orders*: Tel: 800 263-4374
        905 238-6074)

Australia
Blackwell Science Pty Ltd
54 University Street
Carlton, Victoria 3053
(*Orders:* Tel: 03 9347 0300
        Fax: 03 9349 3016)

A catalogue record for this title
is available from the British Library

ISBN 0-632-03603-6

Library of Congress
Cataloging-in-Publication Data
Tyldesley, Barbara.
    Muscles, nerves, and
  movement: kinesiology in
  daily living/Barbara Tyldesley,
  June I. Grieve. — 2nd ed.
      p.   cm.
  Includes bibliographical
  references and index.
    ISBN 0-632-04096-3 (pb)
    1. Kinesiology.
  I. Grieve, June I.
  II. Title.
    QP303.T95   1996
  612.7'6 — dc20   96-13775
                        CIP

Contents

Preface to the second edition

In this second edition of *Muscles, Nerves and Movement* we have retained the same general approach to the study of normal movement. Some additions have been suggested by our readers. We have introduced other changes which aim to link human biology with the medical sciences of neurology and orthopaedics.

· The need was recognized for more specific information on the structure of the joints of the body. These have been incorporated in the relevant sections on joint movements, and the diagrams from Appendix 2 of the first edition have been included in the body of the text.

The addition of 'clinical note-pads' gives relevance to the study of the musculo-skeletal and neuromuscular systems and explains the clinical features that are observed in the clients referred for therapeutic intervention.

In Section 3, Integration of Movement, the order of presentation of some of the sections has been changed, particularly in relation to the influence of the brain stem, basal ganglia and cerebellum on motor performance.

The learning objectives at the end of each chapter have been reviewed and expanded. A clearer indication is given of how the complexity of detail in neurology increases as the book progresses.

Many of the diagrams have been improved or modified for greater clarity. To maintain the cost of the book at a reasonable price, we were advised to present the diagrams in monochrome. We have done our best to ensure that no essential detail has been lost in the process.

We hope that we have continued to maintain a satisfactory balance between structural detail and relevant function in daily living. Our aim is to facilitate a link between the understanding of normal movement and the identification of some of the problems observed in clients by the therapist.

Acknowledgements

We would like to thank Miranda Bailey DipCOT, Department of Occupational Therapy, The National Hospital for Neurology and Neurosurgery, for her comments and suggestions for the 'clinical note-pads' in neurology. At Blackwell Science, Lisa Field gave us encouragement to start the second edition, and Janet Prescott worked patiently with us on the preparation of the manuscript and the figures. We give special thanks to Janet for her cooperation and her understanding of what we wanted to achieve.

Barbara Tyldesley
June Grieve
1996

Section 1 Introduction to Movement

FUNCTIONAL UNITS, TERMINOLOGY, COMPONENTS OF THE NERVOUS SYSTEM

1 / Functional Units: Components of the Musculoskeletal and Nervous Systems

The study of movement of the body as a whole must include some understanding of its basic components. The unit of structure is the *cell*, which is studied in detail by the histologist, biochemist, pharmacologist and geneticist. In movement studies, it is our concern to appreciate how cells and tissues are organised to produce a moveable joint, a contractile muscle, an active nerve fibre, and how some connective tissues limit movement. With this in mind, the unit of structure of the cell, and the organisation of cells into the functional units of the musculoskeletal and nervous systems will be considered.

1.1 The cell and basic tissues

Every cell has an outer limiting *membrane* which supports the cell and controls what substances will enter and leave it. The cell membrane is largely composed of fat and protein molecules. The fat is usually arranged in two layers, with protein molecules peppered in between (Fig. 1.1). The fatty layers (in the form of phospholipids, glycolipids and sterol cholesterol) play a structural role, and the protein assists transport of substances across the membrane, i.e. in and out of the cell. Some substances pass through the membrane by diffusion, and small particles, e.g. ions, will pass through with greatest ease. All cell membranes are selectively permeable, and the presence of enzymes in the protein part of the membrane allows larger particles to move in or out. In addition, the presence of enzymes allows

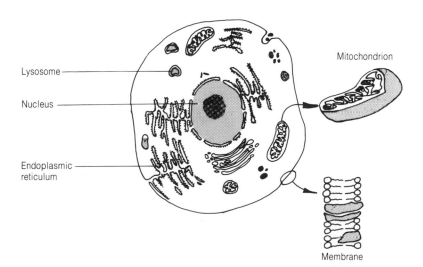

Lysosome

Nucleus

Endoplasmic reticulum

Mitochondrion

Membrane

Fig. 1.1. A typical cell, membrane and mitochondrion enlarged.

3

some particles to move against the tide of diffusion, i.e. against the concentration gradient, by active transport. For example, some of the protein in the cell membrane acts as an enzyme to continuously transport sodium ions out of the cell. This active transport, known as the 'sodium pump', removes sodium that would be harmful to the internal function of the cell.

Inside the cell lies the nucleus embedded in cytoplasm. *Organelles*, each with their own membrane, are found within the cytoplasm. Some examples of organelles are as follows.

(1) **Endoplasmic reticulum** is an elaborate system of tubes which extends from the cell membrane to the nuclear membrane. It provides a conducting system for the movement of substances inside the cell and divides the cell into compartments, with sites, known as *ribosomes*, for production of protein. In muscle cells, the endoplasmic (sarcoplasmic) reticulum stores calcium ions, which play an essential role in the contractile mechanism.

(2) **Mitochondria** are the 'power houses' of the cell where energy rich compounds, e.g. adenosine triphosphate (ATP), are stored and carbohydrate (glycogen) is broken down to release energy. Each mitochondrion has a double membrane, the inner one is thrown into folds, giving a large surface area for chemical reactions to occur (Fig. 1.1). Cells with high energy requirements, such as muscle cells and neurones have a large number of mitochondria. The aerobic reactions in the release of energy occur in the mitochondria. Pyruvic acid enters the mitochondria to be broken down to carbon dioxide and water, under the action of enzymes. Different parts of the process take place in specific areas of the mitochondria.

(3) **Lysosomes** are organelles with a single membrane, varying in size and shape, and form the disposal units of the cell. Lysosomes are important in cell growth and repair when cell molecules are broken down before being removed from the cell. They also break down toxins, bacteria and viruses that have entered the cell. The resultant products are either excreted to the exterior of the cell or absorbed into it.

Cells are collected together to form a *tissue*, a collection of similar cells lying in an intercellular substance. Each tissue has a particular function. Three basic tissues play important roles in movement: *connective tissue*, *muscle* and *nerve*.

1.2 Connective tissues in the musculoskeletal system

The overall function of connective tissue is to unite or connect structures in the body, and to give support. Bone is a connective tissue which provides the rigid framework for support. Where bones articulate with each other dense fibrous connective tissue, rich in collagen fibres, surrounds the ends of the bones, allowing movement to occur while maintaining stability. Cartilage, another connective tissue, is also found associated with joints, where it forms a compressible link between two bones, or provides a low friction surface for smooth movement. Connective tissue attaches muscles to bone, either in the form of a cord (tendon) or a flat sheet (fascia). The three connective tissues which play a major role in movement will be described below.

1.2.1 Dense fibrous tissue

Dense fibrous connective tissue unites structures in the body while still allowing movement to occur. It has high tensile strength to resist stretching forces. This connective tissue has few cells and is largely made up of fibres of collagen and elastin – protein strands that give the tissue great strength. The fibres are produced by fibroblast cells that lie in between the fibres (Fig. 1.2). The toughness of this tissue can be felt when cutting through stewing steak with a blunt knife. The muscle fibres are easily sliced, but the covering of white connective tissue is very tough. Examples of this tissue are as follows.

(1) The **capsule** surrounds the moveable (synovial) joints, binding the bones together (see Fig. 1.8).

(2) **Ligaments** form strong bands which join bone to bone. Ligaments strengthen the joint capsules in particular directions and limit movement.

(3) **Tendons** unite the contractile fibres of muscle to bone.
In tendons and ligaments, the collagenous fibres lie in parallel in the direction of greatest stress.

(4) **Aponeurosis** is a strong flat membrane, with collagen fibres that lie in different directions to form sheets of connective tissue. Aponeuroses can form the attachment of a muscle, such as the oblique abdominal muscles, which meet in the midline of the abdomen (see Fig. 10.6). In the palm of the hand and the sole of the foot an aponeurosis lies deep to the skin and forms a protec-

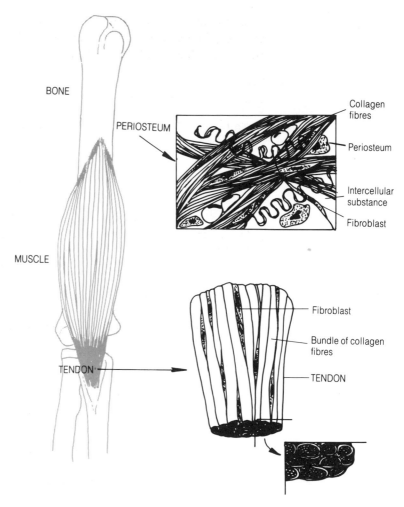

Fig. 1.2. Dense fibrous connective tissue seen covering bone as periosteum, and forming the tendon of a skeletal muscle.

tive layer for the tendons underneath (see Chapter 3, Section 6.4.1, and Fig. 8.22b).

(5) **Retinaculum** is a band of dense fibrous tissue which binds tendons of muscles and prevents bowstring during movement. An example is the flexor retinaculum of the wrist, which holds the tendons of muscles passing into the hand in position (see Fig. 6.13).

(6) **Fascia** is a term used for the large areas of dense fibrous tissue that surround the musculature of all the body segments. Fascia is particularly developed in the limbs, where it dips down between the large groups of muscles and attaches to the bone.

In some areas, fascia provides a base for the attachment of muscles, for example the thoracolumbar fascia gives the posterior attachment for the abdominal muscles (see Fig. 10.6f).

(7) **Periosteum** is the protective covering of bones. Tendons and ligaments blend with the periosteum around bone (see Fig. 1.2).

(8) **Dura** is thick fibrous connective tissue protecting the brain and spinal cord (see Fig. 3.23).

Clinical note-pad 1A: Contracture

Fibrous connective tissue loses its strength and elasticity when there is loss of movement for any reason over a period of time. When muscles and tendons remain the same length for any length of time, e.g. due to muscle weakness in stroke, or joint pain in rheumatoid arthritis, permanent shortening occurs (contracture) which leads to joint deformity. Also see Dupuytren's contracture, clinical note-pad 6B.

1.2.2 Cartilage

Cartilage is a tissue that can be compressed and has resilience. The cells (chondrocytes) are oval and lie in a ground substance that is not rigid like bone. There is no blood supply to cartilage so there is a limit to its thickness. The tissue does have a great resistance to wear, but cannot be repaired when damaged.

Hyaline cartilage is commonly called gristle. It is smooth and glass-like forming a low friction covering to the articular surfaces of joints. In the elderly, the articular cartilage tends to become eroded or calcifies, so that joints become stiff. Hyaline cartilage forms the costal cartilages which join the anterior ends of the ribs to the sternum (Fig. 1.3). In the developing foetus, most of the bones are formed in hyaline cartilage. When the cartilaginous model of each bone reaches a critical size for the survival of the cartilage cells, ossification begins.

- *LOOK at some large butcher's bones to see the cartilage covering the joint surfaces at the end. Note that it is bluish and looks like glass.*

Fibrocartilage consists of cartilage cells lying in between densely packed collagen fibres (Fig. 1.3). The fibres give extra strength to the tissue while retaining its resilience. Examples of where fibrocartilage is found are: (a) the discs between the bones of the

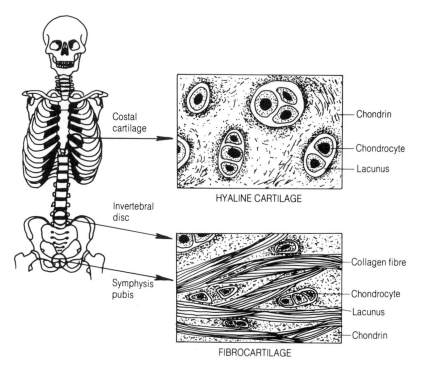

Fig. 1.3. Microscopic structure of hyaline and fibrocartilage, location in the skeleton of the trunk.

vertebral column; (b) the pubic symphysis joining the two halves of the pelvis anteriorly; and (c) the menisci in the knee joint.

1.2.3 Bone

Bone is the tissue that forms the rigid supports for the body by containing a large proportion of calcium salts (calcium phosphate and carbonate). It must be remembered that bone is a living tissue composed of cells and an abundant blood supply. It has a greater capacity for repair after damage than any other tissue in the body, except blood. The strength of bone lies in the thin plates (lamellae), composed of collagen fibres with calcium salts deposited in between. The lamellae lie in parallel, held together by fibres, and the bone cells (*osteocytes*) are found in between. Each bone cell lies in a small space or lacuna, and connects with other cells and to blood capillaries by fine channels called canaliculi (Fig. 1.4a).

In **compact bone**, the lamellae are laid down in concentric rings around a central canal containing blood vessels. Each system of concentric lamellae (known as an Haversian system or an osteon) lies in a longitudinal direction. Many of these systems

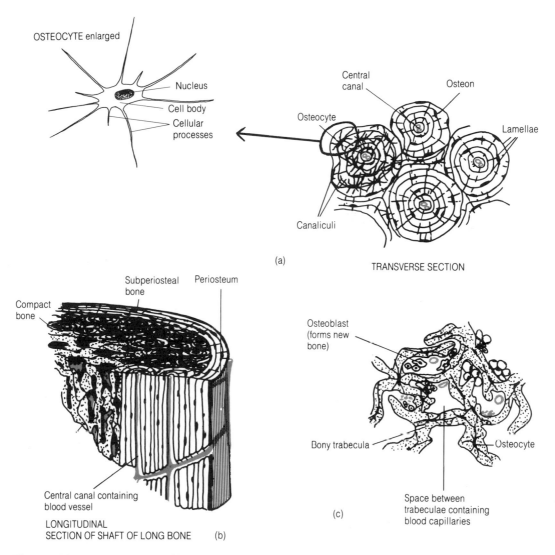

OSTEOCYTE enlarged

Nucleus
Cell body
Cellular processes

Central canal
Osteon
Osteocyte
Lamellae
Canaliculi

(a)

TRANSVERSE SECTION

Subperiosteal bone
Periosteum
Compact bone

Osteoblast (forms new bone)

Bony trabecula
Osteocyte

Central canal containing blood vessel

Space between trabeculae containing blood capillaries

(c)

LONGITUDINAL SECTION OF SHAFT OF LONG BONE
(b)

Fig. 1.4. Microscopic structure of bone: (a) an osteocyte (enlarged), and the organisation of osteons in compact bone seen in transverse section; (b) a section of the shaft of long bone; (c) cancellous bone showing trabeculae with osteocytes.

are closely packed to form the dense compact bone found in the shaft of long bones (Fig. 1.4b).

In **cancellous** or **trabeculate bone**, the lamellae form plates arranged in different directions to form a mesh. The plates are known as trabeculae and the spaces in between contain blood capillaries. The bone cells lying in the trabeculae communicate with each other and with the spaces by canaliculi (Fig. 1.4c). The expanded ends of long bones are filled with cancellous bone covered with a thin layer of compact bone. The central cavity of

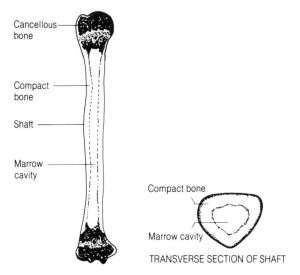

Cancellous bone

Compact bone

Shaft

Marrow cavity

Compact bone

Marrow cavity

TRANSVERSE SECTION OF SHAFT

Fig. 1.5. Gross structure of a long bone; longitudinal and transverse sections.

the shaft of long bones contains bone marrow. This organisation of the two types of bone produces a structure with great rigidity without excessive weight (Fig. 1.5). Bone has the capacity to remodel in shape in response to the stresses on it, so that the structure lines of the trabeculae at the ends of the bone follow the lines of force on the bone. For example, the lines of trabeculae at the ends of weight bearing bones, such as the femur, provide maximum strength to support the body weight against gravity. Remodelling of bone is achieved by the activity of 'bone forming' cells known as osteoblasts, and 'bone destroying cells' known as osteoclasts; both these types of cell are found in bone tissue. The calcium salts of bone are constantly interchanging with calcium ions in the blood, under the influence of hormones (parathormone and thyrocalcitonin). Bone is a living, constantly changing connective tissue, that provides a rigid framework on which muscles can exert forces to produce movement.

- *LOOK at any of the following examples of connective tissue that are available to you:*

(1) *Microscopic slides of dense fibrous tissue, cartilage and bone, noting the arrangement of the cellular and fibre content.*

(2) *Dissected material of joints and muscles which include tendons, ligaments, aponeurosis and retinaculum.*

(3) *Fresh butcher's bone – note the pink colour (blood supply), and central cavity in the shaft of long bones.*

(4) *Fresh red meat to see fibrous connective tissue around muscle.*

1.3 Articulations

Where the rigid bones of the skeleton meet, connective tissues are organised to bind the bones together, and to form *joints*. It is the joints which allow movement of the segments of the body relative to each other. The joints or articulations between bones can be divided into three types based on the particular connective tissues involved. The three main classes of joint are *fibrous*, *cartilaginous* and *synovial*.

1.3.1 Fibrous joints

Here the bones are united by dense fibrous connective tissue.

The **sutures** of the skull are fibrous joints which allow no movement between the bones. The edge of each bone is irregular, and interlocks with the adjacent bone, a layer of fibrous tissue linking them (Fig. 1.6a).

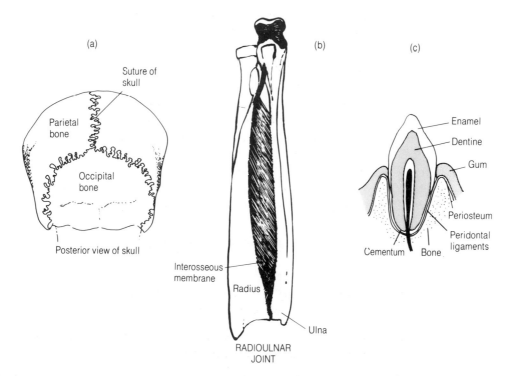

Fig. 1.6. Fibrous joints: (a) suture between bones of the skull; (b) syndesmosis between the radius and ulna; (c) gomphosis – tooth in socket.

A **syndesmosis** is a joint where the bones are joined by a ligament or fibrous membrane which allows some movement between the bones. A syndesmosis is found as an interosseous membrane between the shafts of the radius and ulna (Fig. 1.6b).

A **gomphosis** is a specialised fibrous joint which fixes the teeth in the sockets of the jaw.

1.3.2 Cartilaginous joints

In these joints the bones are united by cartilage.

A **synchondrosis** is a joint where the union is composed of hyaline cartilage. The articulation of the first rib with the sternum is by a synchondrosis. During growth of the long bones of the skeleton, there is a synchondrosis between the ends and the shaft of the bone, where temporary cartilage forms the epiphyseal plate. These plates disappear when growth stops and the bone becomes ossified (Fig. 1.7a).

A **symphysis** is a joint where the joint surfaces are covered by a thin layer of hyaline cartilage and united by a disc of fibrocartilage. This type of joint allows a limited amount of movement between the bones by compression of the cartilage. The bodies of the vertebrae articulate by a disc of fibrocartilage. Movement between two vertebrae is small, but when all the intervertebral discs are compressed in a particular direction, considerable movement of the vertebral column occurs (Fig. 1.7b). Little movement occurs at the pubic symphysis, the joint where the right and left halves of the pelvis meet. Movement is probably increased at the pubic symphysis in the late stage of pregnancy and during childbirth, to increase the size of the birth canal.

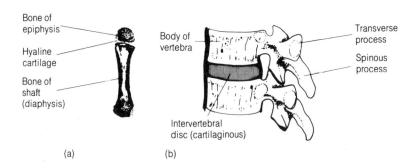

Bone of epiphysis

Hyaline cartilage

Bone of shaft (diaphysis)

Body of vertebra

Transverse process

Spinous process

Intervertebral disc (cartilaginous)

Fig. 1.7. Cartilaginous joints: (a) synchondrosis in child's metacarpal, as seen by X-ray; (b) symphysis between the bodies of two vertebrae.

(a)

(b)

1.3.3 Synovial joints

Synovial joints are the mobile joints of the body. There are a large number of these joints, which show a variety of form and range of movement. The common features of all of them are shown in the section of a typical synovial joint (Fig. 1.8).

The ends of the two articulating bones are covered by *hyaline* (articular) *cartilage* to give low friction in the movement between them.

Surrounding the joint like a sleeve is the *capsule* of dense fibrous tissue, which is attached at the articular margins, or some distance away, on each bone. The capsule binds the bones together while allowing movement to occur between them. In the embryo, the capsule is attached to the site of the epiphyseal plates.

There is a *joint cavity* inside the capsule which allows free movement between the bones.

The capsule is strengthened by *ligaments*, some of which blend with the capsule, while others are found attached to the bones close to the joint.

A *synovial membrane* lines the joint capsule and all the non-articular surfaces inside the joint, i.e. any structure within a joint not covered by hyaline cartilage. The synovial membrane secretes a viscous fluid, known as synovial fluid, which fills the joint cavity.

One or more *bursae* are found associated with some synovial joints at a point of friction where a muscle tendon or the skin rubs against bony structures. A bursa is a closed sac of fibrous

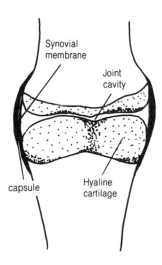

Fig. 1.8. Typical synovial joint.

tissue lined by a synovial membrane and containing synovial fluid. The cavity of the bursa sometimes communicates with the joint cavity. Pads of fat, liquid at body temperature, are also present in some joints. Both structures have a protective function.

All the large moveable joints of the body, for example the shoulder, elbow, wrist, hip, knee and ankle, are synovial joints. The direction and the range of their movements depend on: (a) the shape of the articular surfaces; and (b) the presence of ligaments and muscles close to the joint. The different types of synovial joint are described in Chapter 2, Section 2.3, when the directions of movement at joints are described.

> ### Clinical note-pad 1B: Osteoarthritis and rheumatoid arthritis
>
> Osteoarthritis is a degenerative disease occurring in the middle aged and elderly. There is progressive loss of the articular cartilage in the weight bearing joints, usually the hip and the knees. Bony outgrowths occur and the capsule becomes fibrosed. The joints become stiff and painful.
>
> Rheumatoid arthritis is a systemic disease which can occur at any age (average 40 years) and it is more common in women. The peripheral joints (hands and feet) are affected first, followed by the involvement of other joints. Inflammation of the synovial membrane, bursae and tendon sheaths leads to swelling and pain which is relieved by drugs. Deformity is the result of erosion of articular cartilage, stretching of the capsule and the rupture of tendons.

1.4 Skeletal muscle

The special feature of muscle tissue is its ability to actively contract. The connective tissues already described have elasticity, they can be stretched and return to the original length. Muscle cells can also be passively stretched, but they have the additional capacity to actively shorten.

The function of skeletal muscle is to: (a) shorten to produce movement of the body at joints; and (b) to resist active stretching by external forces acting on it. For example, if a weight and/or gravity is acting on a body part, as in holding a full glass in the hand, active muscle tissue prevents the hand from falling by resisting stretching, and muscle can also lift the weight by shortening.

- *HOLD a glass of water in the hand and feel the activity in the muscles above the elbow as they resist stretching.*

- *LIFT the glass to the mouth and feel the muscle activity in the same muscles as they shorten.*

Skeletal muscle is only active when nerve impulses reach the muscle through the nerve supplying it. If the nerve supply is damaged, the muscle is unable to function. Details of the way in which nerve impulses arrive at the muscle cells will be discussed in Section 1.5.

1.4.1 The muscle fibre – gross and microscopic structure

The muscle fibre, the unit of structure of a skeletal muscle, is an elongated cell with many nuclei surrounded by a strong outer membrane, the *sarcolemma*.

A muscle fibre can just be seen with the naked eye. If one fibre is viewed under a light microscope, the nuclei can be seen close to the membrane around the fibre. The chief constituent of the fibre is several hundreds of *myofibrils*, strands of protein, extending from one end of the fibre to the other (Fig. 1.9). The arrangement of the two main proteins, actin and myosin, that form each myofibril present a banded appearance. The light and dark bands in adjacent myofibrils coincide, so that the whole muscle fibre is striated.

The electron microscope reveals the detail of the cross striations in each myofibril. A repeating unit, known as the *sarcomere*, is revealed along the length of the myofibril. Each sarcomere links to the next at a disc called the Z line. The thin filaments of actin are attached to the Z line and project towards the centre of the sarcomere. The thicker myosin filaments lie in between the actin strands. The darkest bands of the myofibril are where the actin and myosin overlap in the sarcomere.

The arrangement of the myosin molecules in the thick myosin filaments forms cross bridges which link with special sites on the active filaments when the muscle fibre is activated. The result of this linking is to allow the filaments to slide past one another, so that each sarcomere becomes shorter. This in turn means that the myofibril is shorter, and since all the myofibrils respond together, the muscle fibre shortens. The initiation of the active state in the myofibrils depends on the release of calcium from the endoplasmic reticulum of the muscle fibre. During relaxation of the fibre, the calcium returns to the tubules of the endoplasmic reticulum.

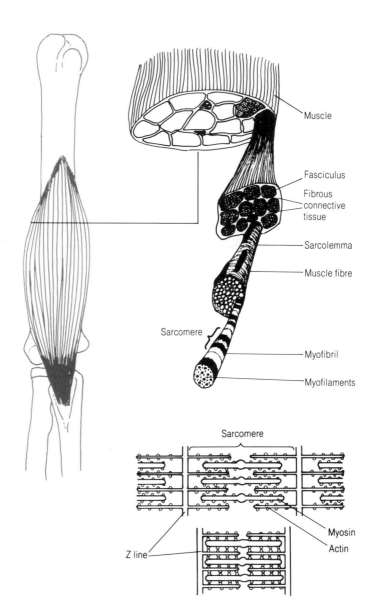

Muscle

Fasciculus

Fibrous connective tissue

Sarcolemma

Muscle fibre

Sarcomere

Myofibril

Myofilaments

Sarcomere

Myosin

Actin

Z line

Fig. 1.9. Skeletal muscle; the organisation of muscle fibres into a whole muscle, and of the sarcomeres (seen by an electron microscope) in the myofilaments.

- *LOOK closely at Figure 1.9 to see clearly how: (a) sarcomeres lie end to end to form a myofibril; (b) myofibrils are packed tightly together inside a muscle fibre; and (c) the sarcolemma encloses the myofibrils in a muscle fibre.*

All cells contain high energy compounds (mainly adenosine triphosphate) in the mitochondria which provide the *energy* for cell activity. Muscle cells have a higher level and rate of energy output than other cells, supplied by ATP and a 'back up' of another high energy compound, phosphocreatine. The store of ATP is replenished by chemical reactions in the mitochondria

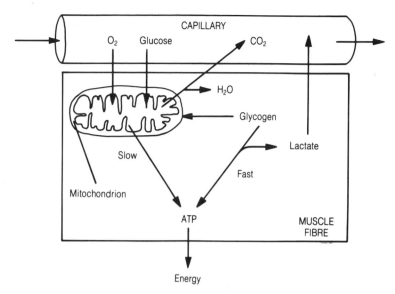

Fig. 1.10. Energy for muscle contraction (simplified). The 'slow' pathway predominates in Type I fibres when ATP is replenished by aerobic reactions to provide energy for long periods of low level activity. The 'fast' pathway predominates in Type II fibres when glycogen provides energy without oxygen for short bursts of high level activity.

using oxygen and glucose brought by the blood in the network of capillaries surrounding muscle fibres (Fig. 1.10). In this way, the muscle fibres have a continuous supply of energy, as long as the supply of oxygen is maintained (aerobic metabolism).

Glycogen is another source of energy that is stored in muscle fibres. When there is insufficient oxygen to replenish ATP by oxidative reactions, energy released from breakdown of glycogen is also used to maintain ATP levels, during a short burst of high level muscle activity.

Types of muscle fibre

Different types of fibres in a muscle have been identified by the relative amounts of oxidative and glycolytic reactions used to produce energy.

- *LOOK at the muscle seen in chicken meat to see the white muscles of the breast (glycolytic), and the more vascular red muscles of the legs (oxidative).*

In human muscle, the distinction is not so marked, and all muscles contain fibres of each type, but the proportion depends on the function of the muscle.

Red slow muscle fibres, known as Type I, are specialised for slow sustained activity, and they are resistant to fatigue. Postural muscles contain more red slow oxidative fibres. They are red because they contain myoglobin which stores oxygen, like the haemoglobin in the blood, and they are also surrounded by many capillaries.

White fast muscle fibres, known as Type II, are found in muscles which have rapid intense bursts of activity. Energy for contraction is supplied by anaerobic (without oxygen) breakdown of glucose and stored glycogen. These fibres fatigue quickly when the limited glycogen stores are used up.

Most muscles are involved in both postural and phasic activity at the same or at different times. There is evidence that in response to training, some Type II fibres become more like Type I, and the muscle can then perform over longer periods of time. The implications of this are important for the athlete who wants to increase his/her endurance. The energy capacity of a given muscle fibre is not fixed, and the proportions of Types I and II can change in response to the type of activity performed by the muscle.

1.4.2 Shape and form of skeletal muscle

The structure of a whole muscle is the combination of muscle and connective tissues, which both contribute to the function of the muscle when it is active. In a whole muscle, groups of contractile muscle fibres, of varying diameter, are bound together by fibrous connective tissue to form *fasciculi*. Further coverings of connective tissue bind the fasciculi together and an outer layer surrounds the whole muscle (Fig. 1.9). The total connective tissue element lying in between the contractile muscle fibres is known as the *parallel elastic component*. The tension that is built up in muscle when it is activated depends on the tension in the muscle fibres and in the parallel elastic component. The fibrous connective tissue which links the whole muscle to bone, e.g. the tendon, is known as the *series elastic component*. The initial tension that builds up in an active muscle tightens the series elastic component and then the muscle can shorten. A model of the elastic and contractile parts of a muscle is shown in Figure 1.11. If the connective tissue components lose their elasticity, through lack of use in injury or disease, a muscle may go into contracture. Lively splints are used to maintain elasticity and prevent contracture while the muscle recovers.

The individual muscle fibres lie within a muscle in one of two

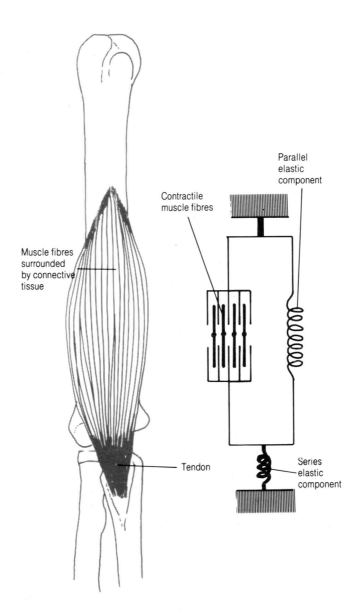

Parallel
elastic
component

Contractile
muscle fibres

Muscle fibres
surrounded
by connective
tissue

Tendon

Series
elastic
component

Fig. 1.11. Elastic
components of muscle.

ways: (a) parallel, or (b) oblique, to the line of pull of the whole muscle.

Parallel fibres are seen in *strap* and *fusiform* muscles illustrated in Figure 1.12a and b. These muscles have long fibres which are capable of shortening over the entire length of the muscle, but the result is a less powerful muscle.

Oblique fibres are seen in *pennate* muscles. The muscle fibres in these muscles cannot shorten to the same extent as parallel fibres. The advantage of this arrangement, however, is that more muscle fibres can be packed into the whole muscle, so that

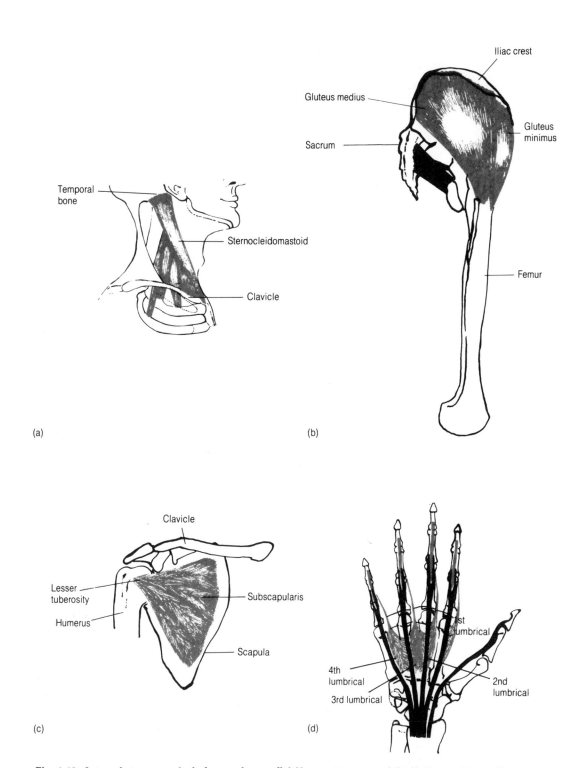

Fig. 1.12. Internal structure of whole muscle: parallel fibres – (a) strap and (b) fusiform; oblique fibres – (c) multipennate and (d) unipennate and bipennate.

greater power can be achieved. These muscles are known as unipennate, bipennate or multipennate, depending on the particular way the muscle fibres are arranged (Fig. 1.12c and d).

Some of the large muscles of the body combine parallel and oblique arrangements. The deltoid muscle of the shoulder (Fig. 5.4a) has one group of fibres that are multipennate, and two groups that are fusiform, which combines strength to lift the weight of the arm with a wide range of movement. The form of a particular muscle reflects the space available and the demands of range and strength of movement.

Strength and flexibility

The strength of a muscle is the maximum force it can develop in a particular direction. Increase in strength can be achieved by exercising the muscle against gradually increasing loads. The muscle responds by an increase in the size of individual muscle fibres; there is no change in the total number of fibres in the muscle. Fitness programmes, and the re-education of weak muscles after injury, include weight training.

Increase in strength alone may result in shortening of the muscle and loss of range of movement at the joint. It is important for the muscle to remain flexible to allow the joint to move with a wide range and speed of movement for the needs of the particular person. Flexibility depends on the elasticity of, not only the muscle fibres, but also all the connective tissue in the muscle and the joint on which it acts. Stretching exercises are designed to elongate or extend the length of a muscle. Flexibility training reduces the incidence of torn muscles.

Some muscle stretching can be achieved by the positioning of a body part. For example, if one arm is straightened and the weight of the trunk is supported on it while the other arm is used to do an activity, the muscles of the supporting arm will be stretched.

Active stretching of muscles involves slowly moving the joint through its maximum range, holding it, and then letting go. Here one group of muscles is active to stretch the opposing group. For example, moving the leg backwards in this way actively stretches the muscles and ligaments on the front of the hip. The muscle fibres of the stretching muscles must be relaxed, then the connective tissues of the muscle and the ligaments of the joint yield to the prolonged stretch.

The muscles of each individual have unique properties of strength and flexibility related to his or her daily activities.

Efforts to improve muscle function must include increase in both strength and mobility.

Muscle is a highly specialised tissue which is adapted to the demands of the movement it performs. A muscle has a limited capacity for repair, although a small area of damage to muscle fibres may regenerate. In more extensive damage, the connective tissue responds by producing more collagen fibres and a 'scar' is formed. An intact nerve and adequate blood supply is essential for muscle function; if these are interrupted the muscle may never recover. Movement can then only be restored by other muscles taking over the functions of the damaged muscles.

Clinical note-pad 1C: Myopathies

Neuromuscular disorders that are myopathic originate in the muscle, and may be inherited or acquired. There is muscle weakness in the proximal muscles, which is slowly progressive with muscle wasting.

Duchenne muscular dystrophy is a myopathy which is inherited and affects boys only. There is a rapid progression of muscle weakness that begins in childhood.

Acquired myopathy can result from infections, endocrine disorders or as a complication of steroid drug treatment.

1.5 Nervous tissue

1.5.1 The neurone

The neurone is the unit of structure of the nervous system. Neurones are *excitable*, they generate impulses in response to stimulation. Neurones also *conduct* the impulses from one point to another in the system. Networks of neurones *process* or *integrate* the information before passing it on to other groups of neurones, or to other parts of the body to produce a response.

Each neurone has a cell body and numerous processes extending outward from the cell. The processes are living structures and their membrane is continuous with that of the cell body (Fig. 1.13). (Think of the cell body like a conker with spines projecting out in all directions.) The projections vary in length, some are short , known as *dendrites*, and each neurone has one long process, known as the *axon*. The dendrites are adapted to receive information. *Impulses* are received by the dendrites and passed on to the cell body. Some neurones, particularly in the brain, have a large number of complex branching dendrites, so

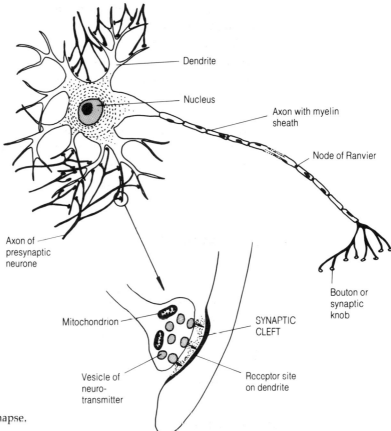

Fig. 1.13. Neurone and synapse. Synaptic cleft enlarged.

that information from many other neurones can be received and processed.

The axon is the output end of every neurone. The length of an axon varies from a few millimetres to up to one metre long. Cell bodies of motor neurones in the spinal cord in the lower back have long axons that extend down the leg to supply muscles of the foot. The axon may be surrounded by a sheath of *myelin*, a fatty material, that increases the rate at which impulses are conducted down it. The myelin is laid down between layers of membrane of Schwann cells that wrap round the axon. Gaps in the myelin occur between successive Schwann cells forming nodes of Ranvier (Fig. 1.13).

The axon branches at its end, and each branch is swollen to form a bouton or synaptic knob. The boutons lie near a dendrite or cell body of another neurone. Axons also terminate on muscle fibres on some blood vessels and in glands.

An *impulse* is a localised change in the membrane of a neurone. When a neurone is excited, the membrane over a small area allows charged particles (ions) to pass across the membrane, a process known as depolarisation, and an impulse is generated. The area of depolarisation then moves to the adjacent area and the impulse travels down the membrane in one direction only. Each impulse is the same size, like a morse code of dots only, but the information carried can be varied by the rate and pattern of the impulses conducted along the neurone. When an impulse arrives at the end of the axon, a chemical, known as a *neurotransmitter*, is released from the boutons (Fig. 1.13). The membrane of the next neurone is depolarised and the impulse is conducted on to this neurone if sufficient transmitter substance is released from the boutons at the end of the axon.

Each neurone has a *threshold* level of stimulation. The level of *excitation* reaching a neurone must be sufficient to depolarise the membrane, so that impulses are generated. Some impulses reaching a neurone affect the membrane in such a way that no impulses are propagated; this is known as *inhibition*. The source of inhibitory effects may be the presence of small neurones, whose activity always produces inhibition, or the release of different transmitter substance from the boutons of the axon. The mechanism of inhibition will be discussed in more detail in Chapter 13.

Clinical note-pad 1D: Multiple sclerosis, MS

In multiple sclerosis, changes in the myelin sheath around axons result in the formation of plaques, which affects the rate of conduction of nerve impulses. Axons in the central nervous system (brain and spinal cord) are affected, while those in the peripheral nervous system are not. The visual system seems to be most sensitive to plaque formation. Disturbance of movement and of sensation occurs. Fatigue and cognitive impairment are other common clinical features that affect function.

The number of plaques, and their sites, vary between individuals, and with time in the same individual, so that the disease sometimes follows a course of relapse and remission. In some patients there is progressive deterioration.

1.5.2 Synapse

A synapse is the junction between neurones, where impulses pass from one neurone to another. Impulses always travel in one direction at a synapse, i.e. from the axon of one neurone to the dendrites and cell body of the next neurone. This ensures the one way traffic in the nervous system.

Each bouton or synaptic knob at the end of the axon lies near to a special receptor site on the cell body or dendrite of the other neurone, but there is a gap in between, the synaptic cleft (Fig. 1.13). A neurone may have as many as 5000 synaptic knobs lying over the cell body and dendrites, so that the variety of input to the neurone is enormous. There is a delay in the conduction of the impulse at the bouton, while the neurotransmitter is released and diffuses into the synaptic cleft. The effect of the transmitter substance is to depolarise the membrane and generate impulses in the next neurone. The transmitter substance is broken down by enzymes, but can be taken up again by the bouton to be reformed into transmitter substance and stored.

Acetyl choline is the neurotransmitter released at most of the synapses in the nervous pathways involved in movement, including those between nerve and skeletal muscle, the *neuromuscular junctions*. Drugs which prevent the release of acetyl choline at synapses are used as relaxants for muscles, e.g. in abdominal surgery.

Motor and sensory neurones

Neurones whose axons carry impulses *away* from the central nervous system to all parts of the body are known as *motor* or *efferent nerve fibres*. Neurones that carry impulses *towards* the central nervous system are known as *sensory* or *afferent neurones*.

Neurones that lie in descending pathways which carry impulses *down* from the brain to the spinal cord are *motor*. The ascending pathways which carry impulses *up* to the brain from the spinal cord are *sensory*.

1.5.3 Motor neurones: the motor unit

The spinal cord has a central H shaped core of cell bodies of neurones called the grey matter. The motor neurones lying in the anterior (ventral) limb of the H are known as 'lower motor neurones' or anterior horn cells. The motor neurones that activate a particular group of muscles lie together and form a *motor neurone pool* (Fig. 1.14). Activity in a particular muscle is generated by impulses from its anterior horn cells, along axons in particular spinal nerves, which branch to form the nerve supply-

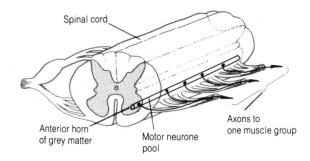

Fig. 1.14. Motor neurone pool in the spinal cord.

ing the muscle. Since there are fewer motor neurones in the pool than muscle fibres in the muscle, each neurone must supply a number of muscle fibres.

A **motor unit** consists of one motor neurone in the anterior horn of the spinal cord, its axon and all the muscle fibres innervated by the branches of the axon (Fig. 1.15). The number of muscle fibres in one motor unit depends on the function of the muscle rather than its size. Muscles performing large, strong movements have motor units with a large number of muscle fibres. For example, the large muscle of the calf has approximately 1900 muscle fibres in each motor unit. In muscles that perform fine precision movements, the motor units have a small number of muscle fibres, (e.g. up to 100 in muscles of the hand). The muscle fibres of one motor unit do not necessarily lie together in the muscle, but may be scattered in different fasciculi. The number of motor units that are active in a muscle at any one time determines the level of performance of the muscle.

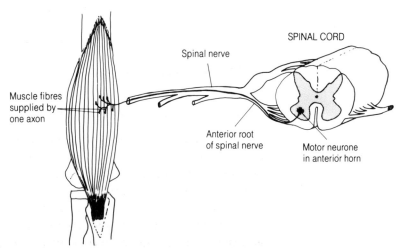

Fig. 1.15. The motor unit.

Types of motor unit

Low threshold motor units supplying slow Type I muscle fibres are involved in the sustained muscle activity that holds the posture of the body. The number of active motor units remains constant, but activity changes between all the low threshold neurones. The slow Type I muscle fibres do not fatigue easily and the activity is maintained over long periods.

High threshold motor units with large diameter axons supplying fast Type II muscle fibres are involved in fast active movements, which move the parts of the body from one position to another. These motor units soon fatigue, but they are adapted for fast strong movements such as running and jumping.

In a strong purposeful movement, such as pushing forwards on a door, the motor units are activated or recruited in a particular order. The slow units are active at the start of the movement and then the fast units become active as the movement reaches its peak.

All muscle activity includes a combination of slow and fast motor units. The slow units contribute more to the background postural activity, while the fast units play a greater part in rapid phasic movements. In manipulative activities the shoulder muscles have sustained postural activity to hold the limb steady, so that the hand can do rapid precision movements, such as writing, sewing or using a tool.

Clinical note-pad 1E: Motor neurone disease

This is a progressive disorder of the motor neurones in the spinal cord. Muscle weakness and fatigue of the muscles of the limbs and the trunk occurs, which may become generalised to affect swallowing and speech. There is no sensory loss. Onset is usually around age 40 years, with rapid deterioration over 3 to 5 years.

1.5.4 Sensory neurones and receptors

The basic units for conduction of nerve impulses *into* the central nervous system are the *sensory neurones*, which lie in all the nerves distributed all over the body. Sensory neurones bring information from all parts of the body, including the muscles, to the central nervous system. Axons of sensory neurones are found in all the spinal nerves that emerge from the spinal cord, and many of the cranial nerves arising from the brain. The cell bodies of these neurones are found in ganglia just outside the spinal cord. There are no synaptic junctions on the cell bodies, and the axon divides into two almost immediately after it leaves the cell. The two long processes formed by this division are: (a) axon or nerve fibre in the spinal nerve and its branches which ends in a specialised sensory receptor; and (b) nerve fibre that enters the spinal cord and terminates in the central nervous system.

Figure 1.16a shows the arrangement of a typical sensory neurone. It is sometimes called 'pseudo unipolar', since it has one axon but appears to be bipolar. Compare this with the multi-polar motor neurone shown in Figure 1.13.

Figure 1.16b shows the position of a sensory neurone in relation to the spinal cord, a spinal nerve and its branches. Note the cell body lying in a ganglion (swelling) and the axon entering the spinal cord.

The function of these sensory neurones is to carry information about the external environment, and the internal state of the body, into the central nervous system for processing.

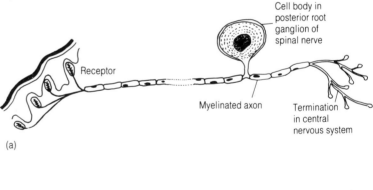

(a)

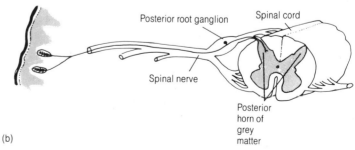

(b)

Fig. 1.16. Sensory neurones: (a) typical sensory neurone; (b) the position of a sensory neurone in a spinal nerve and the spinal cord.

> ### Clinical note-pad 1F: Neuropathies
>
> Neuromuscular disorders that are neurogenic originate in the nerve supply to the muscles, either in the spinal cord, the nerve roots or in the peripheral nerves (see Chapter 4, Section 4.3). Neuropathies of peripheral nerves affect sensory and motor axons, usually commencing distally and are known as 'glove and stocking'. Muscle weakness and sensory loss occur. Peripheral neuropathy can occur as a complication of diabetes which is not under control. Guillain-Barré syndrome is an acute peripheral neuropathy that affects motor axons. It usually follows a viral infection, and the resulting motor weakness involves the trunk and proximal limb muscles, mainly in the lower limbs. Recovery is nearly always complete unless there is severe involvement of the respiratory muscles or axonal damage.

Receptors

Sensory receptors are specialised structures which respond to a *stimulus*, and generate nerve impulses in sensory neurones. The stimulus may originate in the external environment around us, or from changes inside the body.

Many receptors are free branched endings, while others are encapsulated in a variety of ways. Receptors in the sense organs respond to a specific stimulus, for example receptors in the eye respond to light of different intensity, but this specificity does not apply to many other receptors. Some are more sensitive to certain types of stimuli than others. One receptor may respond to more than one type of stimulus, or several different receptors may respond to the same stimulus.

The overall sensation from the body, excluding the sense organs, can be divided into three types: (a) exteroceptive; (b) proprioceptive; and (c) interoceptive. The activity from the interoceptors is largely propagated in the autonomic nervous system (see Chapter 4, Section 4.5), which is entirely reflex and below our conscious awareness. The exteroceptors and proprioceptors provide the major input to the *somatic* or *somatosensory* system (see Chapter 11).

The **exteroceptors** lie mainly in the skin and respond to pain, temperature and various qualities of touch, for example two point discrimination. Figure 1.17 shows two different types of touch receptor and a deep pressure receptor, which are all encapsulated endings found in the skin. A free nerve ending is also shown. Harmful stimuli of various kinds, or changes in temperature, produce changes in the chemical composition of the surrounding tissue fluid which activate free nerve endings. Noci-

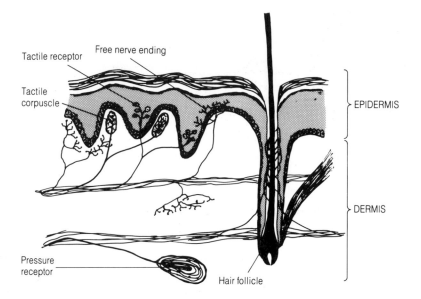

Fig. 1.17. Section of the skin showing exteroceptors.

ceptors are free nerve endings that respond to noxious changes such as an insect bite or local injury to the skin. The encapsulated endings in the skin mainly respond to deformation (mechanoreceptors) which includes touch, pressure and vibration.

The **proprioceptors** lie in skeletal muscles, tendons and joints. They collectively signal the movements and position of body parts from the changes in length of muscles and the angulation of joints during movement. A muscle spindle is an example of a proprioceptor which lies in parallel with skeletal muscle fibres (Fig. 1.19).

The **interoceptors** lie deep in the body, in relation to organs and blood vessels. While some of these receptors respond to deep pain, the majority provide the continuous monitoring of the activity in the internal organs. During movement, receptors in the blood vessels near to the heart respond to changes in the chemical composition of the blood. This information regulates the changes in breathing and circulation required to meet the oxygen demands of the active muscles.

Several receptors of the same type may give input into one sensory neurone. The area covered by all the receptors activating one sensory axon is called a *receptive field*. There may be overlap in receptive fields, so that stimulation of one point may excite more than one sensory neurone (Fig. 1.18). In the finger tips, for example, where the receptive fields are small and there is great overlap, a stimulus such as a pin prick can be very precisely interpreted by the central nervous system.

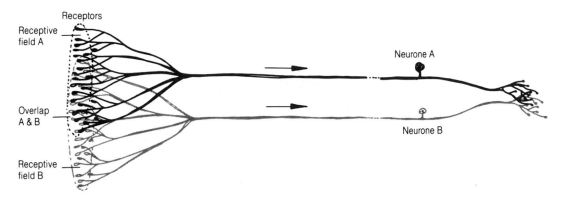

Fig. 1.18. Receptors: receptive fields of two neurones.

When a receptor is stimulated, the membrane of the receptor ending is depolarised and impulses are generated. If the same stimulus continues for some time, the rate of firing of impulses falls and may stop, even though the stimulus is still present. This is known as *adaptation of receptors*. Different receptors adapt at different rates.

Slow adapting receptors continue to produce impulses at the same rate all the time the stimulus is applied. The function of these receptors is to give continuous monitoring of background sensory information. We are not aware of most of this activity, it never reaches consciousness. An example of slowly adapting receptors are those lying in between muscle fibres (muscle spindles) which give information about the length of muscles in the body. These will be discussed in more detail in Section 1.6.

Fast adapting receptors generate a short burst of impulses in response to the stimulus, but activity ceases if the stimulus continues at the same level. Sensation from these receptors usually reaches consciousness. Touch receptors in the skin are fast adapting. When we put clothes on, we feel the clothes at first, and then we are no longer aware of them. If the strength of stimulus changes, e.g. a belt becomes tighter, another burst of impulses is generated, and we sense the change.

Adaptation of receptors allows the nervous system to process the changing features of the environment inside and outside the body, while information of unchanging features is reduced.

1.6 The myotatic unit (stretch reflex)

There are sensory neurones in the nerves supplying a skeletal muscle. Muscles are a source of sensation in the body, as well as a mechanism for motor action. The receptors lie in parallel with the muscle fibres and are known as *muscle spindles*. Each of the spindles consists of a capsule of connective tissue enclosing 5 to 14 specialised small muscle fibres known as *intrafusal fibres*. The central part of these intrafusal fibres of the spindle contains the nuclei and it is non-contractile. Wound round this central area is the primary sensory ending, called the *annulospiral ending* (Fig. 1.19). Impulses from the annulospiral ending pass along the sensory neurone into the spinal cord where they excite the motor units of the same muscle. The fibres of the muscle are known as *extrafusal fibres* to distinguish them from those of the spindle. The neurones supplying the extrafusal fibres are large diameter alpha motor neurones or *skeletomotor neurones*. This complete pathway is sometimes called the 'fusimotor loop' and the reflex activity is known as the 'stretch reflex'. The use of the term 'stretch' is misleading since the spindles do not only respond to a muscle increasing in length. The activity of the spindle depends on the balance of forces developed inside the muscle compared with the external forces acting on it. Also a muscle may be responding to prolonged stretch or to a rapid

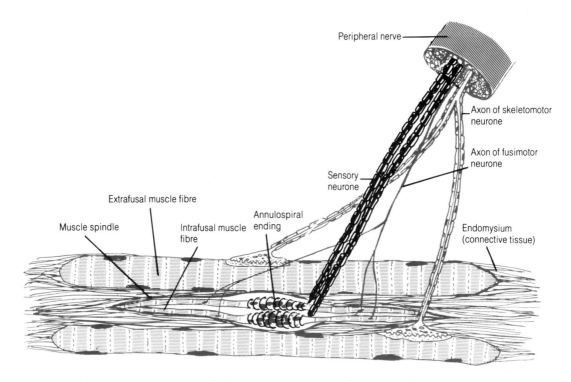

Fig. 1.19. Muscle spindle lying in parallel between two extrafusal fibres.

change in length. In each type of stretch, the response of the spindle is different.

Looking in more detail at the muscle spindle, the intrafusal fibres are themselves contractile and are supplied by small diameter gamma motor neurones originating in the spinal cord. Stimulation of these *fusimotor neurones* makes the intrafusal fibres contract. The spindle then shortens, becomes more sensitive to distortion, and reflex activity is increased. Fusimotor neurones are under the control of descending pathways from the brain; these will be discussed in Chapter 12, Section 12.2.

There are two types of skeletomotor neurones which supply the two types of skeletal muscle fibres described in Section 1.4.1. Large diameter skeletomotor neurones supply the fast Type II muscle fibres active in rhythmic or phasic movements. Smaller diameter skeletomotor neurones supply the slow Type I muscle fibres involved in tonic postural activity. The fusimotor neurones are even smaller in diameter and supply the intrafusal fibres of the muscle spindle. All these motor neurones lie close together in the anterior horn of the spinal cord.

Figure 1.20 shows the myotatic unit, which includes the muscle spindle, the sensory neurone, the skeletomotor and fusimotor neurones, and the extrafusal fibres of the muscle.

Spinal reflex activity in the myotatic units in all the muscles of the body is the basis of *muscle tone*. The level of activity is greatest in muscles holding a body segment against gravity: for example in sitting upright the head is held up by the activity in the muscles at the back of the neck to prevent the head from

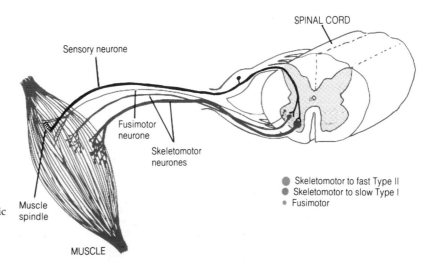

Fig. 1.20. The myotatic unit showing skeletomotor and fusimotor neurones.

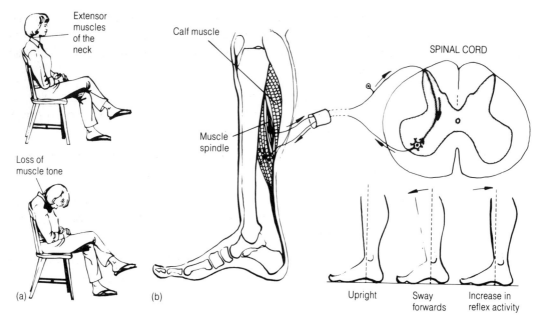

Fig. 1.21. Examples of 'holding a position': (a) the head in sitting; (b) calf muscles in standing.

falling forwards (Fig. 1.21a). In standing, the tendency for the body to sway forwards is counteracted by activity in the muscles of the calf (Fig. 1.21b). Reflex activity in muscles never completely stops: even when the body is asleep some muscle tone is present, except in periods of deep sleep.

- *FEEL the muscles around the shoulder of a partner while the arm is hanging by his or her side. The muscles are not limp, but they are 'lively'. Now ask the partner to lift his or her arm sideways to the horizontal and hold the position. Feel the muscles again, and notice that they are more lively, the tone of the muscles has increased.*

At the end of this chapter, you should be able to:

(1) Explain the functional importance of the connective tissues (dense fibrous, cartilage and bone) in providing support, strength and elasticity in the musculoskeletal system.

(2) Summarise the structure of the three main classes of joints found in the body. Describe the features of a typical synovial joint.

(3) Describe the gross and microscopic structure of skeletal muscle. Distinguish the energy resources of two different types of muscle fibres in relation to their function for slow sustained or fast phasic activity.

(4) Outline the generation and the conduction of impulses in neurones. Describe the role of neurotransmitters in the conduction of impulses at a synapse.

(5) Distinguish the organisational structure and function of motor and sensory neurones. Define a receptive field.

(6) Define a motor unit. Relate the organisation of motor units to the activity of slow and fast muscle fibres in postural or phasic muscle action.

(7) Describe the myotatic unit (stretch reflex). Explain the origin of muscle tone, and the ability to hold a body position.

2 / Movement Terminology and Biomechanical Principles

A vocabulary is needed to communicate to others a useful description of the moving body. The appropriate vocabulary depends on the purpose of the description, and different disciplines have developed their own languages.

Anatomical terminology defines a reference position, and names the direction of movement at each of the joints. For example, in standing up from sitting, we can describe the direction of movement at the hip, the knee and the ankle. A description based on direction alone does not distinguish the difference between rising from a low seat or a high stool, doing it quickly or slowly, staying in balance or losing it. To discuss the dynamic aspects of movement, which involve the forces required and the weights of the body parts, we use terms taken from the vocabulary of mechanics.

The aim of this chapter is to introduce the anatomical terms used in the analysis of daily activities. The application of some simple mechanics to the moving body will also be considered.

2.1 The anatomical position

All movement starts from a posture or position, which must be first defined before proceeding to the changes that follow. We need to use a common reference to describe the positions, relationships and directions of movement.

The reference is the *anatomical position*, standing upright with the palms of the hands facing forwards, the feet parallel and facing forwards (Fig. 2.1). Note that the usual standing position, with the palms of the hands facing the sides, is not used.

- *LOOK at the articulated skeleton to see the difference between the anatomical position and the natural standing position. In the anatomical position, the bones of the forearm are parallel, and the whole of the palm of the hand can be seen from the front.*
- *STAND in a natural position, and then change to the anatomical position. Note the change in position of the forearm and hand. Check that the feet are slightly apart and facing forwards.*

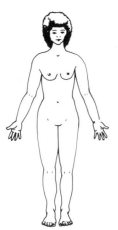

Fig. 2.1. The anatomical position.

2.2 Planes and axes of movement

The reference anatomical position can now be divided into three planes which lie at right angles to each other. The planes are the fixed lines of reference for movement (Fig. 2.2).

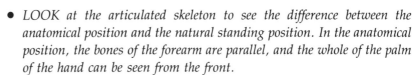

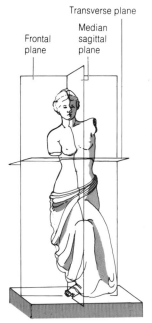

Transverse plane

Median
sagittal
plane

Frontal
plane

Fig. 2.2. Planes of
movement.

2.2.1 Median sagittal plane

The median sagittal plane is a vertical plane which divides the body into right and left halves. Any plane parallel to the median plane, dividing the body into unequal right and left halves is said to be a *sagittal plane*, parallel to the sagittal suture of the skull in the midline of the skull. The terms 'medial' and 'lateral' relate to this plane. A structure nearer to the median plane is medial, and one further away from the median plane is lateral. For example, the medial ligament of the knee is on the inside of the joint, while the lateral ligament is on the outside.

2.2.2 Coronal of frontal plane

This divides the body into front and back halves. Frontal planes are parallel to the frontal suture of the skull across the crown of the head. The terms 'anterior' and 'posterior' relate to this plane. The anterior shaft of the femur is the front of the bone in the anatomical position, the posterior shaft is the back of the bone.

2.2.3 Transverse or horizontal plane

This is parallel to the flat surface of the ground. Planes in this direction divide the body into upper (cranial) and lower (caudal) parts. Crossing the body in this direction, planes are at right angles to the sagittal and frontal planes. The terms 'superior' and 'inferior' relate to this plane. The superior radio-ulnar joint is near to the elbow (i.e. above or towards the head), while the inferior radio-ulnar joint is adjacent to the wrist (below or towards the ground). When the limbs move in different directions, the terms superior and inferior can become confusing, e.g. if the arm is above the head. Another way of identifying structures may then be used. The terms 'proximal' and 'distal' mean nearer to the centre of the body or further away from the centre respectively. The superior radio-ulnar joint can therefore also be named the proximal joint, and likewise the inferior as distal.

The *axis* of movement at a joint is at right angles to the plane. Bending the elbow is a movement in the sagittal plane about an axis passing through the frontal plane at the joint. Turning the head from side to side is a movement in the horizontal plane about a vertical axis through the joint between the first and second vertebrae of the neck. It may help to understand plane and axis if you think of the plane of movement of the wheels of a car, around the axle (axis) at the hub of the wheels.

Movements can be classified in terms of the three planes and axes described. Many functional activities, however, occur in diagonal planes. The leg swing in walking does not occur exactly in the sagittal plane at the hip, but in a diagonal plane between the sagittal and frontal planes, so that the foot comes to the ground near to the midline of the body. Movement at the shoulder which carries the arm forwards and slightly across the body is in a diagonal plane.

2.3 Movements at synovial joints

Most of the movements of the body occur at the synovial joints. See Chapter 1 for the structure of a typical synovial joint.

2.3.1 Classification of synovial joints

The synovial joints are classified by the axes of movement (uniaxial, biaxial, multiaxial) and by structure as follows.

(1) A **hinge joint** allows movement in one direction only, in the sagittal plane. It is a *uniaxial* joint. Examples of a hinge joint are the elbow (Fig. 2.3a) and the ankle.

(2) A **pivot joint** is restricted to rotational movement around a vertical axis in the horizontal plane. It is a *uniaxial* joint. Examples

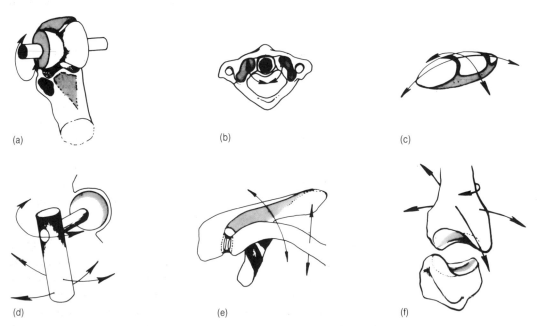

(a) (b) (c)

(d) (e) (f)

Fig. 2.3. Types of synovial joint: (a) hinge; (b) pivot; (c) ellipsoid; (d) ball and socket; (e) plane; (f) saddle.

are the atlantoaxial joint in the neck which turns the head to look sideways (Fig. 2.3b), and the joints in the forearm which allow the hand to turn so that the palm faces backwards.

(3) An **ellipsoid joint** has oval joint surfaces which allow movement in the sagittal and frontal planes, but no rotation. It is a *biaxial* joint. Examples are the radiocarpal (wrist) joint (Fig. 2.3c), and the joints at the base of the fingers (metacarpophalangeal joints).

(4) A **ball and socket joint** allows movement in three planes (Fig. 2.3d). It is a *triaxial* or *multiaxial* joint. Examples are the shoulder and hip joints.

(5) A **plane joint** has flat articular surfaces which allow limited gliding or twisting movement between the bones. An example is the joint between the acromion of the scapula and the clavicle (Fig. 2.3e). Plane joints may be arranged in series, so that the cumulative effect of the limited action at each joint gives considerable movement overall. The synovial joints between the bony arches of adjacent vertebrae are examples of plane joints, which together give the overall movements of the trunk (see Chapter 10, Section 10.3).

(6) A **saddle joint** has a surface which resembles a saddle (a concave-convexity) with a reciprocally curved surface sitting on it. The movements are in two planes with a limited range of rotation as well. The first carpometacarpal joint at the base of the thumb is a saddle joint (Fig. 2.3f).

The **range of movement** possible at each synovial joint depends on three main factors.

(1) The shape of the *bony* articulating surfaces determines both the direction and extent of the movement. For example, the shallow socket of the shoulder joint allows a wide range of movement.

(2) The position, strength and tautness of the surrounding *ligaments* affects range. By regular stretching exercises from an early age, gymnasts and ballet dancers can stretch certain joint ligaments to achieve a greater range of movement.

(3) The strength and size of *muscles* surrounding the joint. Bulging muscles around a joint halt movement when the two moving segments come into contact. For example, bending the elbow is limited by contact of the forearm with the upper arm. Other muscles may restrict movement by their position in relation to a joint. Tight hamstring muscles at the back of the thigh limit bending of the hips in touching the toes.

2.3.2 Terms for movement at synovial joints

Starting from the anatomical position, paired terms are used to distinguish the direction of movement of body segments in the three planes described (Fig. 2.4).

(1) **Flexion** and **extension** are movements in the sagittal plane. Flexion movements bend the body part away from the anatomical position. Extension is movement in the opposite direction back to the anatomical position and beyond into a reversed position (Fig. 2.4a). In flexion, the angle between the bones is usually decreased, e.g. flexion of the elbow bends the forearm forwards and upwards towards the arm, flexion of the knee takes the leg backwards towards the thigh. Flexion movements curl the body into a ball, while extension stretches the body out.

(2) **Abduction** and **adduction** are movements in the frontal plane. Abduction movements carry a body part away from the midline. Adduction is movement in the opposite direction towards the midline (Fig. 2.4b). In the hands and feet, the movements are related to the central axis of the segment. The fingers move away from the middle finger, and the toes move away from the second toe.

- *DO NOT confuse aBduction and aDduction – the letter b comes first in the alphabet, and is followed by d, the return movement being adduction. The prefixes come from latin and you will recognise that 'ab' means 'away from', as in abscond – to escape; and 'ad' means 'towards', as in addition and adherent.*

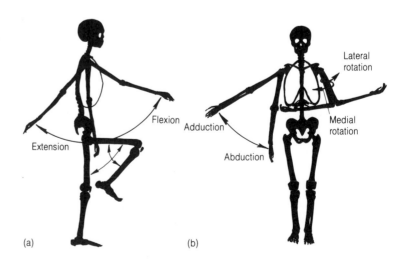

Fig. 2.4. Movements at joints: (a) flexion and extension; (b) abduction and adduction; medial and lateral rotation.

(a) (b)

When the return movement continues beyond the anatomical position, the terms 'hyperextension' and 'hyperadduction' may be used (hyper means 'more than').

(3) **Rotation** is movement in the horizontal plane about a vertical axis. When the bone is rotating away from the midline, or towards the posterior surface, the movement is known as *lateral rotation* (or external rotation). In the reverse movement, the bone turns in towards the midline of the body, and is known as *medial rotation* (or internal rotation) (Fig. 2.4b).

(4) **Circumduction** is a term used to describe a sequence of movements of flexion, abduction, extension and adduction. The bone moves round in a conical shape with the apex of the cone at the moving joint, and the base at the distal end of the bone. True circumduction does not include rotation.

The paired movement terms are also used to name the groups of muscles producing them. Muscles which bend the fingers are known as *flexors* of the fingers, while *extensors* straighten the fingers. The *abductors* of the hip carry the leg sideways.

- *STAND in the anatomical position. Move each of the large joints in turn, e.g. shoulder, elbow, wrist, hip, knee, ankle.*
- *RECORD the movements possible at each of the joints.*

Most body movements do not start at the anatomical position, but they are described with reference to that position. To analyse a movement, the starting position must first be defined. For example, lifting a glass from a table to the mouth starts with the shoulder in a neutral position, the elbow flexed, the wrist extended, and the fingers flexed around the glass. The changes at each joint are then described as the movement proceeds. To drink, the shoulder must be flexed and the elbow flexed further to bring the glass to the lips.

- *OBSERVE some simple everyday activities such as: standing up from sitting, climbing stairs, reaching to a high shelf, and pulling down a blind.*
- *RECORD the starting position, and list the movements made at each of the joints involved.*

2.4 Muscle attachments and group action

Muscles produce movements at joints by pulling on the bones to which they are attached. To describe a muscle, we name its attachments. One end of the muscle is usually fixed, and the attachments at the other end move. The attachment that is usually fixed or held steady is known as the *origin* of the muscle, it is usually more proximal. The moving end is called the *insertion* and is usually more distal. Some muscles can work from either end. For example, the muscle that extends the hip (gluteus maximus) pulls the thigh backwards as in climbing stairs (Fig. 2.5a). On the other hand, if the trunk is flexed forwards, this hip extensor acts in reverse to pull the pelvis upwards and straighten the trunk on the leg (Fig. 2.5b).

Group action in muscles (Fig. 2.6)

No muscle acts alone. All the muscles arranged around a joint are involved in the movement at that joint. In the case of the elbow joint, there are four muscles crossing the front of the joint and two that lie posteriorly. The anterior group are the flexors and the posterior group are the extensors. When the elbow is actively flexed, the flexors are the *prime movers* (or *agonists*), and the extensors become the *antagonists*. The extensors are recipro-

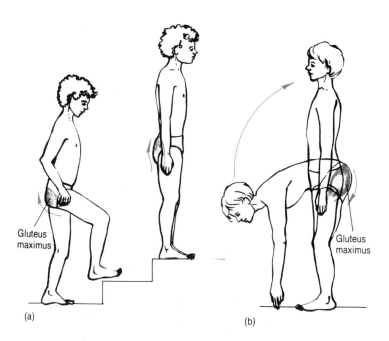

Fig. 2.5. Muscle attachments. Action of the gluteus maximus in extension of the hip: (a) distal attachment moves; (b) proximal attachment moves.

Gluteus maximus

(a)

Gluteus maximus

(b)

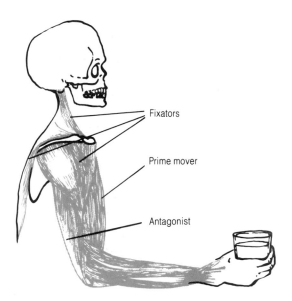

Fixators

Prime mover

Antagonist

Fig. 2.6. Group action of muscles in lifting a glass. Prime mover (biceps), antagonist (triceps), and fixators (muscles attached to the clavicle and scapula).

cally relaxed during elbow flexion, but will act as controllers of the extent and speed of the movement. Other muscles are active to support the proximal joints, these are known as *fixators*. They are able to fix the origin of the prime movers. When the biceps are active as a prime mover, the muscles attached to the trunk, scapula and humerus are active as fixators to fix the origin of the biceps. If the muscles acting as prime movers pass over more than one joint, other muscles known as *synergists* are active to prevent undesirable movements occurring at the other joints. For example, the flexors of the fingers cross the wrist and other joints in the hand. When gripping the handle of a tool or a racquet, the wrist extensors act as synergists to prevent wrist flexion, and allow the finger flexors to exert maximum holding power on the handle.

2.5 Types of muscle action (known as muscle work)

Muscle action is not only used to make a body part *move*, it may also be necessary to *hold* the position of a body part, such as the forearm supporting a book in the hand. Muscles are also used to control the effect of an external force acting on a body part. When moving from standing to sitting down on to a chair, the extensors of the leg work to control the effect of gravity, which is pulling the body down on to the seat. The term 'muscle contraction' may be a misleading one, because muscle action may involve the *shortening* of the muscle, or staying the *same* length, or a controlled *lengthening* of the muscle. For this reason, muscle action (muscle work) is categorised into concentric, eccentric and static work.

Concentric work (now sometimes called isotonic shortening)

This applies to muscles that are shortening to produce a movement. When a saucepan is lifted off a stove, the elbow flexors are working concentrically – they shorten to lift the pan (Fig. 2.7a).

Eccentric work (now sometimes called isotonic lengthening)

An active muscle that is lengthening is doing eccentric work. The muscle activity is controlling the rate and extent of movement as the attachments are drawn apart by external forces, such as gravity. When a saucepan is put down on to a stove, gravity is assisting the movement, so the elbow flexors must work eccentrically to control the movement, allowing the pan to be placed carefully on the hot plate (Fig. 2.7b).

Static work (also called isometric)

The active muscles which remain the same length to hold a position are doing static or isometric work – 'isometric' means same length. If the saucepan is held still over the stove, the elbow flexors are working isometrically to prevent it from dropping down.

Static work is the most tiring form of muscle work and should not be performed for long periods without rest. Fatigue is largely due to poor blood flow and accumulation of waste

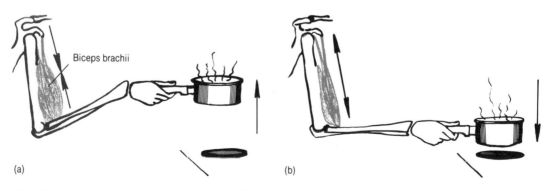

(a) (b)

Fig. 2.7. Types of muscle work: (a) concentric; (b) eccentric.

products in the muscle, partly because the static state reduces the pumping action of contracting muscles on the circulation of the blood. The terms 'isometric' and 'isotonic' were first used by physiologists to distinguish two types of muscle response in isolated frog muscle. Isotonic means 'the same tension', and applies to a muscle that changes in length without a change in the tension within the muscle. In the human body, true isotonic muscle activity rarely occurs, because over the whole range of movement changes in muscle tension occur in response to the changing effects of gravity and leverage (see Section 2.6.3 for discussion of leverage). Isometric work does occur in the body when muscles are not changing length but they are active to hold the position of a body segment and any added load. The term is also used in exercise programmes, when the muscles are working against the resistance of springs or weights.

- *ASK a partner to lift the forearms to a horizontal position and feel the tension in the elbow flexors by palpating the muscles above the elbow.*
- *PLACE a tray in the hands with the forearms in the same position. Note the change in the tension (hardness) of the elbow flexors even though there has been no change in length of the muscles. This is because the elbow flexors are having to develop tension to support the added load of the tray.*

2.6 Biomechanical principles

Mechanical principles that apply to buildings and machines, such as bridges, cranes and trucks, are equally appropriate when applied to the human body and its segments. Therapists commonly use terms such as muscle tension, strength and power in the rehabilitation of weak muscles. In this section, the terms used in biomechanics to describe the mechanical components of muscle action will be defined. Their application to both body movement and to the adaptation of the environment will also be considered.

When a muscle is active, it becomes tense. This *tension* that develops inside a muscle generates a *force* at the point of attachment of the muscle to a bone. The force produces movement at the joint over which the muscle is acting. The work done by the active muscle is the product of the force generated by its action and the distance moved by the body part.

Forces outside the body also produce movement. One external force is *gravity*, which is a constant downward force acting at the centre of a body segment, for example the thigh or the trunk. The whole weight of an object, or of a body segment such as the forearm, acts vertically downwards through the *centre of gravity* of the segment. The position of the centre of gravity of any symmetrical object of uniform density can be found in the following way:

- *TAKE a piece of card of symmetrical shape – square, oblong or circular. Draw diagonals across it. The point where the diagonals meet is the centre of gravity.*
- *THREAD a string through the centre of gravity and note how the card is balanced at this point.*

The *force of gravity* acting on each body segment produces movement at joints. Other external forces acting on a body segment may be: the weight of an object, for example a book held in the hand; or the resistance offered by an object, for example a heavy lid on a box.

What happens to a joint at any instant depends on the net effect of all the *moments of force* acting around it. A moment of force is the product of its *magnitude* and its *distance* from the joint to which it is being applied (force × distance). In the body, moments of force act in different directions around a joint. If they are equal and opposite, they will cancel out and the joint will not move. The joint is then being held actively in a fixed position. If they do not cancel out, movement will occur towards the greatest moment of force. The balance between the opposing moments may be very finely tuned, leading to slow precise movements, for example in finger dexterity. A large difference in the balance of moments of force leads to rapid and accelerative movement, which may be seen at the shoulder when sweeping a floor, or cutting a hedge in the garden.

In bending the elbow (Fig. 2.8), the flexors exert a moment of force which depends on: (a) the force exerted by the muscles; and (b) the distance between the insertion of the muscles on the bones and the centre of the elbow joint. Gravity also exerts a moment of force in the opposite direction which is the product of: (a) the weight of the forearm and hand; and (b) the distance between the centre of gravity of this body segment and the centre of the joint. If the moment of force of the elbow flexors is greater than the moment of force due to the weight of the forearm, movement occurs.

The *power* output of a muscle is a combination of strength and speed of action. High levels of muscle power are needed

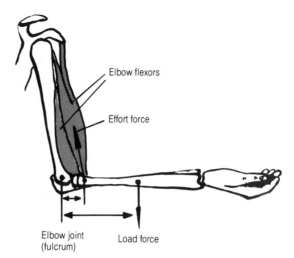

Fig. 2.8. Moments of force at the elbow. Fulcrum (elbow joint); load force (weight of the forearm and hand acting at the centre of gravity); effort force (tension in the elbow flexors acting at the point of insertion into the bones of the forearm).

when the speed of action is crucial to lift heavy loads in a few seconds.

In the process of *rehabilitation* of weak muscles, the upper limb may be supported by a sling, which will allow movement but will reduce the force due to gravity. This encourages weak muscles to perform tasks that may be impossible when the full effect of gravity must be overcome. As the muscles of the upper limb become stronger, movements can be achieved without the extra support.

Adaptation of the environment can reduce the need for using strong muscle forces against gravity. Reaching above the head demands strong muscles around the shoulder. In the kitchen, frequently used items can be placed in cupboards at the level of the elbow when standing, or when sitting in a wheelchair. Chairs with seats at an adequate height reduce the muscle work in the lower limbs required to stand up from sitting, compared with the extra muscle work needed to stand from a low seat.

2.6.1 Stability

An essential feature of all movement is the need to keep the body in stable equilibrium, so that we do not fall over while the body is changing position. We can all imagine the stability problems of a gymnast balancing on a beam, or a ballet dancer poised on the toes, but we take for granted the balance requirements of everyday activities. We do not have to think about balance at each step as we walk, but we may become aware of

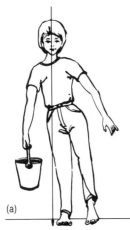

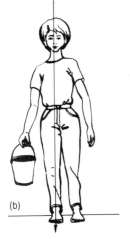

(a)

(b)

Fig. 2.9. Stability in carrying a weight at the side of the body: (a) unstable; (b) stable.

the problem when we are standing on a jolting train or bus. If the nervous system, which automatically makes the adjustments, is not functioning correctly, the balance of the body may become a constant problem and movements are difficult to perform.

The two main factors that contribute to stability are: (a) position of the centre of gravity; and (b) size of the base of support.

Position of the centre of gravity

An object is in stable equilibrium when its centre of gravity lies over its base of support.

- *RETURN to the piece of card used to find the centre of gravity. PLACE the card flat on a table and move it towards the edge of the table. Note when the card falls off the table.*

In the same way, the upright body is only stable when the line of weight from the centre of gravity lies within the foot base. If the line of weight moves outside the foot base as we move around, we will fall over. If the body was rigid like a plaster figure, the addition of a weight on one side would move the centre of gravity to that side and the figure would topple over as soon as the line of weight falls outside the base. In the body, the postural mechanisms of the nervous system make sure this does not happen. Figure 2.9a shows how the added weight of a bucket held in the hand moves the line of weight to the right and beyond the foot base so that the body will fall to that side. Figure 2.9b shows how the body segments alter their position to move the line of weight back over the foot base and the body becomes stable again. This realignment of body segments occurs automatically.

In upright standing, the *centre of gravity* of the body is located just anterior to the upper border of the sacrum (see Chapter 10, Fig. 10.2). This position, low in the trunk and over the feet, offers stability. The centre of gravity changes position during movement. Lifting the arms raises the centre of gravity, bending the knees lowers it.

The important principle to remember is that the stability is greater when the centre of gravity is lower, so it follows that all efforts to help the balance of the body should be directed to positions where the centre of gravity is lowest. If we bend to pick up a child or a box, the knees should be bent and the trunk flexed to move the centre of gravity down and over the feet. A hoist used to move a patient will be most stable if it is adjusted to the lowest position.

Base support

The upright body is least stable when the feet are parallel and close together because in this position the base support is small (Fig. 2.10a). As the feet are moved further apart the base support is increased and we are less likely to fall over (Fig. 2.10b).

The centre of gravity moves horizontally in reaching forwards and to the side in standing. The line of weight from the centre of gravity must be maintained within the foot base to keep the body in balance.

In standing up from sitting, stability can be increased by moving the feet back and leaning the trunk forwards in preparation for standing, see Chapter 8, Figure 8.11c.

Walking aids such as a stick, crutches or pulpit frame all increase the size of the base support and therefore allow more swaying of the body above without falling (Fig. 2.10c). A therapist should stand with feet apart and knees bent to be in a stable position to resist the added weight of the patient he/she is helping to move.

2.6.2 Principles of levers

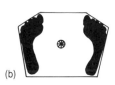

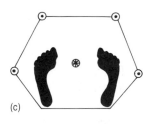

Fig. 2.10. Base support: (a) feet together; (b) feet apart; (c) feet with walking frame.

In the body, the bones form rigid levers and each joint is a pivot or *fulcrum*. The principles of levers therefore apply to all posture and movement in the body.

We have already defined 'moment of force' at the beginning of Section 2.6; it is the product of the force and its distance from the fulcrum. A moment of force is always tending to produce movement, and a lever is only balanced when the moments of force acting around the fulcrum are equal and opposite.

We are all familiar with this principle when sitting on a see saw with a small child. By putting the child at the far end on one side of the see saw, we can balance the see saw by sitting near to the central pivot or *fulcrum*. This shows how a large force at a short distance can balance a small force at a larger distance (Fig. 2.11a). Levers do not always have the fulcrum in the middle, the forces may both be acting on the same side of the fulcrum. A wheel barrow is an example of this type of lever (Fig. 2.11b). The wheel in contact with the ground forms the fulcrum. The load in the barrow is near to the fulcrum, and the effort is applied by the hands to the handles at a greater distance from the fulcrum on the same side.

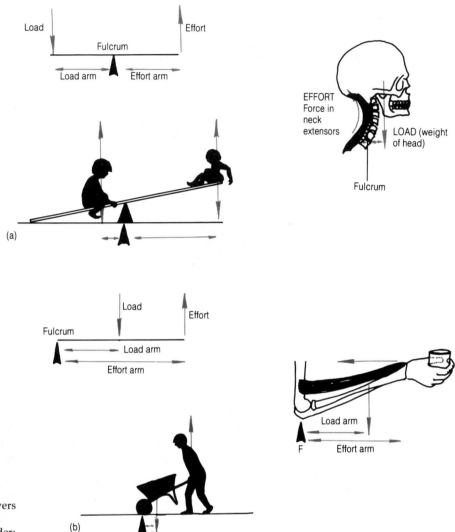

Fig. 2.11. Levers
(a) first order;
(b) second order;

The muscles acting on the joints exert *effort forces* on the bony levers. The part of a lever between the fulcrum and the point of application of effort can be called the *effort arm*.

The total force of the weight of any body segment and any added weight is the *load force*. The part of a lever between the fulcrum and the point of application of the load can be called the *load arm*.

For movement to occur against gravity, the muscle moment (effort force times effort arm) must be greater than the gravity moment (load force times load arm). If either force, or its point of application, is changed, the leverage changes.

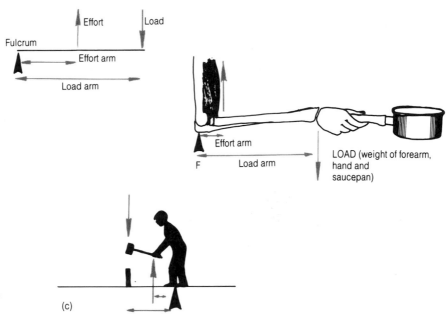

Fig. 2.11. (cont)
(c) third order.

(c)

Levers are classified into first, second and third class. Figure 2.11 shows the arrangement of effort, fulcrum and load in each of the three orders of levers, with examples of each. Most of the muscles of the body act as third order levers since the muscles are attached near to the joint they move. The advantage of this arrangement is that it gives a greater range and speed of movement, which is important in throwing and swinging actions of the upper limb, as well as in walking and running actions in the lower limb. A few muscles, for example brachioradialis in the forearm, act as second class levers (Fig. 2.11b). The tension in this muscle is important to relieve the stress on the bones of the forearm when weights are held in the hand.

The principles of levers can be used to increase the *strength of muscles* by exercise against gradually increasing loads. For example, activities for weak shoulder muscles should first involve gravity assisted movement and then movements with the elbow flexed so that the load arm is short (Fig. 2.12a). As the muscles become stronger, the shoulder can be used to reach with the extended upper limb (load arm longer) (Fig. 2.12b). Eventually, reaching with an object held in the hand (load force larger) can be achieved (Fig. 2.12c).

In weight training programmes, the muscles are exercised against increasing resistance placed at increasing distances from the joint which forms the centre of the movement. If we wish to

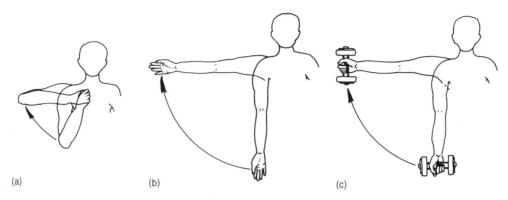

Fig. 2.12. Principles of levers. Increase in effort required to lift the arm sideways: (a) short load arm; (b) long load arm; (c) long load arm plus added object.

increase the strength of abdominal muscles, sit ups are performed first without weights, next with a weight held in front of the chest, and finally with the weight held in the outstretched arms.

In *lifting* and *carrying loads* the effort force of the back muscles acts at the fulcrum in the lower back. This effort force must overcome the moment of force of the trunk plus the added load. Figure 2.13 shows how the length of the load arm (distance between the line of weight and the fulcrum in the lower back) changes in different starting positions for lifting a child. Position (c) requires least effort for the back muscles as the load arm is shortest.

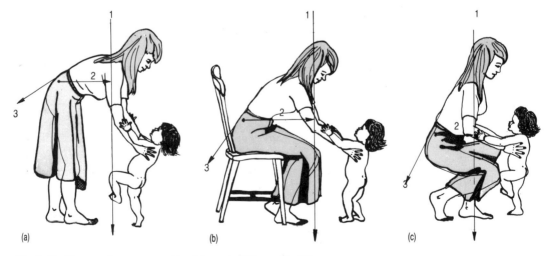

Fig. 2.13. Changes in moment of load force in lifting with different start positions: (a) standing with straight legs; (b) sitting; (c) bent knees. 1 = line of weight; 2 = load arm; 3 = effort force.

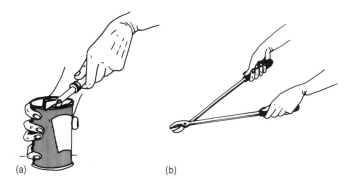

Fig. 2.14. Adaptation of tools to reduce effort: (a) tin opener with extended handle; (b) long handled shears.

(a)   (b)

Leverage is also applied in *adapting tools* used in daily living for people with weak muscles or painful joints. If the lid of a jar is opened by a tool with a long handle then less effort will be required than when grasping the lid itself. Scissors and shears with long handles will be easier to use than those with short handles (Fig. 2.14).

In the adaptation of tools and equipment for use by people with weak muscles it is important to remember two rules.

(1) Put the *load* as *near* to the pivot as possible.

(2) Apply the *effort* as *far* from the pivot as possible.

At the end of this chapter, you should be able to:

(1) Define the anatomical position, and the three major planes and axes of movement of the body.

(2) Describe the classification of synovial joints based on structure, and the movements that occur in each type of joint. Outline the factors that affect the range of movement at joints.

(3) Define the terms for movement in the three planes at the joints of the body.

(4) Appreciate how the attachments of muscles are described. Understand what is meant by the 'group action of muscles'.

(5) Distinguish three types of muscle work: concentric, eccentric and static.

(6) Define the following biomechanical terms: muscle tension, moment of force, centre of gravity (of a body segment and of the whole body) and muscle power.

(7) Explain how the position of the centre of gravity of the body, and the area of base suppport, affect body stability.

(8) Understand the principles of levers applied to: (a) movement resulting from the balance of moments of force acting around a joint; and (b) the adaptation of equipment and tools to reduce the effort required in their use.

3 / Control Systems: The Brain and Spinal Cord

The organisation of the nervous system begins centrally as folds which appear along the back of the 3-week-old embryo. The folds meet to form the neural tube, and the nervous tissue destined to become the central nervous system is laid down. Folding and bending of the cranial (head) section of the tube follows to form the *brain*, whilst simpler growth changes in the remainder of the neural tube form the *spinal cord*. While the adult brain presents a clear superficial appearance, the result of the folding in the embryo is a complex arrangement of the deep brain areas. The 'first look' at the central nervous system in this chapter will be focused on providing the names, location and overall function of the parts of the brain and spinal cord, with particular emphasis on their role in movement.

PART I
THE BRAIN

3.1 Position and relations of the main brain areas

At first glance the brain seems to only be composed of the two cerebral hemispheres (Fig. 3.1). Although they are the largest feature of the brain, they conceal many other important areas. The two symmetrical hemispheres have a folded surface with their inner aspects lying close together in the midline. Underneath the posterior end of each cerebral hemisphere is the *cerebellum*, which also has two hemispheres that are joined together in the midline. Part of the *pons* is visible anterior to the cerebellum; and below the pons, is the cone shaped *medulla oblongata*. The medulla leads down into the spinal cord at the foramen magnum ('large hole') in the base of the skull.

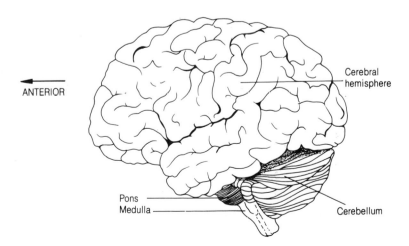

ANTERIOR

Cerebral hemisphere

Pons
Medulla

Cerebellum

Fig. 3.1. External appearance of the brain, lateral view of the left side.

A look at the development of the brain shown in Figure 3.2a will help in the understanding of the position and form of the brain areas in the adult.

The **forebrain** first grows laterally and backwards. It then folds forwards on itself and takes on the appearance of a hand wearing a boxing glove with the thumb touching the palm when

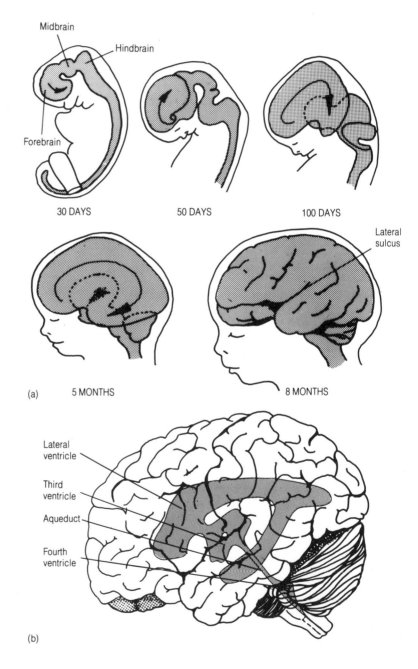

Fig. 3.2. (a) Development of the brain showing folding of the forebrain. (b) Adult brain viewed from the left showing the position of the cavities.

viewed from the side in the adult *cerebral hemispheres*. Hidden by the extensive growth of the cerebral hemispheres, the base of the forebrain develops to form the *basal ganglia, thalamus* and *hypothalamus*. The part of the forebrain known as the *diencephalon* or 'between-brain', containing the thalamus and hypothalamus, provides important links between the cerebral hemispheres and other parts of the central nervous system for both sensory and motor activity. The cavity in the centre of the diencephalon is a thin slit between the two thalami, called the third ventricle.

The **midbrain** continues in the same position during development, increasing in total size, but obscured in the external view of the brain by the lower temporal lobes of the cerebral hemispheres. In the adult, the midbrain looks like the 'waist' area with the expanded forebrain above and hindbrain below. Find the midbrain in the sagittal section of the brain (Fig. 3.3). The midbrain provides routes for pathways carrying impulses up or down to various levels of the central nervous system and is also important for analysis of information from the eyes and ears.

The *brain stem* is the term used to describe the brain areas below the diencephalon, which include the *midbrain*, and the *pons* and *medulla* of the **hind brain**. The *cerebellum* grows out posteriorly from the hind brain to lie below the posterior part of the expanded cerebral hemispheres. If the outgrowths of the cerebral hemispheres and the cerebellum are removed from the

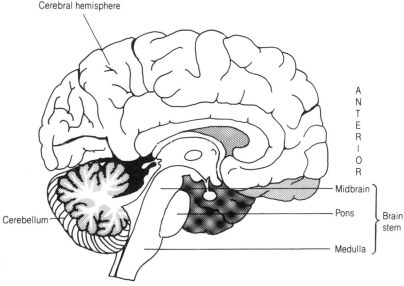

Fig. 3.3. Median sagittal section of the brain.

brain, the complete brain stem can be seen with the diencephalon above. The functional importance of the brain stem in movement is the regulation of all the automatic adjustments to changes in posture which maintain the balance of the body.

The developing brain retains an internal cavity which forms the ventricular system containing cerebrospinal fluid. The cavity within each cerebral hemisphere follows the shape of the half clenched hand and is known as the lateral ventricle. The cavity in the centre of the diencephalon is a thin slit between the two thalami, called the third ventricle. The central cavity of the midbrain is a narrow canal called the aqueduct which leads down into the fourth ventricle, the cavity of the midbrain. The fourth ventricle lies behind the pons and upper part of the medulla, with the cerebellum forming the roof of the cavity. Figure 3.2b shows the cavities of the brain in position in the adult brain.

- *LOOK at a model of the brain, and diagrams of sections through the brain in anatomy textbooks to identify the position and relationships of the following brain areas: cerebral hemispheres, thalamus, basal ganglia, midbrain, pons, cerebellum and medulla oblongata.*

3.2 Cerebrospinal fluid

Cerebrospinal fluid is found in all the cavities of the brain, and in the central canal of the spinal cord. The same fluid is also found surrounding the brain and spinal cord, in between two of the three layers of protective connective tissue known as the meninges. (The meninges of the spinal cord are described in Section 3.13.) The main function of the fluid is to act as a shock absorber. It also carries nutrients and other essential substances to the nerve tissue. Figure 3.4 shows a sagittal section of the brain and part of the spinal cord to illustrate the way in which the cerebrospinal fluid circulates through the central cavities and around the outside of the central nervous system. The fluid is secreted from special patches of blood capillaries called choroid plexuses situated in each of the ventricles of the brain. The ventricles are found in the areas of greatest growth and expansion during development. Cerebrospinal fluid is formed by a process of filtration from the capillaries of each choroid plexus at the rate of 500 ml per day. Follow the arrows in Figure 3.4 to see how the fluid flows downwards in the brain and then through openings in the roof of the fourth ventricle into the space between the coverings of the brain. The absorption of cerebrospinal fluid

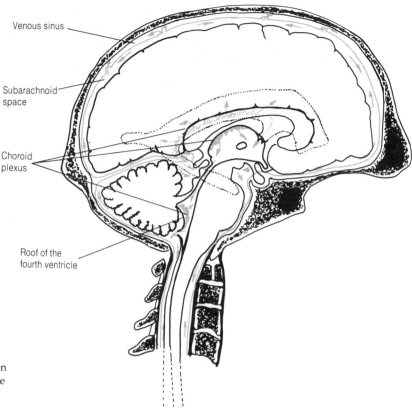

Venous sinus

Subarachnoid space

Choroid plexus

Roof of the fourth ventricle

Fig. 3.4. Sagittal section of the brain to show the circulation of cerebrospinal fluid.

into the blood takes place mainly in the venous sinus between the two cerebral hemispheres, known as the superior sagittal sinus.

3.3 Organisation of grey and white matter

The basic structure of neurones has been described in Chapter 1. Surprisingly, half the volume of the central nervous system is not made up of neurones, but of *neuroglia* which are special support cells found in between neurones, and of capillaries which supply the high oxygen demands of nerve tissue. The neuroglia act as transporting and insulating cells, and also cooperate in the function of the neurones.

All the *cell bodies* and dendrites of the *neurones* form the core of the central nervous system known as *grey matter*. In the brain the core is not continuous, but the cells are collected together for a particular function to form many *nuclei* of grey matter. For example, the thalamus is a nucleus of grey matter where sensory neurones synapse and project to other areas. The *axons* of the neurones lie in the *white matter* surrounding the nuclei in the brain stem. In the cerebral hemispheres and cerebellum an additional layer of grey matter, known as the *cortex*, lies outside the white matter. The cell bodies of the cortical neurones are laid down in layers in an organised way. The cortical grey matter is folded to greatly increase the surface area. Each raised part seen on the surface is known as a *gyrus*. Each depression in between the gyri is called a *sulcus* (Fig. 3.5a). A very deep sulcus is sometimes called a *fissure*. In the white matter the bundles of axons lie in particular directions which are classified into four different functional categories, shown in Figure 3.5b.

(1) Short association fibres connect groups of adjacent gyri. They form 'U' shaped bands which bend around the sulci.

(2) Long association fibres are found lying deeper, and connect one part of the surface grey matter with another within the same hemisphere.

(3) Commissural fibres connect cortical cells from one hemisphere with those of the opposite hemispheres. These fibres come together to form the major bridges between the right and left hemisphere. The main bridge lies above the diencephalon and is

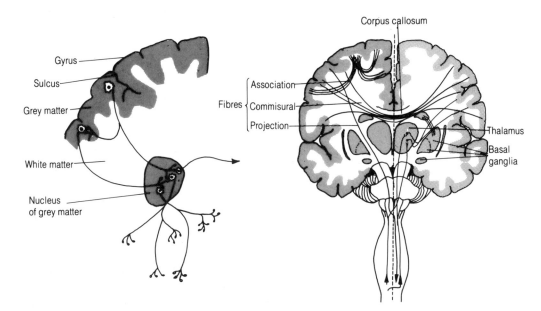

Fig. 3.5. (a) Small area of cortex of grey matter to show gyrus and sulcus, nucleus of grey matter. (b) Frontal section of the brain showing projection, association and commissural fibres.

known as the *corpus callosum*. It contains an estimated one million nerve fibres. There are also smaller groups of commissural fibres located adjacent to the corpus callosum.

(4) Projection fibres convey information between the surface grey matter and lower centres of the brain stem and spinal cord. Each of the projection fibres carries impulses in one direction only, either upwards or downwards.

- *LOOK at a brain model and sections of the brain to identify:*

(1) *The cortical layer of grey matter in the cerebral hemispheres and cerebellum – it forms the outer surface like the skin of a fruit.*

(2) *The nuclei of grey matter in the brain stem and at the base of the cerebral hemispheres and cerebellum.*

(3) *The white matter found below the layers of cortex, and also surrounding the nuclei in the brain stem.*

It is important to build up a three dimensional picture of the shape, position and relations of the areas of the brain. Diagrams of sections taken through the brain at different levels can be compared with slices in various directions of a Swiss (jelly) roll or a piece of marble. Each slice shows one particular colour in a different way, but the shapes can be put together to determine the three dimensional shape inside. This task is not easy, but can be achieved with practice.

3.4 Cerebral hemispheres

The expansion of the cerebral hemispheres (or cerebrum) to envelop nearly all other brain areas distinguishes the primates, especially man, from other animals. It is, therefore, not surprising that the surface of the hemispheres (cerebral cortex) has been studied extensively for over two centuries. The microscopists of the mid-nineteenth century noted variations in the basic cellular architecture in different regions of the cerebral cortex. The result of these studies was a detailed mapping into 52 areas, numbered by Brodman (1909) and used clinically to this day for purposes of description (Fig. 3.6). Meanwhile evidence from brain damage was accumulating to suggest that different areas of the cerebral cortex have particular functions. In 1848, an American railroad worker named Phineas Gage survived an iron bar piercing right through the front of his brain. He could still move, eat and talk normally without a large area of cerebral hemisphere. His friends

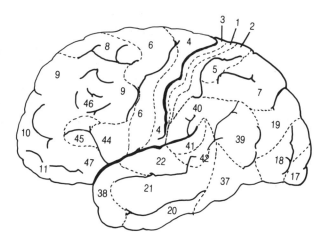

Fig. 3.6. Cerebral hemispheres with examples of Brodman areas.

commented that his personality had changed. A few years later in 1861 Broca identified a particular area in the left hemisphere concerned with speech from the post-mortem examination of a patient with a severe motor speech defect. Evidence from head injuries in soldiers in the trenches in World War 1, and studies of the electrical activity of the surface of the brain during surgical intervention led to the identification of distinct motor and sensory areas related to particular parts of the body. The remaining 'silent' parts of the cortex were described as association areas for interpretation and integration of the activity in the primary areas. A map of functional areas of the cerebral cortex was developed which is still used as a diagnostic tool in damage and disease of the central nervous system.

Each cerebral hemisphere is divided into four lobes named after the skull bones which cover them (Fig. 3.7a). In each hemisphere the lobes are separated by two deep sulci – the central sulcus and the lateral sulcus.

(1) The **frontal lobe** lies anterior to the central sulcus and above the lateral sulcus.

(2) The **parietal lobe** lies behind the central sulcus.

(3) The **occipital lobe** is at the posterior end of the hemisphere, above the cerebellum at the base of the skull.

(4) The **temporal lobe** lies below the lateral sulcus.

Each lobe continues on to the medial surface of the hemisphere, shown in Figure 3.7b, and is separated from the opposite hemisphere by the median sagittal sulcus (Fig. 3.7c).

It is important to realise that the surface of the cerebral hemispheres extends from the level of the eyebrows in front, to

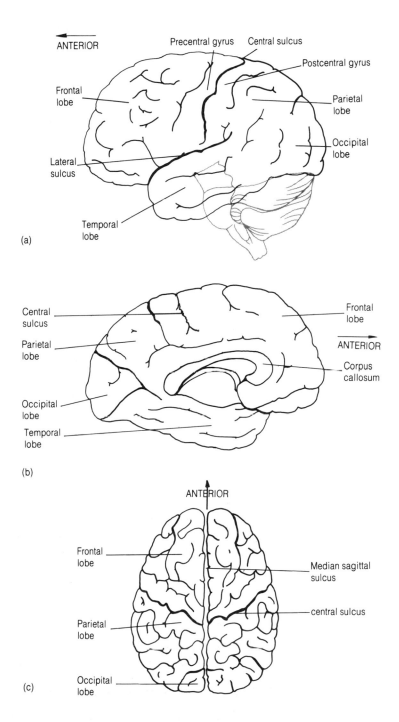

Fig. 3.7. Cerebral hemispheres to show the position of the lobes: (a) lateral view; (b) medial view; (c) view from above.

the base of the skull at the back of the head, and down to the level of the ears at the side. This becomes obvious when a life size model of the brain is placed inside the cranial cavity of the skull.

Clinical note-pad 3A: Cerebral vascular accident (CVA)/ stroke

A CVA is focal damage to brain tissue, which develops rapidly. It is vascular in origin and may be caused by a cerebral haemorrhage or a thrombus or embolus. The resulting damage to brain tissue is known as a lesion, which can be identified by the modern imaging techniques of X-ray, CT scanning and magnetic resonance imaging (MRI). The overall loss of function, including the pattern of motor and sensory loss, depends on the size and the location of the lesion. The effects are contralateral (on the opposite side of the body) to the lesion site in the brain. Bilateral lesions can occur in stroke.

See clinical note-pad 3G for a summary of the effects of lesions.

The overall functions of each lobe of the cerebral hemispheres will be described in turn. It is important to stress that the numerous interconnections between the four lobes means that no individual lobe functions alone.

3.4.1   Frontal lobe

The frontal lobe is a large part of the cerebral hemisphere found underneath the frontal bone of the skull. The part of the frontal lobe particularly concerned with the performance of movement lies more posteriorly in the lobe, leading up to the central sulcus. The larger anterior part of the lobe, which lies above the orbit of the eyes (supraorbital area), is involved in planning and problem solving aspects of both movement and behaviour. This part of the frontal lobe is also called the prefrontal lobe.

The posterior band of grey matter lying immediately in front of the central sulcus (precentral gyrus) is the **primary motor area**, which is concerned with the performance of movement in the whole of the opposite side of the body (Fig. 3.8a). The cell bodies of the neurones in the motor cortex do not project to individual muscles, but to functional groups of muscles. Direct links to the small muscles of the hands, the feet and the face are particularly important, and damage to the motor cortex results in loss of precision movements.

There is representation of half of the body in an 'upside down' position in each primary motor cortex. The head is represented in the lower cortex on the lateral side, then the upper limb and trunk above, and finally the lower leg and feet in the cortex on the medial surface of the lobe. In Figure 3.9, a vertical section through the cerebral hemisphere at the level of the primary motor area is shown (frontal section). Note that the

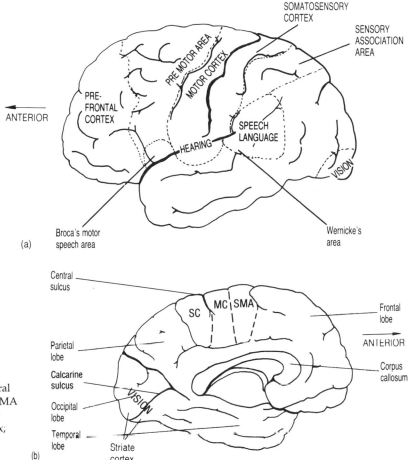

(a)

(b)

Fig. 3.8. Cerebral hemispheres, main functional areas: (a) lateral view; (b) medial view. SMA = supplementary motor area; MC = motor cortex; SC = somatosensory cortex.

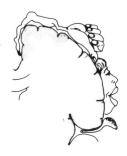

Fig. 3.9. Frontal section through precentral gyrus (motor cortex) to show representation of body parts.

size of the body parts are not in normal proportions. The body parts that move with the greatest degree of precision have larger areas of representation, so that the face and hand are large, while the trunk and leg are small. A figure constructed with these dimensions has a head like a hippopotamus, the hands of a giant and the trunk and legs of a dwarf – it is known as the 'motor homunculus'.

The **premotor area** lies in front of the primary motor area on the lateral surface of the lobe (Fig. 3.8a). Neurones project from this area to the primary motor area on the same and the opposite side. Projection fibres from the premotor area descend directly to the spinal cord, or indirectly via the primary motor cortex. The premotor cortex has a role in the coordination and the execution of learned bilateral movements such as walking.

The **supplementary motor area** also lies anterior to the primary motor area, but mainly on the medial side of the frontal lobe (Fig. 3.8b). This area of cortex is active immediately before the execution of movement, which suggests a role in the planning of movement.

The **motor speech area** identified by Broca lies in the lower part of the frontal lobe in the lip of the lateral sulcus (see Fig. 3.8a). The function of this area, usually only found in the dominant hemisphere, is in the production of fluent speech.

The **prefrontal** (or supraorbital) **area** occupies the large anterior area of the frontal lobe and connects with all the other lobes of the cerebral hemispheres, the thalamus, the limbic system and many other brain areas. The functions of the prefrontal cortex are complex, and our current knowledge is based largely on the observations of the effects of damage to this area. It is concerned with the planning of movement and behaviour to reach a particular goal, and in modifying the plan in response to any changes which may originate internally or externally. The prefrontal cortex seems to determine the way we react to other people and to changes in the environment from day to day.

Clinical note-pad 3B: Frontal lobe lesion

(1) Primary and premotor cortex. Lesion on one side leads to muscle weakness in the muscles of the opposite side of the body, known as hemiplegia. Muscle tone may be low (flaccid) or high (spastic). Fine skilled movements of the extremities are particularly affected.

(2) Prefrontal cortex. Frontal lobe damage may lead to problems in planning movement and in reviewing it during progress. This has implications for safety. Loss of insight into movement performance may be a major factor in the poor prospect of successful rehabilitation. There may be inability to monitor social behaviour.

3.4.2   Parietal lobe

The parietal lobe lies posterior to the frontal lobe and beneath the parietal bone of the skull. The overall function of the parietal lobe is the processing of sensory input from receptors in all parts of the body and also from the special sense organs (eyes and ears). This gives us awareness of the position of the parts of the body during movement, and spatial awareness of the environment around us.

The **somatosensory** (somaesthetic) **area** is the primary area, which lies immediately behind the central sulcus in the post-central gyrus (Fig. 3.8a). Pathways from receptors in the skin, muscles and joints of the opposite side of the body connect with the primary sensory cortex via the thalamus. The areas of the body are represented in an 'upside down' position in the same way as in the primary motor cortex. The area of cortex representing the hand is large, particularly the palmar surface of the thumb and index finger. The lips also have a large area of representation for the complex sensory input required for speech and the mastication of food.

Posterior to the somatosensory area is the **sensory association area** where further processing of the sensory information occurs. An object, such as a key, held in the hand and moved about, can be recognised even with the eyes closed. Information about the size, shape, weight, temperature and texture arriving at the cortex can be integrated with reference to memory, so that the exact nature of the object can be identified. This ability is known as *stereognosis*.

In the parietal lobe, the processing of sensory information from the joints and muscles monitors the position of all body segments at every moment during movement. The parietal lobe also receives input from visual and auditory areas of the cortex so that objects and sounds in the area around the opposite side of space can be located and identified. This spatial information processed by the parietal lobe is essential for the ability to move and find our way around in the environment.

Clinical note-pad 3C: Parietal lobe lesion

There is loss of somatic sensation on the opposite side of the body, particularly in the distal parts of the limbs. The main features are inability to: (a) appreciate position sense of the limbs; (b) judge the weight of objects; (c) localise tactile information; or (d) appreciate degrees of warmth or cold. Inability to recognise objects without vision is known as astereognosis.

Loss of body and spatial awareness on the left side occurs in right parietal lesion. This is known as unilateral neglect, when the patient may ignore one side of the body, or objects in one side of space.

3.4.3 Temporal lobe

The temporal lobe, found beneath the temporal bone of the skull, is the 'hi-fi' area concerned with the reception, recording and replay of sound. The temporal lobe also plays a part in long-term memory.

Sound falling on the ear is transmitted by nerve impulses from the cochlea of the inner ear to the **primary auditory area** below the lateral sulcus in the temporal lobe (see Fig. 3.8a). The pathway is mainly crossed to the opposite temporal lobe, but each auditory area receives some impulses from both ears. The primary area links with auditory association areas in the superior temporal gyrus, which interpret the sound frequencies. In the dominant hemisphere, the extension of the auditory association area around the tip of the lateral sulcus and into the parietal lobe is known as *Wernicke's area* (Fig. 3.8a), which plays a role in receptive aspects of speech and language. Visual and auditory input from the written and spoken word are integrated in this area.

Clinical note-pad 3D: Temporal lobe lesion

If the primary auditory area is affected on one side, slight loss of hearing occurs in both ears, but the loss is greatest in the opposite ear.

More posterior lesions on the left side affect receptive aspects of language. The patient is unable to understand spoken or written words.

3.4.4 Occipital lobe

The occipital lobe lies beneath the occipital bone of the skull. All visual information transmitted from the eye is first processed by the occipital lobe.

The primary visual area, known as the **striate cortex**, lies at the posterior pole of the occipital lobe and extends mainly on to the inner or medial surface, on either side of the calcarine sulcus (Fig. 3.8b). Sections of the primary visual area reveal a horizontal stripe of white matter, hence the name striate cortex.

Impulses from the retina of both eyes arrive in each striate cortex. Information from the left half of the visual field for both eyes is processed in the right striate cortex. Conversely, the right half of the visual field for each eye is relayed to the left striate cortex.

The **prestriate cortex** is an association area which surrounds the primary area on the medial surface of the lobe (Fig. 3.8b). Further processing of the visual information occurs in the prestriate cortex. Links to the parietal and temporal lobes are involved in the recognition of objects and faces, and in the understanding of the written word.

Sensory information from the eyes plays a major role in movement. Vision is required for both the ability to place the foot accurately on the ground in locomotion, and to place the hand in a functional position with objects.

> ### Clinical note-pad 3E: Occipital lobe lesions
>
> (1) Hemianopia. Damage to the primary visual area on one side may result in loss of sight in an area of the opposite half of the visual field of each eye. In small lesions, there may be apparent normal central vision known as macula sparing. Patients usually compensate by turning the head so that objects are viewed in the normal half of each visual field.
>
> (2) Visual agnosia. Damage to the prestriate cortex leads to loss of the ability to recognise objects seen in the opposite side of space, even though the objects can be seen clearly. Bilateral damage results in severe visual recognition problems for objects and faces.

A **summary** of the main functions of the lobes of the cerebral hemispheres can now be made.

(1) **Frontal lobe**: planning and performance of movement; modifying movement and behaviour in response to changes in the environment; motor speech.

(2) **Parietal lobe**: sensation in the skin, the joints and the muscles; stereognosis; awareness of body position and of the spatial relations of the external environment.

(3) **Temporal lobe**: hearing; receptive speech and language; memory.

(4) **Occipital lobe**: vision.

> ### Clinical note-pad 3F: Traumatic brain injury
>
> In brain injury resulting from trauma to the head, multi-lesion sites occur. The clinical signs are complex, variable and related to more than one cerebral lobe, frequently frontal and occipital, or temporal. Mechanical stress on axons produces diffuse axonal injury.

3.4.5 Right and left hemispheres

The functional asymmetry of the right and left hemispheres, first recognised by Broca in the mid-nineteenth century, gained new

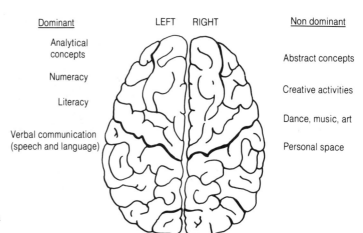

Fig. 3.10. Lateralisation of function in the right and left hemispheres.

interest from 'split brain' studies by Sperry in the 1970s. Sperry devised an experiment using two screens placed in positions so that information could be presented to only one of the visual fields at a time. This in turn meant that only one hemisphere received the information. These experiments showed that each hemisphere processes particular types of information, verbal on the left and spatial on the right.

Both sides of the normal brain receive the same basic input, so that any differences between the two must lie in their capacity to process different types of information. The *dominant* hemisphere (usually the left) contains the areas for speech and language, and this side is particularly concerned with analytical functions. The *non-dominant* hemisphere plays a greater role in non-verbal, creative activity requiring spatial processing (Fig. 3.10).

> **Clinical note-pad 3G: Summary of effects of stroke**
>
> (1) Left hemiplegia (right side lesion). Motor and/or sensory loss on the left side of the body. Visual and spatial problems.
>
> (2) Right hemiplegia (left side lesion). Motor and/or sensory loss on the right side of the body. Receptive and expressive language problems. Anxiety and depression.
>
> (3) Anterior lesions (frontal lobes). Impairment of cognitive function that affects the planning of movement and monitoring of its execution.
>
> (4) Posterior lesions (occipital lobes). Sensory and perceptual problems, inability to recognise objects and faces.

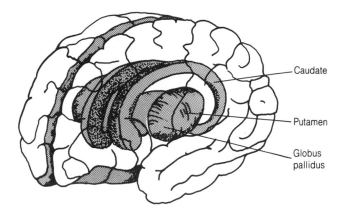

Fig. 3.11. Basal ganglia in position at base of cerebral hemispheres.

3.5 Basal ganglia

The basal ganglia (or basal nuclei) are found at the base of the cerebral hemispheres and in the midbrain. Figure 3.11 has made the lateral cerebral cortex appear to be transparent to reveal three of the basal ganglia: the *caudate*, *putamen* and *globus pallidus*. (The caudate and putamen are sometimes called the *corpus striatum*. The putamen and the globus pallidus are sometimes called the *lentiform nucleus*.) Two other basal nuclei are the *subthalamic nucleus* and the *substantia nigra*. The latter is in the midbrain.

Nerve fibres linking the individual nuclei with each other form a complex interdependent system, which functions as a whole. Most of the input to the basal ganglia is from the motor areas of the cerebral cortex, and the basal ganglia project back to these areas of the cortex via the thalamus (Fig. 3.12). The main influence of the basal ganglia on movement is via the motor cortical areas and their output to the motor neurones of the spinal cord in the planning and execution of movement.

There is evidence that sensory information, specifically related to action, is also processed by the basal ganglia. For example, when walking across the threshold of a door the visual input from the surroundings is integrated with the correct movements to negotiate the space.

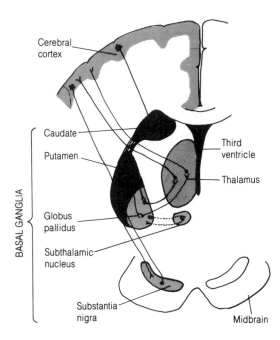

Fig. 3.12. Frontal section to show how the basal ganglia form links with the thalamus and the cerebral cortex.

Clinical note-pad 3H: Parkinson's disease

The progressive degeneration in the neurones of the substantia nigra, which project to other basal nuclei, leads to a reduction of dopamine (neurotransmitter) in the system of basal ganglia. The resulting effects include: (a) a resting tremor in distal joints that disappears during movement; (b) cogwheel rigidity in muscles; and (c) difficulty in the initiation and production of movement.

Other diseases of the basal ganglia include: *hemiballismus*, characterised by uncontrollable purposeless actions; and *Huntingdon's chorea*, an inherited condition that also shows involuntary movements.

Multisystems atrophy (MSA) involves all the basal ganglia and the general deterioration is accelerated.

3.6 Thalamus

The thalamus lies in the diencephalon, at the base of the forebrain and enveloped by the cerebral hemispheres. The slit-like third ventricle lies in the midline, and each thalamus is an oval mass of grey matter on either side of it. Figure 3.12 shows the thalamus on one side of the brain with the third ventricle medially and the basal ganglia laterally.

The thalamus is a complex mass of grey matter made up of

many nuclei. Sensory information arrives at the thalamus from all the sensory systems in the body except smell. The output from the thalamus radiates out to the cerebral cortex of the same side (ipsilateral) like the spokes of an umbrella with the thalamus at its centre.

Some of the nuclei are **specific**, receiving somatosensory information, such as the pressure from the skin of the hand grasping a handle, or the position of a limb from receptors in joint capsules. The thalamus processes this information, and activity is relayed to motor centres in the brain stem and to the cortex.

Non-specific sensory information arrives at the thalamus mainly from the reticular formation, which is a diffuse network of neurones found along the length of the brain stem (Fig. 3.18). The reticular formation, which acts to sift most of the sensory activity originating in the spinal cord, regulates the level of activity in the thalamus.

The overall function of the thalamus is to act as a centre for sensation which is passed on to the cerebral cortex for further processing. The thalamus also has important links with the basal ganglia and cerebellum. The role of the thalamus during movement will be considered in Chapters 11 and 12.

3.7 Internal capsule

The internal capsule is an area of *white matter* containing the projection fibres to and from the brain stem and cerebral cortex. Figure 3.13 is a sagittal section through one cerebral hemisphere showing the corona radiata of projection fibres all converging at

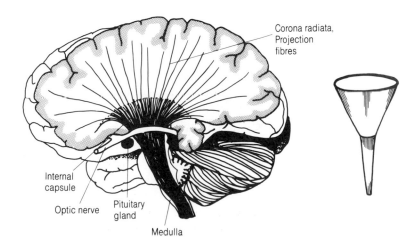

Fig. 3.13. Sagittal section to show the projection fibres converging into the internal capsule like a funnel.

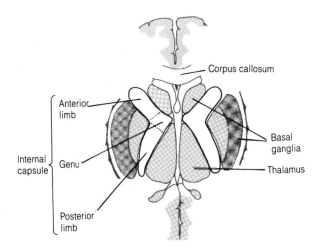

Fig. 3.14. Horizontal section at the level of the internal capsule.

the base of the hemisphere to form the internal capsule. The same fibres continue in the midbrain as the cerebral peduncles (Fig. 3.17a). The narrow pathway of the internal capsule lies between the putamen and globus pallidus laterally, with the thalamus and caudate nucleus medially. Figure 3.14 is a transverse section across the internal capsule to see its position in relation to these masses of grey matter in the diencephalon. Notice that in this view, the internal capsule is shaped like a boomerang. The fibres converge below to become the cerebral peduncles of the midbrain. The internal capsule is composed of motor and sensory nerve fibres supplying the muscles, skin and glands of the opposite side of the body. The term 'capsule' is a misleading one. The internal capsule is like the flattened stem of a funnel through which all the fibres to and from the cortex pass. Because of this convergence of nerve fibres into a narrow area, damage to the internal capsule has more extensive effects than a similar area of cortical damage.

3.8 Hypothalamus and limbic system

The **hypothalamus** is smaller than the thalamus and lies beneath it in the floor of the third ventricle (Fig. 3.15a). Like the basement of a house with thermostats and stopcocks, the hypothalamus contains groups of neurones for the control of body temperature and body water. The output from the hypothalamus is to the autonomic division of the peripheral nervous system (see Chapter 4, Section 4.5) which controls: (a) the diameter of blood vessels; (b) the secretion of sweat glands; and (c) the release of hormones from the pituitary gland.

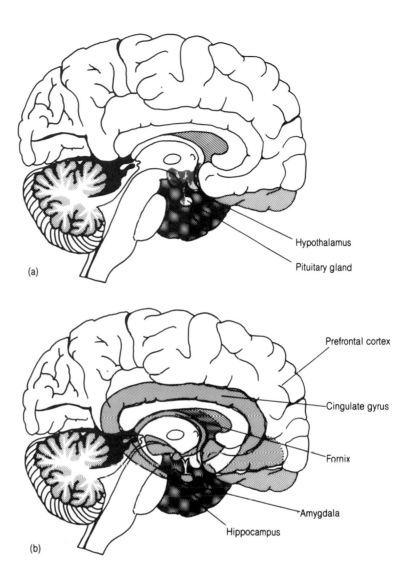

Hypothalamus

Pituitary gland

(a)

Prefrontal cortex

Cingulate gyrus

Fornix

Amygdala

Hippocampus

(b)

Fig. 3.15. Medial view of the left side of the brain to show the position of: (a) hypothalamus; (b) limbic system.

The hypothalamus is the highest control area for all the mechanisms that maintain homeostasis in the body. This area can be referred to as the 'visceral brain'.

The **limbic system** as a whole is a complex series of inter-connected structures lying in the forebrain and midbrain linked by a large cable of white matter known as the fornix. The limbic forebrain includes an area of cerebral cortex (cingulate gyrus) lying medially above the corpus callosum, and the hippocampus lying buried in the temporal lobe (Fig. 3.15b).

The loss of long-term memory associated with damage to the temporal lobe indicates that the hippocampal part of the limbic system has a function in the retention of memory. The limbic system, by its connections with the prefrontal cortex and the hypothalamus, is sometimes called the 'emotional brain'. Feelings of pleasure and anger produce physiological responses via activity in the hypothalamus to the autonomic nervous system (Chapter 4). Links between the limbic system and the motor system, particularly the basal ganglia, have been identified and suggest a function in affective aspects of movement performance.

3.9 Brain stem

When the cerebral hemispheres and the cerebellum are removed from the brain, the whole of the *brain stem* is revealed (Fig. 3.16). From above downwards, the brain stem consists of: *midbrain*, *pons* and *medulla oblongata*, with the *reticular formation* continuous through all three areas. The white matter of the brain stem contains bundles of fibres that form direct routes between the cerebral cortex and the spinal cord. Some of these routes branch to link with nuclei of grey matter in the brain stem and with the cerebellum. This can be compared with a system of roads with direct motorways and branch routes to other areas.

The grey matter of the brain stem includes motor nuclei which act as a unit in regulating the balance of the body during movement. Adjustments in the body position are coordinated in response to changes in visual and auditory input, and to the position of the head (see Chapter 11, Section 11.3 and Chapter 12, Section 12.2.1).

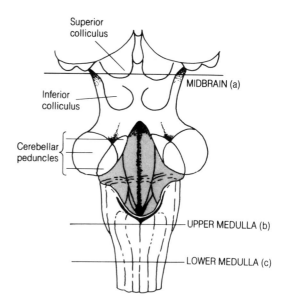

Fig. 3.16. Posterior view of the brain stem. Sections (a), (b) and (c) are shown in Fig. 3.17.

The **midbrain** is the upper part of the brain stem joining the diencephalon above to the pons below. The substantia nigra, one of the basal ganglia described in Section 3.5, is a prominent area of grey matter seen in the section of the midbrain in Figure 3.17a. The remainder of the anterior and lateral part of the midbrain is known as the cerebral peduncles, which contain ascending and descending fibres linking the cerebral cortex with the pons and the spinal cord below.

The **pons** can be easily identified on the anterior side of the brain stem where a bulge is formed by the transverse fibres linking the two halves of the cerebellum. The pontine nuclei form a relay station for fibres from the motor cortex to enter the opposite cerebellar cortex (see Section 3.10, Fig. 3.19 and Chapter 12, Fig. 12.7).

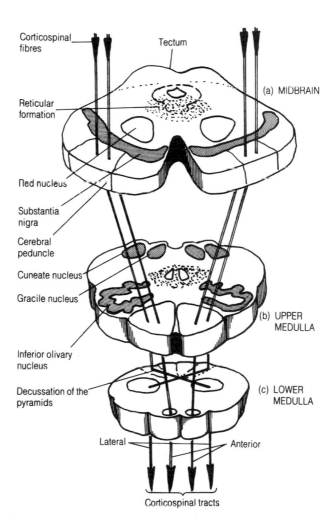

Fig. 3.17. Transverse sections through: (a) midbrain; (b) upper medulla; (c) lower medulla.

The **medulla oblongata** is the cone shaped lower end of the brain stem that leads down into the spinal cord. The white matter of the medulla contains ascending and descending pathways between the cerebral cortex and the spinal cord. Some of these routes cross to the opposite side in the medulla. The descending fibres of the corticospinal tracts cross on the anterior surface of the medulla forming a raised triangular area, the decussation of the *pyramids* (Fig. 3.17c). Posteriorly, an ascending sensory pathway from the spinal cord, the posterior column, ends in the *gracile* and *cuneate nuclei* (Fig. 3.17b) and then crosses to the opposite side in the brain stem to reach the thalamus (see Chapter 11, Fig. 11.2).

Reticular formation

The reticular formation is a diffuse network of neurones in the core of the brain stem extending from the midbrain to the medulla. Some groups of neurones are collected together in nuclei, but in general the reticular formation, unlike other brain areas, consists of scattered cell bodies with the fibres lying in between. The network receives branches from the ascending pathways through the brain stem. Descending tracts from the reticular formation affect the activity of the lower motor neurones which supply the muscles of the trunk and the proximal muscles of the limbs, see Chapter 12, Section 12.2.1.

Neurones of the reticular formation in the midbrain project to all areas of the cerebral cortex and form the ascending reticular activating system (ARAS) shown in Figure 3.18. The activity in these neurones affects our level of arousal and attention. The ARAS controls the 'body clock' which alternates the cycles of sleeping and waking.

The reticular formation forms the link system with the 'visceral brain' (hypothalamus and limbic system). In the lower pons and medulla it contains the 'vital centres' which control the heart from the cardiac centre, the blood pressure from the vasomotor centre and breathing from the respiratory centres. These vital centres respond to changes in blood composition and the activity in sensory nerves from receptors in blood vessels and the lungs. Continuous or intermittent activity in the centres results in stimulation of the muscle of the heart, the walls of blood vessels and muscles involved in breathing such as the diaphragm.

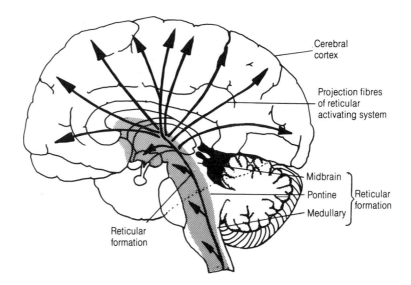

Fig. 3.18. Sagittal section to show the position of the reticular formation in the right side of the brain.

3.10 Cerebellum

The cerebellum is formed from a posterior outgrowth of the brain stem in development, and it lies below the occipital lobe of the cerebral hemispheres in the posterior cranial fossa of the skull. The overall function of the cerebellum is the control of the performance of smooth, coordinated movements with the correct timing and sequence.

The cerebellum has two halves which are connected by a central area known as the *vermis*. The outer layer of grey matter of the cerebellum is folded into uniform narrow gyri. The inner white matter forms a tree shape with the folded grey matter as the leaves. This was called the arboretum vitae (the tree of life) by the early neuroanatomists.

The cerebellum also has a number of deep nuclei, the largest being the *dentate nucleus*. Three pairs of stalks of white matter, known as *peduncles*, connect the cerebellum to the brain stem as follows: (a) the superior peduncles with the midbrain; (b) the middle peduncles with the pons; and (c) the inferior peduncles with the medulla. Figure 3.19 shows diagrammatically the cerebellum and the three cerebellar peduncles linking it to the brain stem.

The cerebellum cannot initiate movement, but it coordinates and regulates muscle activity on the same side of the body based on the input from three sources. Firstly, information about the position of the head reaches the cerebellum from the vestibule of the ear (see Chapter 4, Section 4.4.2, Fig. 4.12). Secondly,

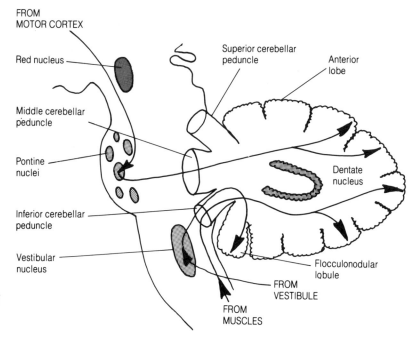

FROM
MOTOR CORTEX

Red nucleus

Middle cerebellar
peduncle

Pontine
nuclei

Inferior cerebellar
peduncle

Vestibular
nucleus

Superior cerebellar
peduncle

Anterior
lobe

Dentate
nucleus

Flocculonodular
lobule

FROM
VESTIBULE

FROM
VESTIBULE

FROM
MUSCLES

Fig. 3.19. Three main pathways bringing information *into* the cerebellum: from the muscles, the vestibule of the ear and the motor cortex.

the position of all the body segments is relayed from the proprioceptors in muscles and joints via the spinal cord to the cerebellum. Thirdly, input from the motor cortex concerning intended movement also reaches the cerebellum via the pons.

There is no direct output from the cerebellum to the spinal cord. The influence of the cerebellum in movement is via output to the primary motor cortex and to the brain stem. The cerebellum plays a major role in the coordination of movement by making appropriate adjustments in muscle activity during its progress from the start to the finish, and by maintaining the background posture.

Clinical note-pad 31: Cerebellar dysfunction

The performance of movement (on the same side of the body) is uncoordinated, clumsy or jerky, known as ataxia. Movements often overshoot or undershoot the intended goal (dysmetria), for example in walking on a narrow base, turning suddenly, or touching the nose with a finger. Muscle tone is usually decreased. Tremor occurs in proximal muscles during purposeful movement.

Friedreich's ataxia is an inherited disorder which begins before 20 years of age.

3.11 Summary of brain areas: function in movement

(1) **Motor areas of the cerebral cortex**: performance of movement. (a) *Primary motor area*: execution of movement. (b) *Premotor area*: learned bilateral movements. (c) *Supplementary motor area*: planning of movement.

(2) **Sensory areas of the cerebral cortex**: somatosensory information from the skin, muscles and joints about the external environment and the position of the body; visual and auditory information from the environment.

(3) **Thalamus**: sensory input to the cerebral cortex.

(4) **Basal ganglia**: planning and execution of movement via the motor cortex.

(5) **Hypothalamus** and **limbic system**: behavioural and visceral aspects of movement.

(6) **Cerebellum**: coordination, start and stop movements, balance and equilibrium.

(7) **Brain stem**: postural background for movement.

(8) **Reticular formation**: arousal and attention level during movement.

PART II
THE SPINAL CORD

The spinal cord appears to be a simple structure by comparison with the brain, but its role in the function of the central nervous system is nevertheless very important. Basic movement patterns of the limbs and trunk are integrated in the spinal cord. Most of the body's sensory information is received by the spinal cord and is passed on to higher levels in the brain.

3.12 The position and segmentation of the spinal cord

The embryonic neural tube grows in diameter and length with the bony vertebrae developing round it. The internal cavity of the tube remains as a small central spinal canal containing cerebrospinal fluid. A pair of spinal nerves grow out from the developing spinal cord between adjacent vertebrae. The segment of the cord that gives rise to each pair of spinal nerves is named in relation to the corresponding vertebra, for example the segment lying under the first thoracic vertebra is known as T1. There are 31 segments in the spinal cord, named as follows: eight cervical (C1 to C8), twelve thoracic (T1 to T12), five lumbar (L1 to L5), five sacral (S1 to S5) and one coccygeal.

There are eight cervical segments. The first pair of cervical nerves lie between the skull and the first cervical vertebra, and C1 to C7 all emerge above the corresponding vertebra.

The eighth pair of cervical nerves emerges between the seventh cervical and first thoracic vertebrae, so that all the nerves below C7 emerge below the corresponding vertebra.

The vertebral column grows in length more rapidly than the spinal cord, so that in the adult the lower end of the spinal cord lies at the level of the disc between the first and second lumbar vertebrae. The lower end tapers to a point and is attached by a strand of connective tissue (filum terminale) to the lower end of the sacrum and to the coccyx.

- *LOOK at an articulated skeleton, or the individual vertebrae loosely strung together. Put a piece of plastic tubing 45 cm long into the vertebral canal and note where the lower end lies. The tubing should be thicker towards the upper and lower ends to truly represent the spinal cord. Note that the vertebral canal is larger in the cervical and upper*

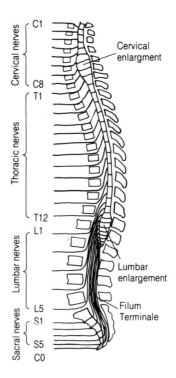

Fig. 3.20. The position of the spinal cord and the spinal nerves in relation to the vertebral column.

lumbar regions to accommodate the cervical and lumbar enlargements of the spinal cord.

- *IDENTIFY the intervertebral foramina between adjacent vertebrae where the spinal nerves emerge. Starting at the skull, see how the spinal segment and pair of spinal nerves C8 appear.*
- *LOOK at Figure 3.20, a sagittal section through the spinal cord and vertebral column with the spinal nerves emerging from the cord. The cervical and lumbar enlargements accommodate the large number of neurones that supply the upper and lower limbs respectively.*
- *LOOK at Figure 3.21 to see a transverse section of the spinal cord lying in position surrounded by the bony vertebra. The right and left sides of the spinal cord are symmetrical and are separated by two longitudinal sulci, one anteriorly and one posteriorly.*

3.13 Spinal meninges

The spinal cord is protected externally by three membranes of connective tissue which are also continuous over the surface of

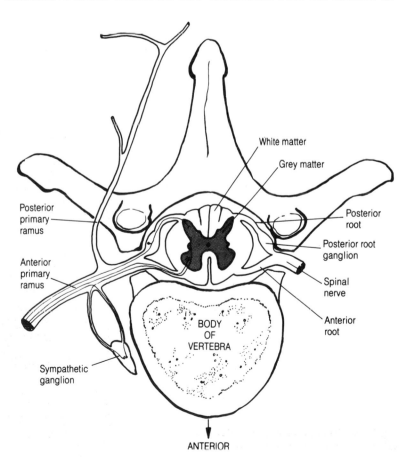

Fig. 3.21. Transverse section of the spinal cord surrounded by the corresponding vertebra.

the brain. The three layers, from superficial to deep, are the dura mater, arachnoid mater and pia mater (Fig. 3.22).

The **dura mater** is a thick layer densely packed with collagen fibres and some elastin which lines the cranial vault of the skull and the vertebral canal of the spine as far down as the level of the second sacral vertebra.

An **epidural space** lies between the dura mater and the periosteum and ligaments of the vertebral column. Anaesthetics injected into the epidural space of one spinal segment may spread upwards or downwards to affect the spinal nerves emerging from adjacent segments.

The **arachnoid mater** is a thin membrane lying in close contact with the dura mater, separated by a thin film of fluid. Deep to the arachnoid mater is the subarachnoid space containing cerebrospinal fluid. The arachnoid mater ends at the level of the second sacral vertebra. This means that between the third lumbar vertebra (where the spinal cord ends) and the second sacral vertebra, cerebrospinal fluid can be extracted for examination without risk of damaging the spinal cord. This procedure, a 'lumbar puncture', is usually done by inserting a blunt needle between the laminae of the third and fourth lumbar vertebrae (Fig. 3.23).

The **pia mater** is a loose membrane of connective tissue which covers the whole surface of the brain and spinal cord, and dips down into all the sulci. There is a rich network of blood vessels associated with the pia mater providing a major part of the blood supply to the brain and spinal cord.

The meninges protect the spinal cord and brain from infection, and the cerebrospinal fluid acts as a shock absorber.

3.14 Organisation of grey and white matter

The internal structure of the spinal cord is organised into an H shaped central core of grey matter with anterior and posterior

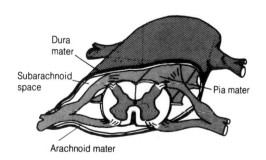

Fig. 3.22. Meninges surrounding the spinal cord.

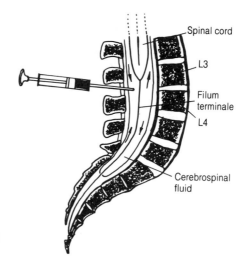

Fig. 3.23. Lower end of the spinal cord showing the position for a lumbar puncture.

horns, surrounded by white matter. Transverse sections of the spinal cord at different levels can be seen in Figure 3.24. The anterior horn is large in the cervical and lumbar regions where the lower motor neurones supplying muscles of the limbs are found. The grey matter in all the thoracic segments, the lumbar segments 1 and 2 and sacral segments 2, 3 and 4, has a lateral horn where the cell bodies of neurones which form part of the autonomic nervous system supplying organs, glands and blood vessels are found. The white matter containing groups of nerve fibres carries impulses up (*ascending tracts*) or down (*descending tracts*) the spinal cord (Fig. 3.25b).

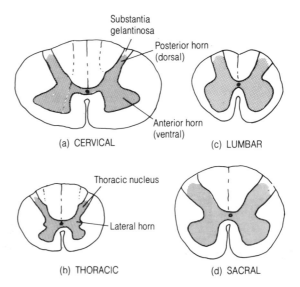

Fig. 3.24. Transverse sections of the spinal cord: (a) cervical; (b) thoracic; (c) lumbar; (d) sacral.

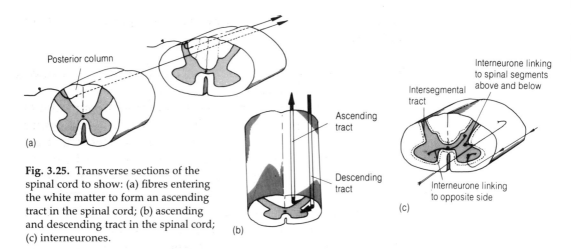

Fig. 3.25. Transverse sections of the spinal cord to show: (a) fibres entering the white matter to form an ascending tract in the spinal cord; (b) ascending and descending tract in the spinal cord; (c) interneurones.

The white matter of the spinal cord is largest at the upper end and smallest at the lower end. Fibres leave the descending tracts at each segment to enter the grey matter. Sensory neurones in spinal nerves link, either directly or after synapsing in the posterior horn, into the ascending tracts of the white matter at every level. Figure 3.25a shows how the posterior column of white matter increases in size as it receives fibres from successive spinal nerves.

3.14.1 Grey matter

The nerve cells which form the grey matter can be divided into the following.

(1) **Motor cells** whose axons are distributed to all parts of the body including the muscles. The motor nerve cells are largely found in the *anterior* (ventral) horn and include the alpha and gamma motor neurones described in Chapter 1.

(2) **Tract cells** which receive impulses from the *sensory* neurones entering the cord at all levels from the skin, muscles and joints. The tract cells are found in the *posterior* (dorsal) horn, and their axons enter the ascending tracts of the white matter.

(3) **Interneurones** lie in the intermediate area between the posterior and anterior horns. The interneurones receive impulses from sensory neurones entering the posterior horn, and from descending tracts in the white matter from the brain. In bilateral activities, interneurones which link across the cord are important. All the segments of the spinal cord are connected by interneurones whose fibres lie in the intersegmental tract (see Section

3.14.2), so that activity can spread to other spinal levels above and below.

Figure 3.25c shows the position of the different types of interneurones in the spinal cord.

The motor neurones of the **anterior horn** are organised into pools of neurones (see Fig. 1.14) which supply particular groups of muscles acting on one joint. There is some evidence that the neurones supplying more distal muscles in the limbs lie lateral and posterior to those supplying proximal muscles. The mapping of neurone pools in the human spinal cord is still uncertain.

The **posterior horn** has been divided into areas based on collections of nerve cells that are histologically distinct. Two of these areas have specific functions which relate to the type of information transmitted to the ascending pathways to the brain. The *substantia gelatinosa* is a broad band around the apex of the posterior horn, where incoming information from the exteroceptors of the skin (see Chapter 11, Section 11.2.3) relays. The thoracic nucleus is present below T1 in the spinal cord and is absent in the cervical cord.

3.14.2 White matter

The white matter is divided for description into three columns or funiculi: posterior (dorsal), lateral and anterior (ventral). The ascending and descending tracts form the white matter. Each tract links two particular areas of the central nervous system and is usually named after these two areas. For example, the spinothalamic tract is an ascending pathway that links the spinal cord with the thalamus, the corticospinal tract is a descending route from the cerebral cortex to the spinal cord. Figure 3.26 shows the position of the main tracts, with the ascending tracts in Figure 3.26a and the descending tracts in Figure 3.26b. It must be remembered that all the tracts are present on both sides of the spinal cord. Details of the function of these tracts will be discussed in Chapters 11 and 12. At this stage you should appreciate the general way in which the white matter is organised. Each tract is rather like a cable of wires, but evidence indicates that there is some overlap of function.

A narrow band of white matter surrounds the whole of the central core of grey matter. The fibres of this band, known as the *fasciculus proprius* or *intersegmental tract*, connect different segments of the spinal cord (Fig. 3.25c and 3.26b). The fibres vary in length, some pass from one segment to another and

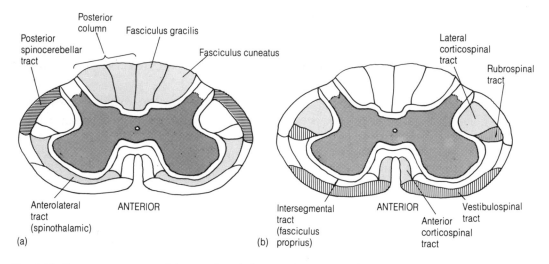

Fig. 3.26. Transverse sections of the spinal cord showing the position of the main tracts in the white matter: (a) ascending tracts; (b) descending tracts.

others pass nearly the whole length of the cord, branching up, down and across the cord.

3.14.3 Spinal reflex movements

A spinal reflex action is one that is initiated by the stimulation of receptors in the skin or the muscles or joints. Impulses pass into the spinal cord in sensory neurones and relay to spinal motor neurones that produce a response in movement or in change in muscle tone. The stretch reflex described in Chapter 1 is an example of a spinal reflex when change muscle tone occurs. In other spinal reflexes, several groups of muscles are active in the response and movement of a limb occurs. In this case, there is spread of impulses to more than one spinal segment. The intersegmental tract of the spinal cord is then involved. An example is the *flexor (protective) reflex*, which flexes a limb away from a painful stimulus. In this reflex, the whole of the damaged limb is flexed and impulses are sent to several muscles via interneurones (Fig. 3.27). This is different from the stretch reflex where the response occurs in only one muscle via a monosynaptic pathway, see Chapter 1, Figure 1.20.

Interneurones also carry impulses across to the opposite side of the spinal cord in the *crossed extensor reflex*, when there is activation of the extensor muscles of the opposite limb to prevent the body from falling over when one leg is flexed. If the activity

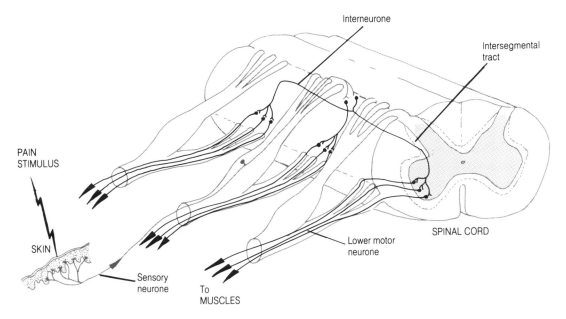

PAIN
STIMULUS

SKIN

Sensory
neurone

To
MUSCLES

Interneurone

Intersegmental
tract

Lower motor
neurone

SPINAL CORD

Fig. 3.27. Flexor reflex. Arrangement of neurones to show spread of activity to three spinal segments.

spreads to the upper limbs, the arm on the same side extends and that on the opposite side flexes. This pattern of movement seen in spinal reflex action forms the background to normal movement.

The spinal cord alone is concerned with basic movement responses to external stimuli. These movements can be seen in the newborn baby when the influence from higher levels of the nervous system has not yet developed. As the control of activity by higher centres in the nervous system develops, these basic movements are modified and more complex movements are possible. Nevertheless, the spinal cord remains as the centre for the final pathway to the muscles, and for processing the information from basic spinal reflexes.

At the end of this chapter, you should be able to:

PART I

(1) Identify the main areas of the brain as seen in (a) external appearance and (b) median sagittal section to reveal the medial aspect of one half of the brain.

(2) Name the lobes of the cerebral hemispheres and the principal gyri associated with each lobe. Outline the function of the individual lobes and the lateralisation of function between the right and left hemispheres.

(3) Recognise the individual components of the basal ganglia. Briefly state the function of the independent basal ganglia system.

(4) Identify the position of the thalamus, the internal capsule, the hypothalamus and the limbic system. Appreciate the importance of the thalamus in the processing of sensory information and its projections to the cerebral cortex.

(5) Identify the parts of the brain stem (midbrain, pons and medulla) and the location of the reticular formation. Outline the function of the brain stem as a unit.

(6) Describe the position of the cerebellum and its structural links with the brain stem. Outline the incoming pathways of information to the cerebellum. Briefly state the function of the cerebellum in normal movement.

PART II

(7) Describe the position of the spinal cord, and the segmentation that relates to the emergence of spinal nerves from the vertebral column.

(8) Describe the arrangement of grey and white matter in the spinal cord seen in transverse section. Name the principal ascending and descending tracts in the white matter.

(9) Outline the arrangement of neurones which form the basis of spinal reflex action, with examples of the flexor and the crossed extensor reflexes. Appreciate the presence of spinal reflexes as a background to movement patterns.

4 / Link Systems: Peripheral Nervous System

The peripheral nervous system provides the link between the central nervous system and all the parts of the body. Links are required to activate muscles for movement, and to monitor ongoing changes in the muscles as movement proceeds. Links from the skin and from the sense organs give information about changes in the environment around the body. Links to blood vessels, glands and organs regulate the internal environment to meet the metabolic demands of the muscles. The peripheral nervous system provides all these links.

The peripheral nerves, containing sensory and motor nerve fibres, are arranged in a bilateral system of paired nerves leaving the central nervous system. Incoming signals are conducted to the brain and spinal cord, and after processing the responses are carried out by outgoing signals in the peripheral nerves.

The axons found in the peripheral nerves can be divided into two functional categories. The *somatic* component consists of all the sensory and motor axons associated with activity in the muscles, the joints and the skin. The *visceral* component is all the axons carrying impulses to the glands, organs and blood vessels. The visceral nerve fibres are part of the autonomic nervous system.

The importance of the peripheral nervous system during movement is to provide the structural framework for the following.

(1) The monitoring of changes in the external environment.

(2) The monitoring of changes in length and tension in the muscles.

(3) The activation of muscles fibres.

(4) The regulation of the internal environment to maintain the oxygen demands of the muscles.

Damage to the nerves of the peripheral nervous system at any point from their origin in the central nervous system to their terminations inside the muscles will result in loss of muscle function. Trophic changes, such as flushing and dryness of the skin, will also occur if the visceral fibres are damaged.

4.1 The position and location of the cranial and spinal nerves

The paired nerves of the peripheral nervous system leaving the central nervous system are divided into the *cranial nerves* leaving the brain; and *spinal nerves* leaving the spinal cord.

The **cranial nerves** consist of 12 pairs of nerves whose cell bodies are located in the brain. Seen most clearly in a ventral view of the brain, the pairs of cranial nerves appear to be formed at irregular intervals. The final position of each pair is a result of the changes in development of the head and neck, and the folding of the embryonic neural tube which forms the brain (Fig. 4.1). The cranial nerves are summarised in Appendix 2, Table A2.1.

The **spinal nerves** consist of the 31 pairs of nerves leaving the spinal cord. Each pair of spinal nerves emerges from the spinal canal of the vertebral column between adjacent vertebrae at the intervertebral foramina. The latter can be seen in the lateral view of a thoracic vertebra in Appendix 1. The lower end of the spinal cord in adults lies at the level of the disc between the first and second lumbar vertebrae. The lower spinal nerves therefore lie in the spinal canal below this level before emerging at their corresponding level. This sheath of lumbar and sacral nerves is known as the *cauda equina*.

- *LOOK at an articulated skeleton and return to Figure 3.21 and Figure 3.22 to revise the emergence of the 31 pairs of spinal nerves from the vertebral column.*

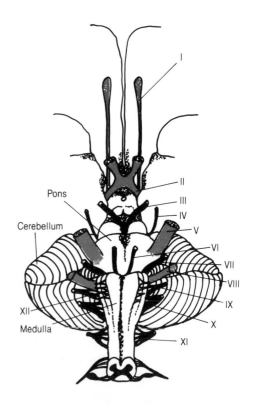

Fig. 4.1. Ventral view of the brain showing the origins of the 12 pairs of cranial nerves.

4.2 Spinal nerves

Each spinal nerve begins at the spinal cord by two roots: the *anterior* (ventral) root and the *posterior* (dorsal) root. Each root consists of a series of rootlets which eventually join. Illustrations of pathways in the nervous system represent the roots as a single trunk for clarity.

The **anterior roots** consist of axons that grow out from multipolar nerve cells in the spinal cord, the lower motor neurones. Axons from the anterior horn cells of the spinal cord are: (a) large diameter alpha fibres which activate skeletal muscle fibres; and (b) smaller diameter gamma fibres innervating the intrafusal fibres of the muscle spindles lying within the skeletal muscles. Motor fibres of the autonomic nervous system are also found in the anterior roots. The cell bodies of these autonomic neurones lie in the lateral horn of certain segments of the spinal cord (see Section 4.5).

The **posterior roots** develop in a different way. A ridge of cells on each side of the neural tube in the embryo forms a pair of ganglia (cells) for each segment of the spinal cord. Fibres grow centrally from each ganglion into the spinal cord, and also laterally to lie alongside the fibres of the anterior root. The fibres of the posterior root are all sensory, carrying information from the receptors in the skin, the muscles and the joints. The cell bodies lie in the posterior root ganglion, isolated from the hundreds of synaptic connections possible for the cell bodies of neurones in the grey matter of the spinal cord. Axons of the sensory neurones enter the spinal cord, branch to segments of the cord above or below, or turn into the posterior white matter to reach the brain stem before synapsing.

The spinal nerve is the common nerve trunk formed by the anterior and posterior roots joining, distal to the posterior root ganglion.

Remember the following:

(1) Anterior roots are motor. Interruption leads to loss of movement.

(2) Posterior roots are sensory. Interruption leads to loss of sensation.

(3) Spinal nerves are mixed; each contains motor and sensory nerve fibres.

4.2.1 Divisions of the spinal nerve

The spinal nerve formed from the two roots is only a few millimetres long and then it gives off a branch posteriorly. This

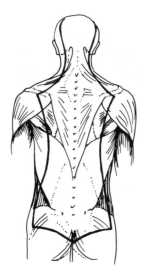

Fig. 4.2. Posterior view of the head and trunk. Area of skin supplied by posterior primary rami of the spinal nerves.

branch is known as the *posterior* (dorsal) *primary ramus*, which passes close to the articular processes of the vertebra. The posterior primary rami of all the spinal nerves together supply the deep muscles of the back and the skin covering them (Fig. 4.2).

Each spinal nerve continues as the *anterior* (ventral) *primary ramus*. These branches of the spinal nerves supply all the skin and muscles other than those innervated by the posterior primary rami.

Visceral nerve fibres of the autonomic nervous system in the anterior primary rami connect with ganglia, which lie on the sides of the bodies of the vertebrae, by grey and white rami. Figure 3.21 shows these connections. The white rami carry preganglionic myelinated fibres from the spinal nerve to the ganglion. Grey rami carry non-myelinated post-ganglionic fibres from cell bodies in the ganglion to the spinal nerve. The autonomic fibres will be considered again in Section 4.5.

The content and distribution of the anterior primary ramus from this point is called the spinal nerve. Each spinal nerve contains all the somatic and visceral nerve fibres which supply the corresponding body segment. The thoracic spinal nerves are like the basic plan described. The other spinal nerves show considerable mixing, branching and joining before passing as peripheral nerves to their destination. This regrouping of nerve fibres occurs in a *plexus*. Some nerve fibres from one spinal nerve may eventually lie alongside those from a different spinal nerve in one peripheral nerve. Figure 4.3 shows how two spinal nerves (C5 and C6) contribute fibres to the peripheral nerve supplying the biceps muscle in the arm.

There are four major plexi formed by the anterior primary rami of the spinal nerves.

(1) Cervical plexus (C1-C4) to the muscles of the neck.

(2) Brachial plexus (C5-T1) to the muscles of the upper limb.

(3) Lumbar plexus (L1-L4) to the muscles of the thigh.

(4) Sacral plexus (L4-S4) to the muscles of the leg and foot.

Figure 4.4 shows the plexi formed by the spinal nerves. The lumbar plexus and the sacral plexus can be considered together as the lumbosacral plexus supplying the whole of the lower limb.

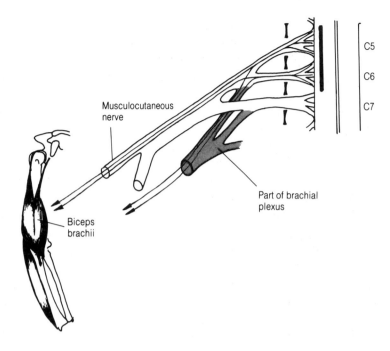

Fig. 4.3. Formation of a peripheral nerve (musculocutaneous) from two spinal segments (C5 and C6).

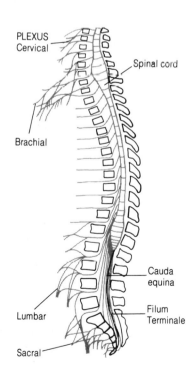

Fig. 4.4. Spinal cord in relation to the vertebral column. Spinal nerves forming the cervical, brachial, lumbar and sacral plexi.

4.2.2 Dermatomes and myotomes

A **dermatome** is an area of skin supplied by all the sensory nerve fibres of one spinal nerve. An example of a dermatome is a band of skin around the trunk innervated by the sensory nerve fibres of the second pair of thoracic nerves. A map of the dermatomes of all the spinal nerves is seen in Figure 4.5. In the trunk, the dermatomes form a series of bands, one for each spinal nerve from T1 to L1 in order. There is some overlap, and each dermatome may receive nerve fibres from three or four spinal nerves. In the limbs, the arrangement of dermatomes is

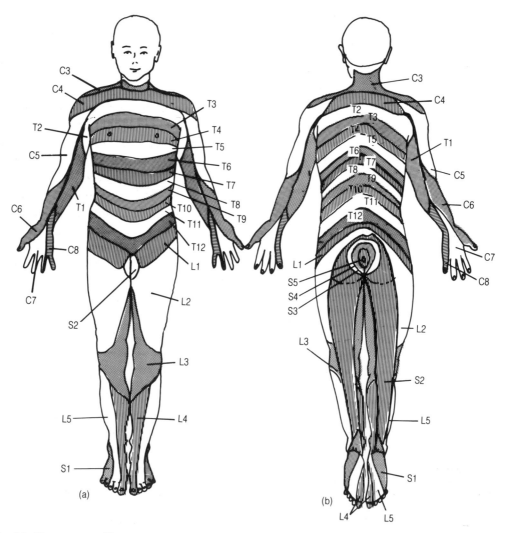

Fig. 4.5. Dermatomes. The cutaneous distribution of the spinal nerves in (a) anterior and (b) posterior view.

more complicated. Each limb develops from a bud, which grows out in the embryo, and some dermatomes are carried to the ends of the limb. C7 and C8 are carried in this way to the hand, while L5, S1 and S2 reach the skin of the foot. From the diagram, you can see that damage to the spinal nerves in the upper part of the neck (C5, C6) will give loss of sensation around the shoulder, while severance of lower roots (C7, C8) will affect sensation in the hand.

Clinical note-pad 4A: Herpes zoster (shingles)

A viral infection with localised cutaneous changes within the distribution of one or more sensory dermatomes. The skin develops painful vescicles over the clearly defined area. The virus is latent in the posterior root ganglion and migrates along the sensory axons to the skin supplied by them.

A **myotome** is all the muscles supplied by one spinal segment and its pair of spinal nerves. For example, nerve fibres from the first thoracic nerve (T1) are distributed to a long finger flexor muscle in the forearm and some of the intrinsic muscles of the hand. Each individual muscle, however, receives fibres from two or three spinal nerves (Fig. 4.3), so that injury to one spinal segment may only have a limited effect on one particular muscle.

The segmental origin of the nerves supplying the muscle groups of the limbs is given in Appendix 2, Table A2.2

Clinical note-pad 4B: Spinal cord damage

Spinal cord injury is associated with spinal fracture due to falls or road traffic accidents. Spinal damage also results from tumours in the vertebrae, the spinal meninges (see Chapter 3, Section 3.13) or, rarely, in the cord itself.

The effects of damage to the spinal cord depend on the level and extent of the injury or disease. Motor and sensory loss, related to the segmental origin of the spinal nerves, occurs below the level of lesion. Appendix 2, and Tables A2.2, A2.3 and A2.4, give summaries of the muscles of the limbs supplied by the segments of the cord. When there is partial damage, imbalance of muscle activity and muscle spasms occur. Complete transection leads to:

C4 – loss of diaphragm and intercostal muscle action.
C4 – T1 – loss of movement in all four limbs, quadriplegia.
T1 – small muscles of the hand affected.
Mid-thoracic – loss of movement in the lower limbs, paraplegia.

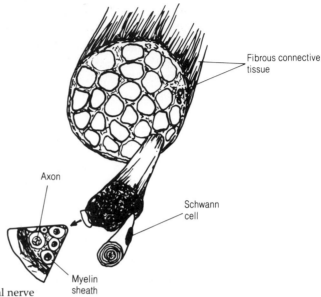

Fig. 4.6. Transverse section of a peripheral nerve showing the connective tissue and axons.

4.3 Peripheral nerves: composition and distribution

Branches of the spinal nerves, and the plexi formed from them, are distributed to all the parts of the body. These branches are known as peripheral nerves. The structure of a peripheral nerve is shown in Figure 4.6. Half of the total bulk of a nerve is connective tissue, surrounding both the nerve and also the bundles of axons within the nerve. Each nerve has its own blood supply, which branches along the length of the nerve in both directions.

Note: peripheral nerves are 'mixed', i.e. contain motor and sensory fibres. The motor fibres include axons of the autonomic nervous system described in Section 4.5.

In their course along a limb, peripheral nerves branch to enter muscles, tendons, joints and blood vessels. Some of the peripheral nerves pierce the deep fascia of connective tissue around the body, deep to the skin. These nerves are *cutaneous nerves* which supply all the structures in the skin.

4.3.1 Muscular branches

The nerves that enter muscles contain motor nerve fibres which supply the muscle fibres; without these motor fibres the muscle cannot function. No reflex or voluntary movement is possible if these motor neurones are damaged (see lower motor neurones in Chapter 12, Section 12.1). The nerves which enter muscles also contain sensory nerve fibres from the proprioceptors in the muscle (see Chapter 1, Section 1.5.4). The proprioceptive fibres provide the central nervous system with information on the length and tension of the muscles, and the angulation of the joints.

4.3.2 Cutaneous branches

The cutaneous nerves contain sensory fibres from the receptors in the skin. One nerve often connects with other cutaneous nerves in the same area, so that severing one cutaneous nerve may reduce sensation in the area, but does not abolish it.

There are also motor fibres in cutaneous nerves which are part of the system supplying blood vessels, sweat glands and the small muscles at the base of hair follicles. Damage to the vasomotor fibres supplying the blood vessels leads to flushing and dryness of the skin.

An example of a cutaneous nerve is the superficial terminal branch of the radial nerve (see Chapter 7, Section 7.3.2). This nerve pierces the deep fascia above the wrist, and branches to supply an area of skin on the back of the hand. Damage to this nerve usually results in a very small area of sensory loss due to overlap from the other cutaneous nerves in the hand.

Clinical note-pad 4C: Peripheral nerve injury

Peripheral nerve injury can have a variety of causes. Fractures and lacerations often involve peripheral nerve damage, but the axons of peripheral nerves are also affected in diseases of the anterior horn of the spinal cord or peripheral neuropathies (see clinical note-pad 1F). The changes in movement and sensation that occur when a peripheral nerve is damaged by trauma may be different in every case.

If the nerve is stretched or crushed, but no axons are actually severed, there may still be some conduction of nerve impulses, but it will be poor due to swelling or haemorrhage (Fig. 4.7a). Some loss of movement and muscle tone occurs, but the sensation of touch and pain remains. Recovery may begin after a few days. If the axons are severed (Fig. 4.7b) there may be complete loss of movement and sensation, as well as flushing of the skin (as a result of loss of vasomotor fibres to blood vessels). Recovery will depend upon the extent of involvement of the sheaths around the axon, Schwann cell sheath and endoneurium (Fig. 4.7b and c). Axons growing into intact sheaths will complete regeneration in a few weeks. If new tubules must be formed by the Schwann cells, recovery may take months.

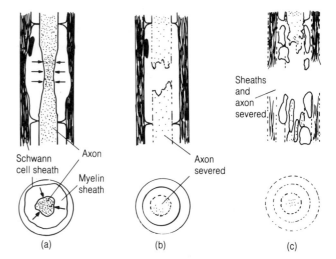

Fig. 4.7. Injury to peripheral nerve:
(a) axon and Schwann cell sheath
intact, swelling of the myelin
sheath;
(b) axon severed, sheaths intact;
(c) axon and sheaths severed.

4.4 Cranial nerves

In general, the components of a cranial nerve are similar to the basic plan of spinal nerves already described. However, not all cranial nerves are 'mixed'; some contain sensory fibres only, for example the optic nerve from the retina of the eye. Some of the cranial nerves contain motor fibres of the parasympathetic division of the autonomic nervous system described in Section 4.5.

All the fibres of one cranial nerve emerge together from the brain either as a single bundle, or as a row of filaments which join together at a short distance from the brain stem. (Note that in each mixed spinal nerve, motor and sensory fibres were separated into two distinct roots leaving the spinal cord.)

Each cranial nerve has one or more nuclei of grey matter in the brain stem, where motor fibres originate and sensory fibres terminate. The sensory fibres of some cranial nerves, particularly from the sense organs, synapse in other brain areas before relaying in the nucleus of the specific cranial nerve. The nuclei of the cranial nerves are not found in an orderly sequence in the brain stem. Migration of these nuclei occurs in development from the primary segments to a final position in the mature brain.

The **functions** of the cranial nerves include the following.

(1) Conduction of sensory information from the special senses – the eyes, ears, organs of balance, nose and tongue – to the brain for processing.

(2) Providing the pathways for *brain stem reflexes* essential for the orientation of the head, movement of the eyes, and other reflexes such as sneezing and coughing.

(3) Conduction of motor information which controls the size of the pupil of the eye, the muscle of the heart, and the activity of the digestive organs (motility and secretion).

A summary of the 12 pairs of cranial nerves is given in Appendix A2.1. The cranial nerves particularly concerned with movement and posture will now be described in outline.

4.4.1 Movement and sensation of the face

The facial VII and trigeminal V nerves cooperate in movements of the face and the mouth for the expression of mood and emotion (Fig. 4.8), the production of speech, and in mastication.

The **facial nerve** contains motor fibres to the muscles of facial expression. Descending corticobulbar (corticonuclear) fibres from the opposite motor cortex of the brain, synapse in the motor nucleus of the nerve in the pons. The facial nerve emerges from the pons and leaves the skull through a foramen in the temporal bone close to the middle ear. The nerve then passes through the parotid salivary gland just in front of the ear and divides into five branches like the digits of a goose's foot (Fig. 4.9a). Between them the branches supply all the muscles of the scalp and face, except the muscles of mastication, which receive motor fibres of the *trigeminal nerve*. Movements of the lips and tongue, essential for speech, are made by coordination of activity in the facial nerve with the *hypoglossal nerve* to the muscles of the tongue.

Figure 4.9c shows the position of the main muscles of the face. Combining in different ways, they produce all the movements involved in facial expression, in speech and in the mastication of food.

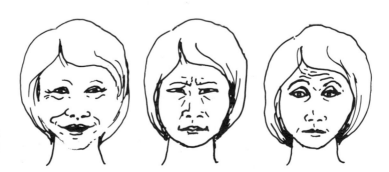

Fig. 4.8. Facial expressions resulting from activity in various muscles of the face.

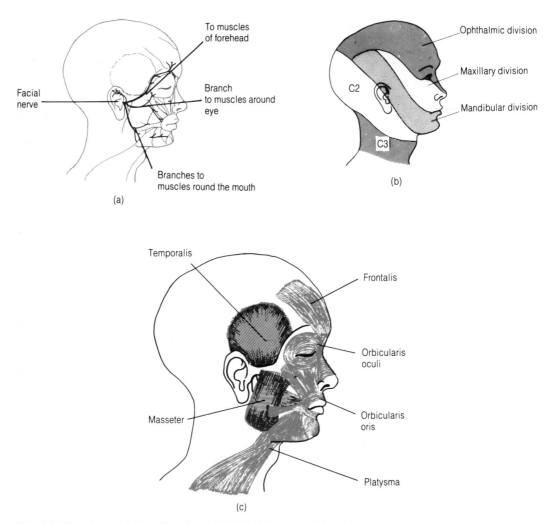

Fig. 4.9. Side view of the head to show: (a) the facial nerve and branches to the muscles of the face; (b) the distribution of the three divisions of the trigeminal nerve, (c) the muscles of the face.

Clinical note-pad 4D: Bell's palsy

Bell's palsy is a facial nerve disorder of unknown origin. It frequently follows exposure to cold on one side of the face, or a mild viral respiratory infection. Facial paralysis occurs on one side affecting the eyelid, forehead and the muscles moving the lips. Recovery from Bell's palsy is usually spontaneous.

The **trigeminal nerve** is important for sensation in the skin of the face. The three divisions of this nerve supply particular areas

(Fig. 4.9b). The ophthalmic branch enters the orbit and then branches to the skin of the forehead and the front of the scalp. The maxillary branch passes through the floor of the orbit and then turns downwards to the skin over the cheek and to the teeth of the upper jaw. The mandibular branch supplies the skin over the side of the head and the lower jaw. Loss of sensation in the face leads to difficulty in activities such as shaving and putting on make up. Motor branches of the nerve supply the temporalis and masseter muscles used in the mastication of food (Fig. 4.9c).

4.4.2 Movement of the head and eyes

Cranial nerves form the sensory and motor pathways of *brain stem reflexes* involved in movement of the head and eyes.

The **vestibular nerve** is a sensory nerve which is one division of the eighth cranial nerve. The nerve conducts information into the brain stem from the part of the inner ear that responds to the position of the head. The receptors lie in the utricle, saccule and semicircular canals of the inner ear (see Chapter 11, Section 11.3), and the vestibular nucleus lies in the pons and medulla. Changes in the position of the head in relation to gravity are signalled via the brain stem to the spinal cord (Fig. 4.10). Appropriate changes in postural muscle activity are then made to keep the body in equilibrium.

Turning the head changes the pattern of impulses in the two vestibular nerves, and this is relayed via the brain stem to the three motor cranial nerves which supply the muscles at the back of the eye. This pathway (Fig. 4.10), known as the *vestibulo-ocular reflex*, keeps an object in view as the head turns during movement. As the head turns to one side, the eyes are turned in the opposite direction to keep a constant image on the retina. If the head continues to turn, the eyes will move rapidly in the same direction of head movement to focus on a new fixed point. The combination of slow eye movement in the opposite direction followed by a rapid movement in the same direction is known as *nystagmus*. The same eye movements occur when the body remains still and the field of view is moving, for example looking out of a window while sitting in a moving train.

4.5 Autonomic nervous system

The autonomic nervous system innervates smooth muscle, cardiac muscle and the glands of the body. It is largely a motor

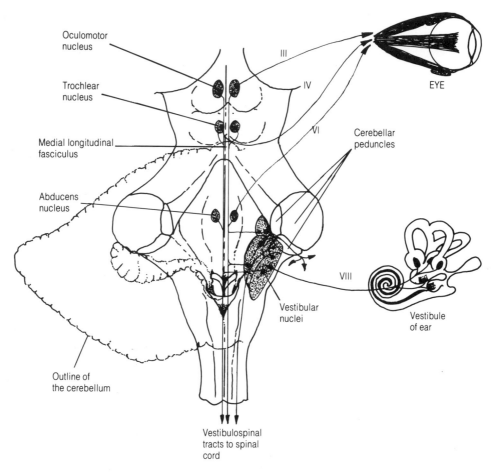

Fig. 4.10. Posterior view of the brain stem showing the components of the vestibulo-ocular reflex.

system, which regulates many important reflexes, for example the vasomotor control of blood pressure and the motor control of the bladder. During movement, autonomic fibres in the peripheral nerves regulate the blood flow to the active muscles, by their effect on the smooth muscle of the walls of blood vessels. The reflex activity of the autonomic nervous system is influenced by centres in the brain, for example the hypothalamus and regions in the brain stem.

Conduction of impulses in the autonomic fibres is slower than in the somatic component of the peripheral nervous system, since the axons are of a smaller diameter. Unlike the somatic motor system, there are two neurones between the central nervous system and the effector organ, so there is delay at the synapse between them. The junction between the two neurones is located in an autonomic ganglion. The preganglionic neurones originate in the brain stem or the spinal cord, and their fibres lie in cranial or spinal nerves.

The autonomic nervous system is divided into two divisions: the **sympathetic** and **parasympathetic**. The two divisions differ in their sites of origin in the brain and spinal cord. Also the neurotransmitter secreted by the post-ganglionic neurones of the sympathetic is noradrenalin (norepinephrine) while all the other neurones are cholinergic. Many of the organs and glands are innervated by fibres of both the sympathetic and parasympathetic systems, which frequently have opposing effects. For example, parasympathetic fibres to the heart decrease the heart rate, whereas sympathetic fibres have the opposite effect.

Sympathetic nervous system

Neurones of the sympathetic nervous system originate in the lateral horn of the grey matter of all the thoracic segments and the first two lumbar segments of the spinal cord. These pre-ganglionic fibres lie in the spinal nerves T1 to L2 and synapse in one of the sympathetic ganglia lying on the bodies of the vertebrae (Fig. 4.11). The post-ganglionic fibres link to the same spinal nerve, or pass up or down to other spinal levels via the chain of sympathetic ganglia located on either side of the vertebral column, from the base of the skull to the coccyx. This means that stimulation of the sympathetic nervous system can have a widespread effect in all regions of the body.

Stimulation of the sympathetic nervous system prepares the body for action in the following ways.

(1) Stimulation of cardiac muscle to increase the heart rate and the force of contraction.

(2) Constriction of the smooth muscle of blood vessels to regulate the blood pressure.

(3) Relaxation of the smooth muscle of the walls of the bronchioles of the lungs to increase the ventilation volume.

(4) Liver glycogen is mobilised to raise the glucose level of the blood.

(5) Dilation of the pupil of the eye to allow more light to enter.

(6) Stimulation of sweat glands in the skin to lose the extra heat generated from the muscles, and to keep the body temperature constant.

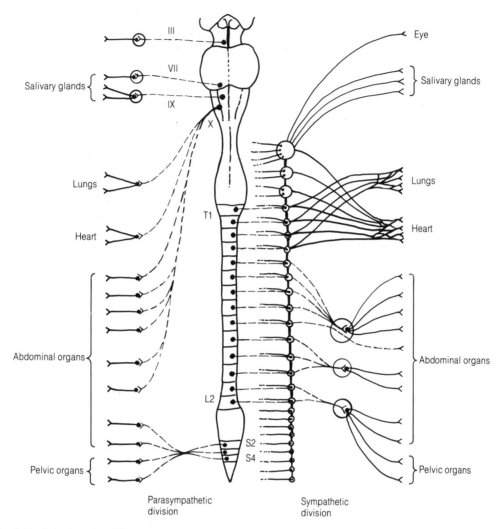

Fig. 4.11. Spinal cord and brain stem. General plan of the autonomic nervous system. Sympathetic division on the right, and parasympathetic division on the left of the diagram. – – – = preganglionic neurones.

The hypothalamus and the limbic system control activity in the sympathetic system in response to changes in the external and the internal environment (see Chapter 3, Section 3.8). Sympathetic responses to emotional changes such as fear, anxiety and stress are also mediated via the hypothalamus.

Parasympathetic nervous system

The parasympathetic system acts in localised regions of the body, unlike the widespread response of the sympathetic system. The pre-ganglionic parasympathetic fibres are long and the ganglia are found near to the structure supplied. The post-ganglionic fibres are short and multibranching. There are two widely separated parts of the parasympathetic nervous system:

(1) The cranial division originates in motor fibres of the cranial nerves III, VII, IX and X.

(2) The spinal segments S2 to S4 contain pre-ganglionic neurones in the lateral horn of the grey matter. Their axons form the **pelvic splanchnic nerves** which supply the descending colon and rectum, the bladder and the reproductive organs.

The parasympathetic division conserves and restores energy in the body in the following ways.

(1) Decrease in the heart rate and in the force of contraction.

(2) Constriction of the smooth muscle of the respiratory bronchioles.

(3) Constriction of the pupil of the eye in response to bright light.

(4) Stimulation of the smooth muscle and the glands of the digestive system.

At the end of this chapter you should be able to:

(1) Summarise the functions of the peripheral nervous system as the link between the central nervous system and all the parts of the body. Distinguish between somatic and visceral components of peripheral nerves.

(2) Describe the origin, formation and divisions of a typical spinal nerve. Identify the major plexi formed by spinal nerves (cervical, brachial, lumbar and sacral). Define a dermatome and a myotome.

(3) Describe a peripheral nerve. Distinguish the features of cutaneous and muscular branches of peripheral nerves.

(4) Describe the origin and formation of cranial nerves. Summarise the functions of cranial nerves.

(5) Outline the nerve supply to the skin and the muscles of the face.

(6) Describe the coordination of the movements of the head and the eyes to keep an object in focus on the retina, the vestibulo-ocular reflex.

(7) Summarise briefly the structural and functional differences between the somatic and the autonomic parts of the peripheral nervous system.

(8) Distinguish between the functions of the sympathetic and parasympathetic divisions of the autonomic nervous system.

Further Reading for Section 1

Galley P.M. & Forster A.L. (1987) *Human Movement*. Churchill Livingstone, Edinburgh.

Gilman S. & Winans Newman S. (1992) *Manter & Gatz's Essentials of Clinical Neuroanatomy and Neurophysiology*. FA Davies, Philadelphia.

Gowitzke B.A. & Milner M. (1988) *Understanding the Scientific Basis of Human Movement*. Williams & Wilkins, London.

Hay J.G. & Reid J.G. (1988) *The Anatomical and Mechanical Bases of Human Motion*. Prentice-Hall, Hemel Hempstead.

Lamb J.F., Ingram C.G., Johnston I.A. & Pitman R.M. (1992) *Essentials of Physiology*. 3rd edn., Blackwell Science, Oxford.

Loewy A.G. & Siekevitz P. (1991) *Cell Structure and Function*. Holt, Rinehart & Winston, New York.

MacKinnon P. & Morris J. (1986) *Oxford Textbook of Functional Anatomy*, Vol. 1, Oxford Medical Publications, Oxford.

McClintic J.R. (1985) *Basic Anatomy and Physiology*. John Wiley & Sons, Chichester.

Mitchell L. (1989) *Simple Relaxation – The Mitchell Method for Easing Tension*. John Murray, London.

Netter F.H. (1983) *The Ciba Collection Of Medical Illustrations. Vol 1, Parts 1 & 2: Nervous System*. Ciba, New Jersey.

Seeley R., Stephens T. & Tate P. (1992) *Anatomy & Physiology*. 2nd edn., CV Mosby Co., St. Louis.

Tortora G. & Grabowski S.R. (1993) *Principles of Anatomy & Physiology*. 7th edn., Harper-Collins College Publishers, New York.

Wirhed R. (1984) *Athletic Ability and the Anatomy of Motion*. Wolfe Medical, London.

Section 2 The Anatomy of Movement

ORGANISATION AND COOPERATION
IN DAILY LIVING

5 / Positioning Movements: The Shoulder and Elbow

PART I
MOVEMENTS OF THE SHOULDER

5.1 Functional movements of the shoulder

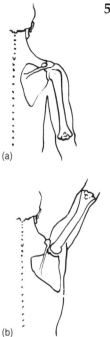

(a)

(b)

Fig. 5.1. Posterior view of the right scapula and humerus: (a) anatomical position; (b) abduction of the humerus with lateral rotation of the scapula.

The shoulder forms a foundation from which the whole of the upper limb can move. Acting like the cab of a crane, the shoulder allows the hand to be placed in all directions around the body, in the same way as the jib of a crane places its load. The wide area that can be covered in positioning the hand is due largely to the movement at the **glenohumeral joint** between the head of the humerus and glenoid cavity of the scapula. Range is further increased by movement of the scapula on the chest wall in the same direction as the humerus, which allows the humerus to move further. Figure 5.1 shows the combined movement of the humerus and scapula in abduction of the arm to reach the vertical position.

- *PLACE the hand on the scapula of a partner. Feel the movement of the scapula in the same direction as the humerus, while your partner moves the arm to place the hand all around the body.*

The muscles arranged around the shoulder not only perform the wide range of movement, but also anchor the arm to the trunk, supporting the weight of the upper limb as it moves. When the hand performs precision movements, the shoulder muscles hold the arm steady.

All the muscles involved in movements of the shoulder region are attached to the humerus, scapula and clavicle. The proximal attachments of the larger muscles extend on to the sternum, ribs and vertebral column.

The pectoral girdle

The bony clavicle and the scapula form the pectoral girdle which provides the link between the upper limb and the trunk. Two articulations are involved in this link: (a) the *sternoclavicular joint* between the medial end of the clavicle and the clavicular notch on the manubrium of the sternum (Fig. 5.2a); and (b) the *acromioclavicular joint* between the lateral end of the clavicle and the acromiom process of the scapula (Fig. 5.2b). The sternoclavicular joint is stabilised by the strong costoclavicular ligament, and by an intra-articular disc attached to the clavicle above and to the first costal cartilage below. This disc gives

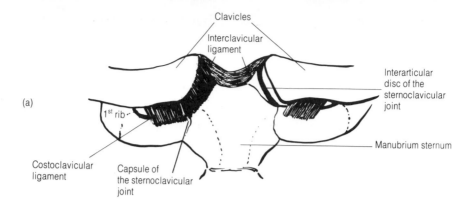

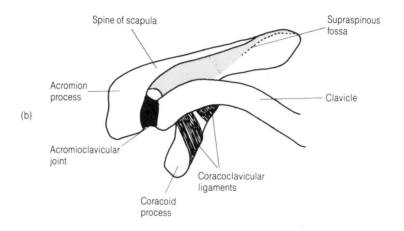

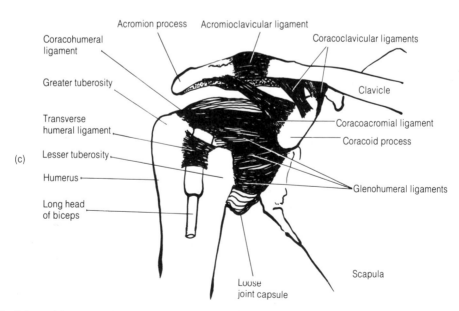

Fig. 5.2. Joints of the pectoral girdle and the shoulder: (a) sternoclavicular joints, anterior view (left joint with capsule removed); (b) right acromioclavicular joint, superior view; (c) right glenohumeral joint, anterior aspect.

added range of movement to the sternoclavicular joint. The medial end of the clavicle rocks on the disc, and the disc moves on the clavicular notch of the sternum.

- *PALPATE the sternoclavicular joint on a partner and feel the rocking action of the clavicle on the sternum during the shrugging of the pectoral girdle and the movement of the point of the shoulder forwards and backwards. Then feel the much reduced adjustment that takes place at the acromioclavicular joint during these same movements.*
- *PALPATE the sternoclavicular joint while the arm moves at the shoulder in all directions. Note that movement at the sternoclavicular joint occurs each time the humerus moves.*

The muscles that move the shoulder girdle and the glenohumeral joint can be divided into three.

(1) The muscles stabilising the glenohumeral joint.

(2) The muscles acting on the glenohumeral joint.

(3) The muscles moving the pectoral girdle.

Remember that the muscles in each section do not act in isolation, but combine in various ways, grouping and regrouping as the movement proceeds. The division into three sections is for the purpose of description only

5.2 The glenohumeral joint and the muscles stabilising it

The bony articulation of the *glenohumeral joint* occurs between the head of the humerus and the shallow glenoid fossa at the lateral aspect of the scapula (Fig. 5.2c). The head of the humerus is approximately one-third of a sphere, but only one-third of its surface area is in contact with the glenoid fossa during movement. The fibrous joint capsule is both thin and loose. The shape of the bony surfaces and the loose capsule both provide for a wide range of movement at the joint, but they present a poor prospect for stability. Two ligaments give some support. The *coracohumeral ligament* extends from the coracoid process to the upper aspect of the greater tuberosity of the humerus. This ligament assists in holding the head of the humerus up to the glenoid fossa, but it is not entirely successful in this. The *coracoacromial ligament* is an accessory ligament that extends between the coracoid process and the acromion process. This ligament helps to form a secondary arch over the joint which prevents upward dislocation of the head of the humerus, for example in a fall onto the abducted arm.

The most effective provision of support for the joint is from the four muscles surrounding it and blending closely with the capsule. These muscles are the *supraspinatus*, *infraspinatus*, *teres minor* and *subscapularis*, which act like guy ropes holding the humerus in contact with the scapula, and are known as the 'rotator cuff' muscles (Fig. 5.3). The lesser tuberosity of the humerus receives the subscapularis tendon, covering the joint anteriorly. The other three muscles are inserted into the greater tuberosity, with supraspinatus superiorly, then infraspinatus and teres minor below and posteriorly. The absence of any additional support inferiorly means that dislocation is usually downwards and forwards, under its own weight as the arm hangs by the side, or during abduction movement.

The 'rotator cuff' muscles have weak action as prime movers since their insertions are close to the joint, but they function as stabilisers in all movements of the shoulder joint. Supraspinatus initiates abduction of the shoulder before deltoid can exert its pull on the lateral shaft of the humerus. The other three muscles act as rotators of the humerus, subscapularis medially, infraspinatus and teres minor laterally.

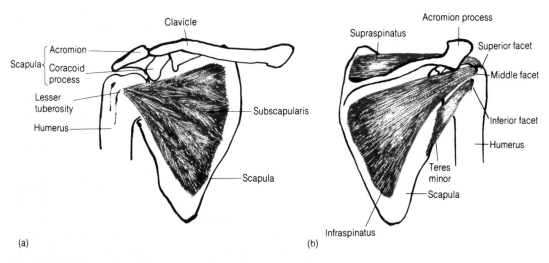

Fig. 5.3. Right scapula and humerus to show the 'rotator cuff' muscles: (a) anterior view; (b) posterior view.

> ### Clinical note-pad 5A: The shoulder joint
>
> Subluxation of the shoulder is when the head of the humerus drops in the glenoid fossa. This may occur in a stroke patient when there is general weakness of all the muscles around the shoulder.
>
> Periarthritis is a painful condition of the shoulder caused by inflammation of the bursa below the acromion or of the synovial sheath in the bicipital groove, or the deposition of calcium in the tendons of one or more of the rotator cuff muscles.
>
> Frozen shoulder usually results if the shoulder is not used due to pain or mild repeated trauma. Pain gradually increases over several months and then subsides leaving stiffness which persists if untreated. All movements at the shoulder joint are limited at first and only return when the stiffness subsides.

5.3 Muscles acting on the glenohumeral joint

Three large muscles, surrounding the glenohumeral joint, move the joint through its wide range. Their attachments cover a wide area of the pectoral girdle and trunk, and converge to insert on to the humerus.

The three muscles are the *deltoid*, the *pectoralis major* and the *latissimus dorsi*. The *teres major* and *coracobrachialis* are two other muscles that will be considered together.

Deltoid

The deltoid muscle gives the rounded shape to the shoulder and has the overall shape of an inverted triangle. The margins of the muscle can be clearly seen in athletes and swimmers. Lack of use after injury may lead to wasting which gives the shoulder a 'squared appearance'.

- *LIFT a saucepan or book down from a high shelf and feel the continuous activity in the deltoid as the arm is raised and then lowered. If the deltoid was relaxed as the arm came down, the movement would be rapid and uncontrolled, and you would probably drop the book on the floor.*
- *PALPATE the origin of the deltoid in a partner with the arm relaxed by the side. Start anteriorly at the lateral end of the clavicle to feel the anterior fibres. Next cross the acromion process of the scapula where the middle fibres arise. Continue along the spine of the scapula to find the posterior fibres. All the fibres converge to insert on the lateral shaft of the humerus about half way down (Fig. 5.4a).*

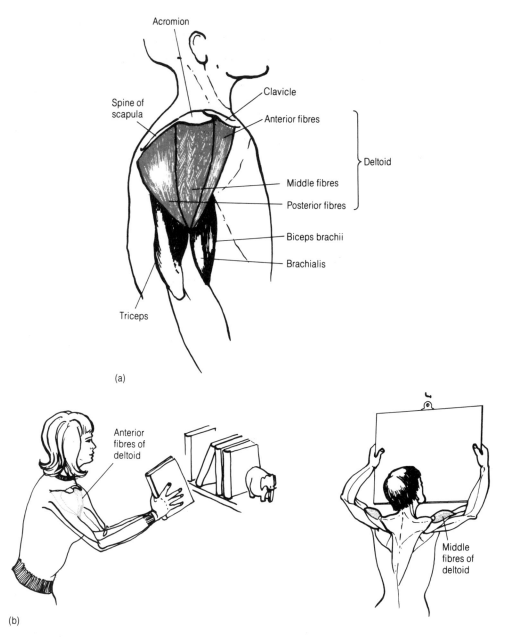

Fig. 5.4. (a) Right shoulder viewed from the side to show the position of the deltoid muscle. (b) Functions of the deltoid: reaching forwards and reaching above the head.

- *INSPECT the skeleton to find the deltoid tuberosity formed by the pull of the deltoid on the humerus.*

The deltoid is a powerful abductor of the arm, lifting the arm sideways and up above the head. It is also active when the arm is lowered back down to the side, working eccentrically to control the effect of gravity. All movements reaching forwards (Fig. 5.4b) and above the head (Fig. 5.4b) demand the deltoid muscle in action.

The anterior fibres flex and medially rotate the glenohumeral joint, while the posterior fibres extend and laterally rotate. Both sets can work together to prevent forwards and backwards movement during abduction of the arm by the strong middle fibres. Part or all of the deltoid is used in most movements of the humerus on the scapula. The muscle also acts as a support sling for the shoulder, especially when the upper limb is carrying heavy loads such as a suitcase or shopping bag.

Pectoralis major

Pectoralis major is a large triangular muscle whose base lies vertically along the midline of the thorax, and the apex is attached to the humerus (Fig. 5.5a). The lower border of the triangle can be felt in the anterior wall of the axilla. The main bulk of the muscle is difficult to observe in women as the breast covers some of its surface.

● *PRESS the hands together in front of the body to put the muscle into action. The muscle can now be palpated in the axilla by a partner.*

The uppermost fibres of pectoralis major arise from the clavicle medial to the anterior fibres of the deltoid. The remainder of the base of the triangle is formed by fibres arising from the anterior surface of the sternum and the costal cartilages of the first six ribs. All the fibres converge to the insertion on the anterior humerus in the groove between the two tubercles (intertubercular sulcus or bicipital groove), with the clavicular fibres lying superficial to the sternocostal fibres.

The clavicular fibres work with anterior fibres of the deltoid to flex the shoulder to a right angle. The lower costal fibres work with the posterior deltoid to pull the arm downwards in extension. Pulling down a window roller blind is an extension movement against resistance. Acting as a whole, pectoralis major is an adductor and medial rotator of the shoulder drawing the arm across to place the hand on the opposite side of the body, as in lifting a saucepan to one side, or moving a pile of books.

Pectoralis major is used to pull the arm forwards in throwing a ball (Fig. 5.5b), javelin or discus. In tennis and squash, the arm

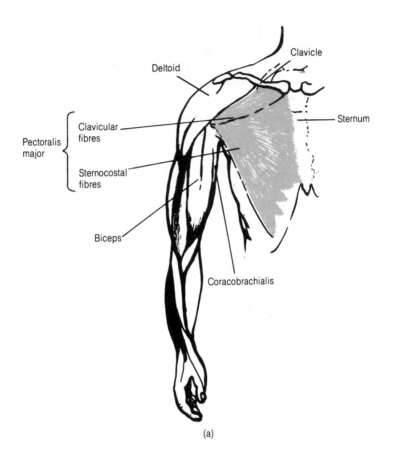

(a)

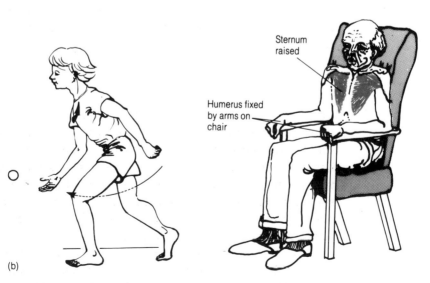

(b)

Fig. 5.5. (a) Right thorax and upper limb showing the position of the pectoralis major. (b) Functions of the pectoralis major: throwing a ball and assisting breathing.

is taken backwards, and pectoralis major draws the racquet forwards to hit the ball in a forehand drive. Another function of pectoralis major is to assist in deep breathing. When the humerus is fixed, the muscle pulls the sternum upwards and outward to enlarge the thorax and draw more air into the lungs. Figure 5.5b shows the position of the arms used to assist breathing while sitting in a chair. (Two of the shoulder girdle muscles, serratus anterior and pectoralis minor, work with pectoralis major in this position to increase the ventilation of the lungs.)

Latissimus dorsi

A shoulder muscle arising from a large origin in the lower back and thorax, latissimus dorsi wraps around the trunk and converges towards the shoulder forming the posterior wall of the axilla. (Note: the pectoralis major forms the anterior wall.) The proximal attachment of latissimus dorsi is by an aponeurosis from the spines of the lower six thoracic, all the lumbar, and the upper sacral vertebrae. Some fibres also arise directly from the posterior half of the iliac crest. The uppermost fibres cross the inferior angle of the scapula holding it down. From the wall of the axilla, the tendon passes underneath the glenohumeral joint to end on the anterior end of the humerus, in the floor of the bicipital groove (Fig 5.6a).

● *HOLD the arm up, palpate the posterior wall of the axilla, and work out how the tendon reaches the anterior aspect of the arm on the humerus.*

The actions of latissimus dorsi are extension, adduction and medial rotation of the shoulder joint. When the hand is above the head, latissimus dorsi (working with the lower fibres of pectoralis major) pulls the arm downwards and backwards against resistance, as in pulling down a blind. Continuation of this movement together with medial rotation takes the hand behind the body, as in tieing an apron (Fig. 5.6b). Working statically, latissimus dorsi adducts the arm against the body to hold a bag or file (Fig. 5.6b). In climbing, the hand is placed above the head, and the muscle works strongly to pull the trunk up towards the arm, and lift the body upwards (Fig. 5.6b).

The latissimus dorsi is an important muscle for anyone with loss of function in the lower limb resulting from weak muscles or stiff joints. If the body cannot be raised from sitting by

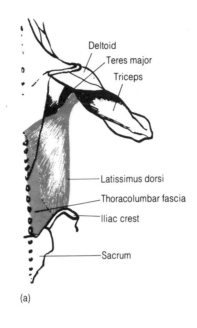

(a)

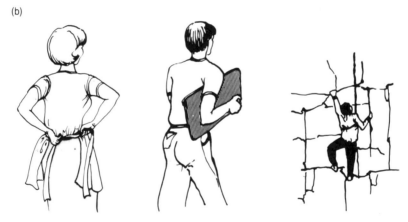

(b)

Fig. 5.6. (a) Posterior view of the right trunk and upper limb showing the position of the latissimus dorsi. (b) Functions of the latissimus dorsi: tieing an apron, holding a document case and rock climbing.

extension of the legs, the hands can be placed on the seat or arms of the chair, and the body lifted off the seat using the adduction action of latissimus dorsi to hitch on the pelvis. Wheelchair patients rely heavily on this muscle to transfer from the chair to a bed or toilet seat. In crutch walking, latissimus dorsi helps to support the weight of the body on the hands. The muscle can also be trained to lift one side of the pelvis, so that the leg clears the ground in the swing phase in walking, known as 'hip hitching', the method used to teach paraplegic patients in long leg calipers to walk.

Teres major and coracobrachialis

These are two strap like muscles with a weaker individual action on the glenohumeral joint.

The teres major is attached to the lower lateral border of the scapula and lies in the posterior wall of the axilla. The insertion is with the tendon of latissimus dorsi on the anterior of the humerus. The two muscles act together on the glenohumeral joint.

The coracobrachialis takes origin from the coracoid process of the scapula and inserts into the rough area on the medial shaft of the humerus. The action of coracobrachialis is flexion of the shoulder from the hyperextended position, i.e. humerus behind the trunk. There is evidence that the muscle functions to swing the arm forwards in walking and running. This muscle also adducts the arm on to the trunk when holding a newspaper or purse under the arm.

5.4 Muscles moving the pectoral girdle

The scapula is a triangular blade of flat bone lying on the posterior wall of the rib cage. Muscles cross the anterior and posterior surfaces of the scapula, and are attached to its borders and processes. The muscles covering the anterior surface are sandwiched between the scapula and the ribs, and are loosely separated by connective tissue and fat, which allows the scapula to move freely on the chest wall. As the scapula is able to follow the direction of movement at the glenohumeral joint, it contributes to the wide range of movement of the upper limb on the trunk.

It is important to understand clearly the position of the scapula in relation to the vertebral column, ribs and walls of the axilla, in order to appreciate the direction of pull of the muscles which turn the scapula in various directions.

Firstly the terms used to describe the movements of the scapula on the chest wall will be described.

(1) **Elevation**: the scapula moves upwards as in 'shrugging the shoulders'.

(2) **Depression**: the scapula moves down to its resting position.

(3) **Protraction**: the scapula moves forwards around the chest wall.

(4) **Retraction**: the scapula moves backwards towards the spine.

(5) **Lateral rotation**: the inferior angle of the scapula moves laterally and the glenoid fossa points upwards.

(6) **Medial rotation**: the inferior angle of the scapula moves medially and the glenoid cavity returns to the rest position.

There are six muscles attached to the triangular scapula that combine to produce these movements. The muscles are the *trapezius, levator scapulae, rhomboid major* and *minor, serratus anterior* and *pectoralis minor*. By pulling together in different combinations, these muscles can elevate, depress, protract, retract and rotate the scapula on the chest wall.

Trapezius (Fig. 5.7a)

The two sides of the trapezius form a kite shaped area of muscle, the most superficial muscle of the back.

Each muscle is a triangle, with its base in the midline from the base of the skull down to the 12th thoracic spine.

The upper fibres originate from the occipital bone of the skull and the ligamentum nuchae, which covers the cervical spines in the neck. The fibres pass downwards and forwards across the neck to the lateral end of the clavicle and continue on to the acromion of the scapula. Acting as a suspension for the pectoral

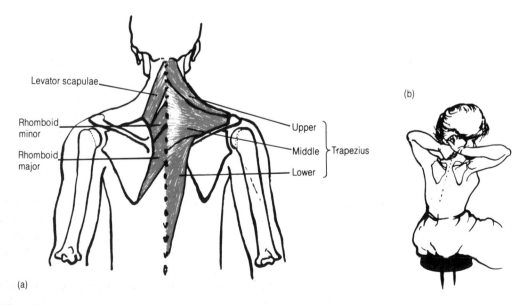

Fig. 5.7. (a) Posterior view of the neck, thorax and arm to show the position of the trapezius, levator scapulae and the rhomboids. (b) Reaching behind the head.

girdle from the skull and neck vertebrae, contraction of these upper fibres lifts the shoulders in *elevation*. In addition, they give support to the shoulders when carrying heavy loads. The static work of the trapezius is felt when carrying heavy luggage or shopping.

The middle fibres pass horizontally from the upper thoracic spines to the length of the spine of the scapula. Contraction of these fibres pulls the scapula towards the spine, the scapula retracts, to reach behind the head. Activities involving this movement include reaching behind the head to comb the hair (Fig. 5.7b) and to grasp a car seat-belt.

The lower fibres pass upwards from the lower thoracic vertebrae into a tendon that inserts into the base (medial end) of the spine of the scapula. Acting alone, these fibres will *depress* the shoulder when it has been raised. More important is the action of the lower fibres with the upper fibres to *rotate* the scapula, turning the glenoid fossa upwards.

Levator scapulae

The transverse processes of the first four cervical vertebrae provide the attachments for levator scapulae, and the fibres descend to the vertebral border of the scapula above the spine (Fig. 5.7a). Levator scapulae lies deep to the upper fibres of the trapezius and works with them to *elevate* the scapula.

Rhomboid major and minor

These two muscles form a continuous layer deep to the middle fibres of the trapezius, originating on the spines of the upper thoracic vertebrae and inserting into the medial border of the scapula (Fig. 5.7a). The rhomboids can be considered as one muscle which pulls the scapula backwards in *retraction*.

Serratus anterior

This has a saw toothed origin from the upper eight or nine ribs, clearly seen in male swimmers and boxers with powerful shoulder muscles. From this wide origin, the fibres wrap around the thorax and underneath the scapula to be inserted in the vertebral border of the scapula (Fig. 5.8a).

The action of the whole muscle pulls the scapula forwards around the chest in *protraction*. This movement increases the forward reach of the upper limb, adds to the force of a punching

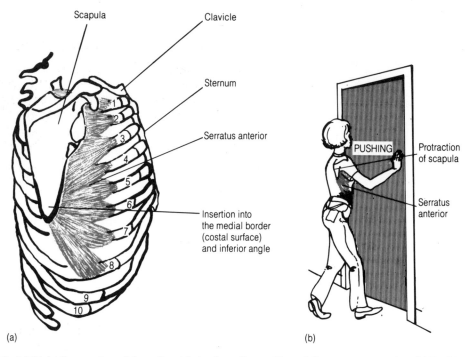

Fig. 5.8. (a) Right thorax viewed from the side to show the position of the serratus anterior. (b) Pushing a door.

action and pushes the arm forwards against a resistance, such as a door (Fig. 5.8b).

The lower fibres of serratus anterior converge on to the inferior angle of the scapula, and their action will *rotate* the scapula laterally to turn the glenoid fossa upwards to allow full abduction of the humerus. In lateral rotation, the serratus anterior works with the upper and lower fibres of the trapezius.

- *LOOK at an articulated skeleton to appreciate the exact position of the serratus anterior. Lying deep to the scapula it separates subscapularis from the chest wall.*

Figure 5.9 shows the serratus anterior and the rhomboids seen in a transverse section across the thorax. Identify the vertebral border of the scapula and note how the serratus anterior and the rhomboids pull on the scapula in opposite directions to protract and retract the scapula respectively.

Pectoralis minor

This is a small muscle lying in the anterior wall of the axilla deep to the pectoralis major, but with no action on the shoulder joint.

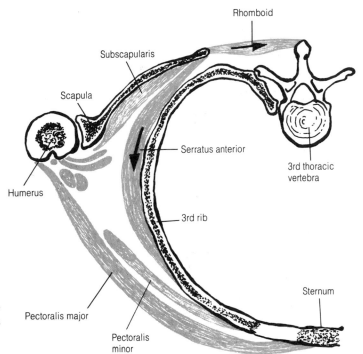

Fig. 5.9. Transverse section through the upper thorax at the level of the third rib. Arrows show the direction of pull of the serratus anterior (protraction) and the rhomboids (retraction).

The fibres of the pectoralis minor ascend from the anterior surface of the 3rd, 4th and 5th ribs, to be attached to the coracoid process of the scapula (Fig. 5.10). By pulling on the coracoid process, the pectoralis minor can *depress* and medially rotate the scapula.

- *LIFT the arm of a partner through the full range of abduction to reach above the head, then full adduction back to the side. Palpate the scapula during this action: lateral rotation can be felt as the arm is raised, then medial rotation as the arm is lowered.*

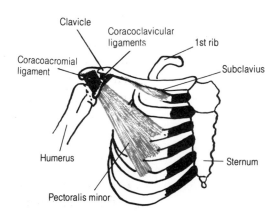

Fig. 5.10. Anterior view of the right upper thorax to show the position of the pectoralis minor and subclavius.

- *MOVE the arm to the horizontal and then round a wide circle forwards and backwards. Palpate the scapula during this action and feel the movement of protraction as the arm swings across the front of the body, and retraction as it swings behind the body.*

All the muscles attached to the clavicle and scapula combine in different ways to produce the movements of the pectoral girdle. The clavicle, spine and acromion of the scapula can be considered as two sides of a triangle, completed by a line across the root of the neck (Fig. 5.11a). This triangle moves in elevation, depression, protraction and retraction, with the sternoclavicular

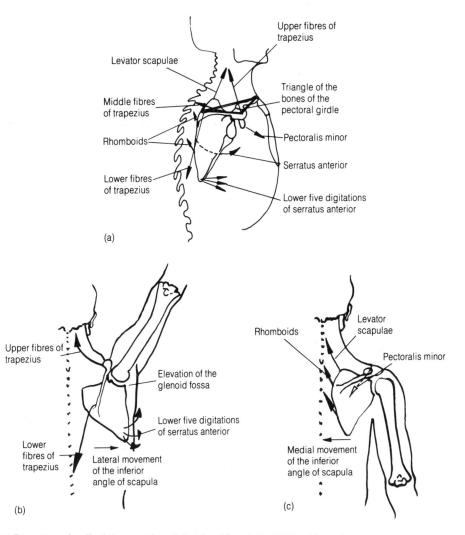

Fig. 5.11. Direction of pull of the muscles of the shoulder girdle: (a) the clavicular scapular and scapular triangles of the pectoral girdle; (b) lateral rotation of the scapula; (c) medial rotation of the scapula.

joint acting as the pivot. The scapula itself is a triangle, which moves in the same directions as the upper triangle when pulled simultaneously at two of its angles. When three angles of the scapula are moved by muscle action, the scapula rotates, either medially or laterally (Fig. 5.11b and c). The axis of rotation lies just inferior to the spine of the scapula, midway along its length.

- *OBSERVE the following functional activities, then record the directions of movement of the scapula and name the muscles involved.*

(1) Reach up to a high shelf.

(2) Push open a door.

(3) Reach behind to grasp a seat belt in a car.

(4) Turn over a page of a newspaper on a table.

(5) Pull open a drawer.

5.5 Summary of the muscles involved in shoulder movement

Many activities involve movements at both the glenohumeral joint and the scapula. The following table summarises the muscles which combine in functional movements of the shoulder.

(1) *Reach and push forwards*
    Flexion of the glenohumeral joint:
        Deltoid – anterior fibres
        Pectoralis major – clavicular fibres
        Coracobrachialis
    Protraction of the scapula:
        Serratus anterior
        Pectoralis minor

(2) *Pull down and backwards*
    Extension of the glenohumeral joint:
        Deltoid – posterior fibres
        Pectoralis major – sternocostal fibres
        Latissimus dorsi and teres major
    Retraction of the scapula:
        Rhomboids
        Trapezius – middle fibres

(3) *Reach sideways and upwards*
    Abduction of the glenohumeral joint:
        Deltoid

Supraspinatus
Lateral (upward) rotation of the scapula:
Trapezius – upper and lower fibres
Serratus anterior
(4) *Pull down to the side*
Adduction of the glenohumeral joint:
Pectoralis major
Latissimus dorsi
Teres major and coracobrachialis
Medial (downward) rotation of the scapula:
Rhomboids
Levator scapulae
(5) *Turn hand and forearm inwards, reach across the body*
Medial rotation of the glenohumeral joint:
Deltoid – anterior fibres
Pectoralis major
Latissimus and teres major
Subscapularis
Protraction of the scapula in reaching across the body:
Serratus anterior
Pectoralis minor
(6) *Turn hand and forearm outwards, reach sideways and backwards*
Lateral rotation of glenohumeral joint:
Deltoid – posterior fibres
Infraspinatus and teres minor
Retraction of the scapula, reaching sideways and backwards:
Rhomboids
Trapezius – middle fibres

PART II
MOVEMENTS OF THE ELBOW

5.6 Functional movements of the elbow

Movement at the elbow brings the hands towards the head and body. The elbow flexors are the 'hand to mouth' muscles. Try splinting the elbow in extension and find out how much we depend on elbow *flexion* for daily activities, such as washing, dressing, eating and drinking. The opposite *extension* movement of the elbow enables the hand to push against resistance, for example a lawn mower, a swing door or a pram. With loss of function of the lower limb, a person relies on elbow extensors to lift the body weight on the hands to rise from a chair or walk with crutches. (Note: the latissimus dorsi and lower fibres of the trapezius are also involved.)

The elbow joint

The elbow is a synovial hinge joint moving through *flexion* and *extension* in the sagittal plane only. The head of the radius and trochlear notch of the ulna articulate with the lower end of the humerus. The pulley shaped trochlear surface at the lower end of the humerus and the trochlear notch of the ulna form the hinge of the elbow joint (Fig. 2.3a). This close fit gives bony stability to the joint. The upper concave surface of the head of the radius slides over the capitulum of the humerus like a ball bearing, allowing the radius to rotate in movements of the forearm at any degree of angulation of the elbow. Collateral ligaments strengthen the capsule and stabilise the joint (Fig. 5.12a and b).

- *WATCH the elbow in action during the following activities.*

(1) *Using a saw or a hammer.*

(2) *Operating a keyboard, e.g. typewriter, micro-computer.*

(3) *Lifting a box or tray from below.*

In all these activities, the forearm as a whole moves like a hinge at the elbow, i.e. about a single axis. The difference in 1, 2 and 3 is the position of the hand, the result of rotation of the lower end of the radius around the ulna carrying the hand with it. The rotation movement of the forearm occurs at the joints between the radius and ulna (see Chapter 6, Fig. 6.3).

Pronation is when the hand turns medially to face backwards from the anatomical position, or downwards when the hand is in front of the body.

Supination is the return movement when the hand turns to face forwards in the anatomical position, or upwards when the hand is in front of the body.

Pronation and supination will be discussed in more detail in Chapter 6, but it is important at this stage to distinguish between forearm and elbow movement, and to note that they often occur together as the hand is used.

● *Look again at the elbow activities 1, 2 and 3, looking this time at the
position of the forearm. In 2 the forearm is in pronation and in 3 it is in*

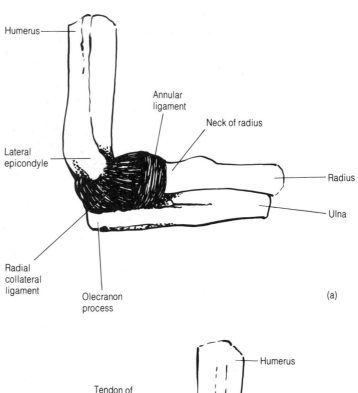

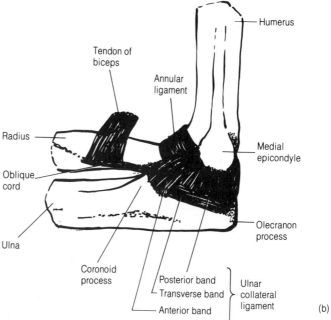

Fig. 5.12. Right elbow
joint: (a) lateral view; (b)
medial view.

supination. In 1 the forearm is in the mid-position between pronation and supination, called mid-prone.

Clinical note-pad 5B: 'Tennis elbow'

Pain occurs in the area of the lateral epicondyle of the humerus, which may radiate widely, and is caused by repeated minor trauma to the muscles originating on the lateral epicondyle (wrist extensors). Flexion and extension of the elbow are normal and painless. Pain occurs in pronation movements.

5.7 Muscles moving the elbow joint

The muscles that move the elbow lie mainly in the arm above the elbow. They are found in anterior and posterior compartments which are separated on the lateral and medial sides by thick sheets of fibrous tissue, known as intermuscular septa. The muscles in these compartments are: the *biceps brachii* and *brachialis* (anterior) (flexors); and the *triceps brachii* and *anconeus* (posterior) (extensors). Two other muscles that are found in the forearm and assist in elbow flexion are *brachioradialis* and *pronator teres.*

5.7.1 Flexors of the elbow

Biceps brachii

The biceps muscle is the bulge in the arm we use to demonstrate our muscle strength. The muscle is easy to see in the relaxed state in those who have done some weight training. The biceps has no attachment to the humerus. The origin of the biceps is by two tendons from the scapula. The long head is a tendon attached to the superior part of the glenoid cavity within the shoulder joint, and emerges from the capsule to lie in the inter tubercular sulcus (bicipital groove) of the humerus. The short head is a tendon from the coracoid process of the scapula, closely connected to the tendon of coracobrachialis. The tendons of the two heads join to form one muscle belly in the lower part of the arm, and the muscle inserts into the tuberosity on the medial side of the radial shaft just below the elbow. The tendon of insertion can be felt when the forearm rests on a table and the muscle is relaxed. A flat band of fibrous tissue, known as the bicipital aponeurosis, extends medially from the tendon and blends with the fascia covering the medial side of the forearm (Fig. 5.13).

The flexor action of the biceps is obvious; contraction draws the radius towards the humerus. The muscle is most effective when the forearm is in supination. Working eccentrically, the biceps controls the lowering of the forearm and hand holding a tool or utensil (see Chapter 2).

The biceps also acts as a powerful supinator, turning the forearm and hand to exert force on (for example) a door handle or screwdriver. Pulling the cork from a bottle with a corkscrew

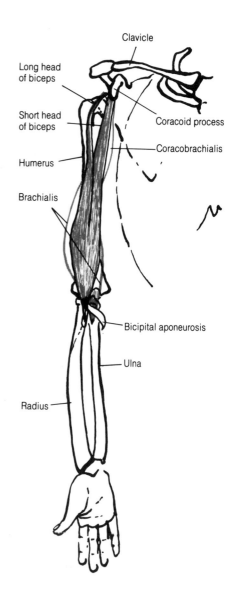

Fig. 5.13. Anterior view of the right upper limb to show the position of the biceps brachii, brachialis and coracobrachialis.

uses both actions of the biceps, supination followed by flexion. Note: the biceps is the 'party muscle'!

- *LOOK at an articulated skeleton and turn the lower end of the radius and the hand into full pronation. Notice how the radial tuberosity has moved posteriorly. The pull of the biceps tendon will now rotate the proximal end of the radius back to the anatomical position, performing an unwinding action of the forearm.*

Brachialis

The brachialis muscle lies deep to the biceps in the lower half of the arm. If the relaxed biceps is lifted and moved from side to side, brachialis can be located below. The fibres of the brachialis arise from the anterior shaft of the humerus below the level of insertion of the deltoid. Passing over the anterior side of the elbow joint, the fibres insert by a broad tendon into the ulnar tuberosity below the coronoid process of the ulna (Fig. 5.13).

The brachialis can flex the elbow efficiently in all positions of the forearm and hand. The ulna does not move in pronation and supination, so the direction of pull of the brachialis tendon always produces flexion. When the elbow flexors increase in size in response to weight training, the brachialis contributes most to the arm bulge.

5.7.2 Extensors of the elbow

Triceps brachii

The posterior compartment contains the three heads of triceps. The long head is a broad tendon attached to the inferior part of the glenoid cavity, outside the capsule, but blended with it. (Note: the long head of the biceps lies inside the joint). The two other heads of triceps arise from the shaft of the humerus. The lateral head takes origin from an oblique line below the greater tuberosity on the posterior shaft. The medial head is deep and attached to the lower posterior shaft of the humerus, corresponding to the origin of the brachialis anteriorly.

The long and lateral heads join to form one layer, which unites with the deep medial head, and all three end as a broad tendon inserted into the olecranon of the ulna (Fig. 5.14a).

All extension movements involve the medial head, the other two heads are recruited when acting against resistance. It is the lateral head that becomes more obvious in the powerful triceps

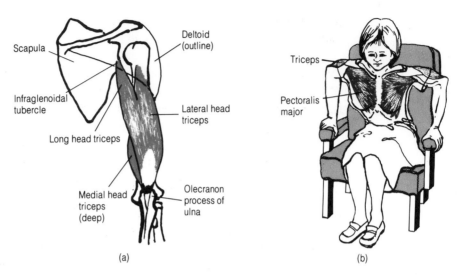

Fig. 5.14. (a) Posterior view of the right scapula and arm to show the position of triceps brachii. (b) Use of the triceps with the pectoralis major and latissimus dorsi to raise the body from sitting.

developed by the gymnast, weight lifter and wheelchair athlete. The triceps provides all the power of the elbow in extension movements to reach above the head, to push forwards and to the side. Figure 5.14b shows the use of the triceps with the pectoralis major to lift the body up from the sitting position if the muscles of the lower limb are weak.

Anconeus

This is the other posterior muscle which extends the elbow. This muscle is small and blends with the lower end of the triceps at the back of the elbow joint. The fibres of anconeus originate on the lateral epicondyle of the humerus, and insert distal to the triceps on the olecranon of the ulna. Anconeus adds little to the total strength of elbow extension, but does contribute to the stability of the elbow joint.

5.7.3 Forearm muscles in flexion of the elbow

Brachioradialis

The brachioradialis is the most superficial muscle on the radial side of the forearm.

- *MOVE the forearm to be at a right angle to the arm.*
  Turn the hand to face medially, i.e. mid-prone position.
  Flex the elbow and offer resistance with the other hand.

- *PALPATE the brachioradialis in position parallel to the long axis of the radius.*

The muscle originates from the ridge above the lateral epicondyle of the humerus. The fibres pass down the lateral side of the forearm, and the tendon inserts into the radius just above the styloid process at the wrist (Fig. 5.15a). In the anatomical position, the muscle can only pull the head of the radius closer to the capitulum of the humerus. When the radius is rotated to bring the styloid process in line with the middle of the elbow joint (the mid-prone position), the brachioradialis is able to flex the elbow in a powerful way. The mid-prone position is frequently adopted to allow the strong leverage to aid flexion, e.g. using a hammer or saw, lifting a baby (Fig. 5.15c) or heavy boxes. Working statically, the brachioradialis holds the elbow in flexion to support books or the handle of a bag over the forearm (for example).

Pronator teres

The pronator teres is another forearm muscle that helps in flexion of the elbow. It arises from the medial epicondyle of the humerus with the wrist and finger flexors. (Note: the brachioradialis origin is above the lateral epicondyle of the humerus with the wrist extensors.) The fibres of the pronator teres cross obliquely below the elbow joint to be inserted into the lateral shaft of the radius about half way down. When the forearm is supinated, the pronator teres gives least power to the elbow flexors. When all the elbow flexors are in action, the pronator teres counteracts the tendency for the biceps to supinate the arm.

Figure 5.15b shows both the brachioradialis and pronator teres, they will be considered again in Chapter 6 with the forearm muscles.

- *WRITE a table of the muscles moving the elbow joint under the following headings: action, muscles involved, function.*

5.8 Positioning movements

The positioning movements of the upper limb involve activity in combinations of groups of muscles around the shoulder and the elbow. Particular combinations that frequently occur together are called movement *synergies*. For example, the flexors of the elbow combine with the flexors, adductors and medial rotators

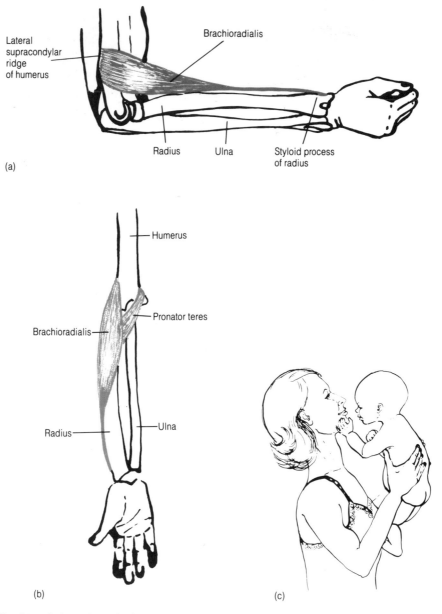

Fig. 5.15. Brachioradialis in the right forearm: (a) lateral view in the mid-prone position; (b) anterior view with pronator teres; (c) lift and hold baby.

of the shoulder, and protractors of the scapula, to bring the hand to the mouth in eating. The same groups combine to position the hand in front of the body and in the central visual field for precision movements of the fingers. Extension movements of the elbow combine with flexion, abduction and lateral

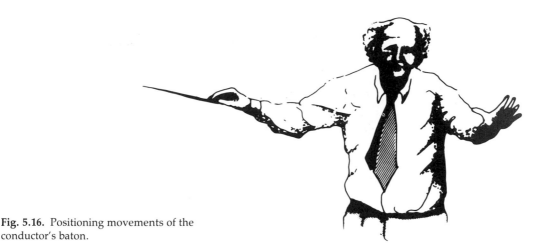

Fig. 5.16. Positioning movements of the conductor's baton.

rotation of the shoulder, and retraction of the scapula, for example in reaching upwards and sideways to move the door of a high cupboard, or pull curtains across.

The wide variety of movements that can be performed by the shoulder and elbow is seen in a conductor of an orchestra moving his baton in all directions (Fig. 5.16).

At the end of this chapter, you should be able to:

PART I

(1) Describe the structure and movements of the joints of the pectoral girdle (sternoclavicular and acromioclavicular), and the shoulder (glenohumeral) joint.

(2) Describe the position, attachments and actions of the muscles that: (a) stabilise the glenohumeral joint; and (b) move the glenohumeral joint in flexion, extension, abduction, adduction, and medial and lateral rotation. Give examples of the use of each of these muscles in daily living activities.

(3) Name the muscles that move the scapula in elevation, depression, protraction, retraction, and medial and lateral rotation.

(4) Appreciate how the combination of movements of the scapula and the humerus allows a wide range of movement at the shoulder in positioning the hand around the body.

PART II

(5) Describe the structure and movements of the elbow joint.

(6) Describe the position, attachments and actions of the muscles that move the elbow in flexion and extension. Define pronation and supination of the forearm. Appreciate how the movements of the elbow and the forearm combine in positioning the hand for manipulative activities.

(7) Summarise the cooperation of muscles around the shoulder and elbow in functional activities of the upper limb.

6 / Manipulative Movements: The Forearm, Wrist and Hand

6.1 Functions of the hand

The complex and intricate movements of the hand are performed by muscles that originate partly in the hand itself (intrinsic muscles) and partly in the forearm (extrinsic muscles), passing over the wrist into the hand. These muscles act on the large number of joints found in the hand to give the *dexterity* of movement in the fingers and thumb.

- *WATCH the finger movements of a musician, keyboard operator or needlewoman.*
- *LOOK at your own hands making a cup of coffee, eating pasta, planting seeds.*

As well as the fine movements of the fingers and thumb used to operate small tools and keyboards, the hand is the mechanism to *grasp* handles and large tools while the upper limb moves them in space. In all gripping movements, the thumb is placed opposite to the fingers in different ways depending on the size and shape of the object. The wrist is also important in gripping by providing a stable base for the hand, and by directing the pull of the tendons of the forearm muscles acting on the fingers and thumb. Our complete ability to grasp includes 'letting go' or 'setting down' as well. These movements involve the opposing group of muscles to those that make the grip.

The hand is also a *sense organ*. The skin of the hand is richly supplied with receptors, and a large area of the somatosensory cortex in the brain (see Chapter 3, Section 3.4.2) processes information from them. Trauma or pathological changes in the bones and joints of the wrist and carpus may damage sensory fibres in the nerves passing over them and affect hand sensation. Response from pain receptors in the skin of the hand is important to protect it from injury. All gripping activities involve the continuous monitoring by the central nervous system of the activity in skin receptors and proprioceptors in the hand. For example in writing, accurate formation of the letters depends on the correct pressure of the fingers on a pen, and the hand on the paper.

- *TRY writing with a pen whilst wearing a thin pair of rubber gloves.*

Further sensory processing of all the sensory information in the brain allows us to 'recognise' objects held in the hand without seeing them. This is known as stereognosis, see Chapter 3, Section 3.4.2.

Finally, the hand is used in *communication* and expression of feelings. Watch how people use their hands as they greet each other or chat in a group. Hands are used to compliment and reinforce the spoken word in a conscious way, or may be used unconsciously in 'body language'.

To summarise, the main functions of the hand are: (a) dexterity; (b) grasp; (c) sensation; and (d) communication.

6.2 Pronation and supination of the forearm in hand function

Movements between the radius and ulna are important to position the whole hand on the forearm, so that gripping and precision movements of the fingers and thumb can occur in a particular direction. Pronation and supination have already been considered in relation to forearm position during flexion and extension movements of the elbow in Chapter 5.

- *FIND handles and rails in different positions, i.e. vertical, horizontal or at an angle. Grip each one and notice how the position of the forearm changes in each position to allow the hand to grip.*
- *GRIP the vertical handle of a teapot or jug and then tip to pour out the contents. Note how the grip remains the same while the tipping is done by pronation and supination of the forearm.*
- *TURN a tap or a round door knob. The fingers and thumb exert pressure on the tap, while the forearm movement provides the power to turn it.*

The importance of the forearm in the use of the hand should now be appreciated.

In the anatomical position, the forearm is supinated and the radius and ulna lie parallel to one another. During pronation, the radius rotates and the lower end crosses over the ulna, carrying the hand with it. The hand then faces downwards when it is in front of the body, or backwards in the anatomical position. In the functional position of the hand the forearm is in the mid-prone position.

Radioulnar joints

The movements of pronation and supination occur at two synovial pivot joints – (a) *proximal* and (b) *distal radioulnar joints*. In between lies the interosseous membrane extending along the length of the shafts of the radius and ulna, which is called the middle radioulnar joint (Fig. 6.1a).

(1) **The proximal radioulnar joint** lies between the head of the radius and the radial notch on the ulna. The joint lies inside the capsule of the elbow joint, but its movements are entirely independent. The annular ligament (lined by a thin layer of cartilage) surrounds the head of the radius and is firmly attached to the margins of the radial notch on the ulna (Fig. 6.1b). The capsule of the elbow joint blends with the annular ligament so that the radius can rotate independently within this ring whatever the angulation of the elbow joint may be (see Chapter 5).

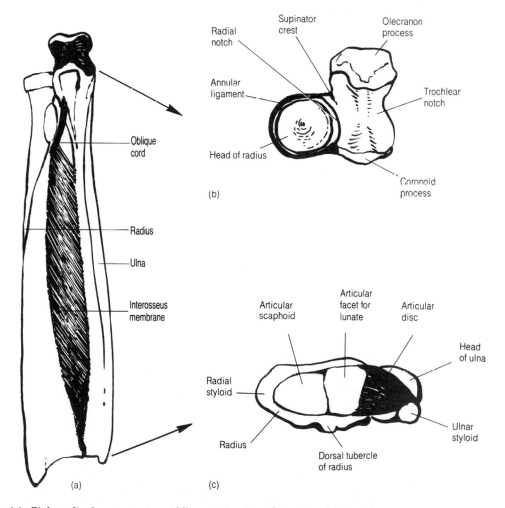

Fig. 6.1. Right radioulnar joints: (a) middle, anterior view; (b) proximal; (c) distal.

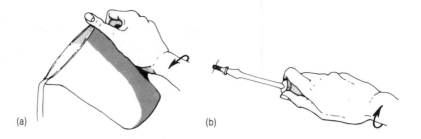

Fig. 6.2. Activities involving pronation and supination: (a) pouring from a jug – pronation; (b) turning a screw – supination.

(a)   (b)

(2) **The distal radioulnar joint**. The lower end of the radius pivots around the head of the ulna, and is held in contact with it by a disc of fibrocartilage. This disc joins the styloid process of the ulna to the ulnar notch of the radius (Fig. 6.1c). The joint has a thin loose capsule, but the bones are also held together by the interosseous membrane.

All the muscles involved in pronation and supination are inserted into the radius, which then moves around the fixed ulna. The supinators, inserted into the radius, can also assist other muscles to move the elbow, e.g. the biceps brachii is also an elbow flexor, and the supinator helps in extension of the elbow.

Pronation puts the palm of the hand flat on a surface, or tips forwards a vessel held in the hand (Fig. 6.2a). Strong pronation and supination movements are needed to use a screwdriver or a corkscrew (Fig. 6.2b). Supination is more powerful than pronation and so most screws have a right handed thread.

The **brachioradialis**, already described with the elbow flexors in Chapter 5, Section 5.7.3, can move the forearm to the mid-prone position from full pronation or full supination.

6.2.1 Muscles producing pronation

Two forearm muscles are active in pronation: the *pronator teres* and the *pronator quadratus*.

The **pronator teres** (Fig. 6.3a), which crosses the anterior forearm from the medial side of the elbow to half way down the lateral shaft of the radius, has already been described in Chapter 5, Section 5.7.3.

The **pronator quadratus** (Fig. 6.3a) is a deep muscle of the forearm just above the wrist. Its fibres pass transversely between the lower anterior shafts of the radius and ulna. The muscle is deep to the flexor tendons which pass into the hand. When force is applied to the outstretched hand in pushing or falling, the pronator quadratus prevents separation of the radius and

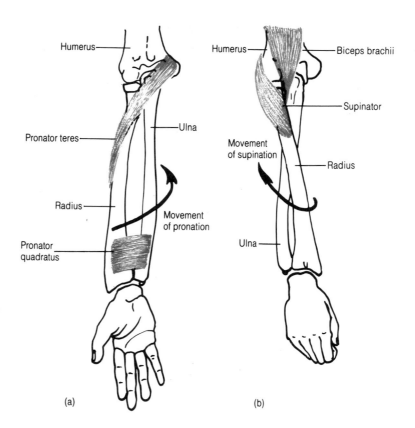

Fig. 6.3. Right forearm and hand: (a) anatomical position, forearm supinated; (b) forearm in pronation, hand turned to face backwards.

(a)

(b)

ulna. Many pronation movements are made with the pronator quadratus alone; the pronator teres is recruited for extra power against resistance.

6.2.2 Muscles producing supination

The two muscles active in supination are the *biceps brachii* and *supinator*.

The **biceps brachii** (Fig. 5.13) makes all supination movements against resistance. Its tendon pulls on the radial tuberosity just below the elbow to rotate the radius to the position parallel with the ulna. The attachments and action of the biceps have already been described in Chapter 5, Section 5.7.1.

Slow, unopposed movements of supination, such as when the arm hangs by the side, are made by a deep posterior muscle of the forearm called the **supinator** (Fig. 6.3b) which is covered by the long extensors of the wrist and fingers. The origin of the supinator is from the lateral epicondyle of the humerus and adjacent areas of the ulna. A short flat muscle, its fibres wrap around the proximal end of the radius close to the bone and insert into the upper end of the shaft.

6.3 Movements of the wrist

The wrist region is concerned with movements of the carpus of the hand on the radius and ulna of the forearm. The range of movement is increased by the movement of the carpal bones on each other, particularly between the proximal and distal rows.

Joints of the wrist

The two main joints of the wrist are the *radiocarpal* and *midcarpal joints*.

The **radiocarpal joint** is formed by the concave distal end of the radius and articular disc over the ulna, with the convexity formed by the three carpal bones in the proximal row, i.e. scaphoid, lunate and triangular (triquetral), see Chapter 2, Figure 2.3c. The articular disc of fibrocartilage covers the distal end of the ulna and forms the medial part of the proximal joint surface.

The **midcarpal joint** lies between the proximal and distal row of carpals, i.e. distal surfaces of scaphoid, lunate and triquetral with proximal surfaces of trapezium, trapezoid, capitate and hamate. The joint cavity is continuous between the two rows of carpals and extends between the individual bones. (Note: the fourth bone in the proximal row, the pisiform, does not take part in either of the joints.)

The capsular ligament of the radiocarpal joint extends to cover the midcarpal joint, and the collateral ligaments continue over medial and lateral aspects of both joints (Fig. 6.4).

The movements at the joints of the wrist are *flexion, extension, abduction* and *adduction*. Abduction is also known as radial deviation, and adduction is ulnar deviation. This avoids confusion between the movements at the wrist when the forearm is pronated or supinated. There is no active rotation of the wrist about a longitudinal axis. Remember that rotation of the hand on the forearm occurs at the radioulnar joints of the forearm, i.e. pronation and supination movements.

Radiographs of the wrist in action show that all the carpals move as well as the radiocarpal articulation. In some movements, the scaphoid, for instance, may move as much as 1 cm. The radiocarpal joint contributes most to extension and adduction, while the midcarpal joint moves further in flexion and abduction.

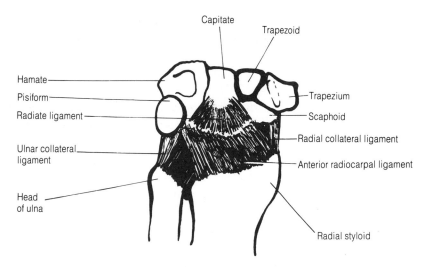

Fig. 6.4. Right wrist (radiocarpal) joint. Anterior aspect.

All the joints act together as a single mechanism for wrist movement.

- *PLACE the supinated hand (palm upwards) on a flat surface in a relaxed position. Notice the slight flexion and deviation to the ulnar side.*
- *LOOK at an articulated skeleton to see the shape of the lower end of the radius extending further on the dorsal side and laterally at the styloid process, which accounts for the position of the hand.*
- *LIFT the hand and move the wrist into flexion, extension, abduction (radial deviation) and adduction (ulnar deviation). Note the range of each of these movements. You will see that the hands move further in flexion than extension, and more easily in ulnar deviation than radial deviation.*
- *COMPARE your own range of these wrist movements with those of other people. Notice the difference in range between individuals, but the relative amounts for each movement are usually the same.*

Since there is a variation in range of movement in normal subjects, the assessment of an injured wrist should be done by comparing it with the normal wrist of the same person and not with the 'average' wrist.

- *LOOK again at the wrist moving in flexion and extension. Notice that in flexion the hand moves slightly towards the ulnar side, and in extension towards the radial side.*

The reason for this difference is the shape of the lower end of the radius, as was noted in the rest position.

- *HOLD a mug of coffee or large tool, e.g. a hammer, in the hand. Note that the forearm is in the mid-prone position and the weight of the mug or tool is tending to pull the wrist into ulnar deviation, so that the abductors of the wrist must work statically to hold the position.*

When the muscles are weak, the unsupported hand falls into flexion or ulnar deviation when holding a load.

Clinical note-pad 6A: Fractures of the forearm and wrist

A common way to fracture the bones of the forearm is a fall onto the outstretched hand, such as slipping on an icy path. This causes:

(1) a Colles fracture when the lower broken ends of bone are displaced backwards; or

(2) a Smith fracture when only the radius is fractured and the distal fragment displaces forwards.

A fall on the hand with the wrist in full extension may fracture the scaphoid. The bone fractures across its waist, and the proximal fragment may die due to poor blood supply. This avascular necrosis may produce persistent pain and weakness of the wrist.

6.3.1 Flexors of the wrist

The two main muscles which flex the wrist are the *flexor carpi ulnaris* and *flexor carpi radialis*. The palmaris longus is another wrist flexor which lies between the other two, but it is absent in 15% of people.

All three muscles have a common origin on the medial epicondyle of the humerus, and lie underneath the skin in the anterior side of the forearm.

The **flexor carpi ulnaris** is attached to the pisiform bone and on to the base of the fifth metacarpal (Fig. 6.5a).

The **flexor carpi radialis** lies deep to the muscles at the base of the thumb as it crosses the wrist and ends at the bases of metacarpals 2 and 3 (Fig. 6.5a).

The palmaris longus has a long thin tendon which inserts into the palmar aponeurosis, a layer of dense fibrous tissue

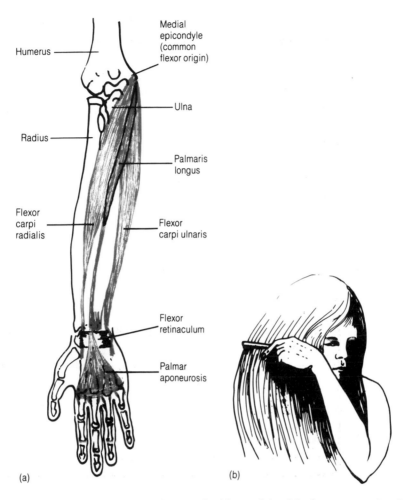

Fig. 6.5. Flexors of the wrist: (a) position in the superficial layer of the right forearm, anterior view; (b) combing the hair.

below the skin of the palm, considered in more detail in Section 6.4.1.

- *MAKE a fist and flex the wrist to see the flexor tendons appear on the anterior aspect. Palmaris longus is in the midline and the flexor carpi ulnaris medial to it, attached to the pisiform. The flexor carpi radialis laterally may be more difficult to find.*

A functional use of the wrist flexors can be seen in Figure 6.5b where they are used to counteract the resistance offered by the hair on the comb.

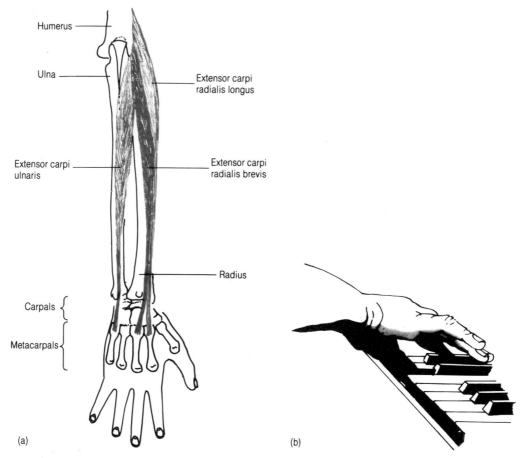

Fig. 6.6. Extensors of the wrist: (a) position in the right forearm, posterior view; (b) the hand held in wrist extension to play the keys of a piano.

6.3.2 Extensors of the wrist

The three muscles that extend the wrist are the *extensor carpi ulnaris* and the *extensor carpi radialis longus* and *brevis* (Fig. 6.6a). The long radial extensor takes origin on the ridge above the lateral epicondyle of the humerus with brachioradialis, already described in Chapter 5. The other two muscles are attached to the lateral epicondyle which is the common extensor origin. All three muscles pass down the posterior side of the forearm and insert at the wrist following the same pattern as the flexors.

(1) Extensor carpi radialis longus into metacarpal 2.

(2) Extensor carpi radialis brevis into metacarpal 3.

(3) Extensor carpi ulnaris into metacarpal 5.

Note: the flexors insert into the anterior or palmar side, and the extensors insert into the posterior or dorsal side.

- *Make a fist and extend the wrist to see the extensor tendons on the posterior side. The extensor carpi radialis brevis is more central and may be difficult to feel, as it is crossed by tendons of muscles passing to the thumb.*

In the use of the pronated hand, e.g. pressing keys of a typewriter or piano (Fig. 6.6b), the wrist extensors are active to lift the weight of the hand against gravity. Weakness of these muscles leads to 'wrist drop'. In strong gripping by the whole hand, the wrist extensors act as synergists to counteract flexion of the wrist by the long finger flexors.

6.3.3 Abduction and adduction of the wrist

If the wrist is viewed in cross section, the flexor and extensor tendons involved in wrist movement can be seen around the oval shape of the carpus (Fig. 6.7). The tendons can combine in different ways, like the strings of a marionette, to produce each movement.

Contraction of the flexor and extensor muscles on the ulnar side will move the hand into adduction, often known as ulnar deviation. Similarly, contraction of the flexor carpi radialis and the extensor carpi radialis longus together will result in abduction of the wrist or radial deviation.

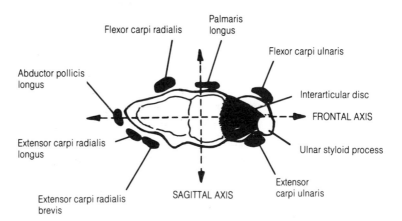

Fig. 6.7. Inferior aspect of the right radius and ulna to show the position of the tendons of the wrist flexors and extensors.

6.4 Movements of the hand

The hand performs complex and precision movements in the manipulation of utensils, tools and equipment in daily living. The increased use of electrically powered equipment in the home and in the work place has reduced the need for the hand to exert great power, but has introduced a greater variety of precision movements required to operate switches and controls.

A large number of muscles, originating in both the forearm and the hand, are inserted into the fingers and the thumb. Most of the tendons of these muscles pass over several joints, and the combinations of different directions of pull of the tendons allow the fingers to move in a variety of ways.

Before describing the muscles moving the hand, it is necessary to learn the terminology used in the description of the hand.

There are five digits numbered 1–5 from lateral (thumb) to medial. The fingers are usually identified by name: index finger, middle finger, ring finger, little finger (Fig. 6.8).

The third metacarpal and the third finger form the central axis of the hand. When the fingers separate, the other fingers move away from the central axis (Fig. 6.10a and b).

Joints of the fingers and the thumb

The positions of the main joints are identified in Fig. 6.8. At the knuckles, the heads of the metacarpals articulate with the

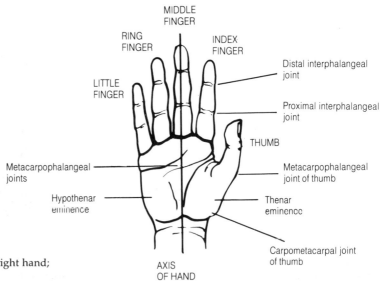

Fig. 6.8. Palmar view of the right hand; location of the joints.

proximal phalanges at the **metacarpophalangeal** or **MCP joints**. In the *fingers* the joints between the phalanges are known as the **proximal interphalangeal** or **PIP joints**, and the **distal inter-phalangeal** or **DIP joints**. The *thumb* has an **MCP joint** and only **one interphalangeal** or **IP joint**.

The **metacarpophalangeal joints of the fingers** are synovial ellipsoid, biaxial joints. The heads of the metacarpals 2 to 5 articulate with oval concavities at the base of the proximal phalanges.

- *LOOK at the palm of your hand to find the MCP joints of the fingers which lie beneath the two horizontal lines of the palm that can be seen below the base of the fingers. Flex the MCP joints and notice that the two lines form deep creases across the palm.*

Each MCP joint of the fingers (Fig. 6.9) has a strong palmar ligament, which is firmly attached to the phalanx but loosely to

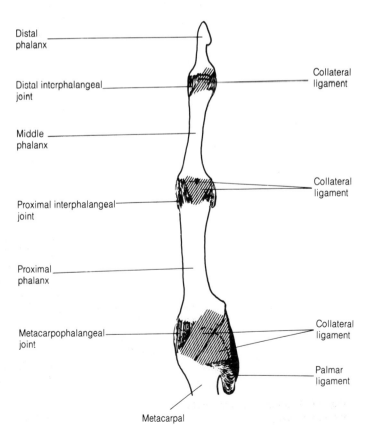

Fig. 6.9. Joints of the finger – lateral aspect.

the metacarpal bone. The palmar ligaments of these four joints are connected by a deep transverse ligament, which holds the heads of the metacarpals together to form the body of the palm of the hand. The collateral ligaments are bands present on each side of the joints. The movements of the MCP joints allow the fingers to flex and extend, abduct and adduct.

The **interphalangeal joints** are all synovial hinge joints, with collateral ligaments (Fig. 6.9). These joints allow flexion and extension movements only.

Movements of the thumb

In the rest position of the thumb, the first metacarpal (thumb) is medially rotated.

- *LOOK at the pad of the thumb when the hand is in a relaxed position on a flat surface. Note that the thumb is facing across the palm at right angles to it.*

With the initial direction of the pad of the thumb facing medially, the movements of the thumb are described at right angles to those of the fingers.

Flexion of the thumb carries it across the palm in a plane at right angles to the thumb nail (Fig. 6.10b).

Extension is the return movement from flexion and continues into the 'hitch a lift' position (Fig. 6.10d). In full extension of the thumb, the oblique pull of the long extensor of the thumb can, in some people, pull the first metacarpal into lateral rotation, so appearing to provide a 'flat' hand.

Abduction takes the thumb away from the palm of the hand and at right angles to it. (Fig. 6.10a).

Adduction is the return movement from abduction, which pulls the thumb back towards the palm of the hand.

The first metacarpal is also able to rotate on the trapezium both medially and laterally. The combined movements of flexion, medial rotation and adduction, which bring the thumb into contact with each of the fingers is known as **opposition**. The thumb can be opposed to the fingers in a variety of ways (see Section 6.5).

The movements of the thumb occur at the **carpometacarpal joint** which is formed between the base of the first metacarpal and the trapezium, the most lateral bone in the distal row of carpals.

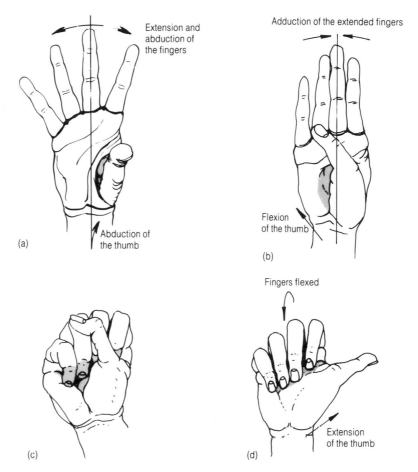

Fig. 6.10. Positions of the right hand seen in palmar view: (a) fingers extended and abducted, thumb abducted – the open hand; (b) fingers extended and adducted, thumb flexed; (c) fingers flexed, thumb in opposition – the closed hand; (d) fingers flexed, thumb extended.

● *LOOK at the back of the wrist area and note the way the lateral (thumb) side of the carpus curves round towards the palm.*

The curved arrangement of the carpal bones forms the floor of the carpal tunnel (see Section 6.4.1), and the trapezium is found on the anterolateral side of the carpal arch. The distal surface of the trapezium is scooped out in two directions to form a unique saddle joint with the base of the metacarpal of the thumb (see Chapter 2, Section 2.3.1, Fig. 2.3f). The shape of this articular surface, combined with a loose capsule, allows the thumb considerable mobility. The capsule is strengthened laterally, anteriorly and posteriorly by ligaments.

- *MOVE the thumb through all the directions described above and feel how all the movement occurs at the carpometacarpal joint.*

The **metacarpophalangeal joint of the thumb** is similar to those of the fingers, but the movements of abduction and adduction are restricted. The main movements are flexion and extension.

The **interphalangeal joint of the thumb** is a hinge joint with movement in only one plane, that is flexion and extension.

- *LOOK at your own hand. Starting at the base of the hand, notice the flexure line of the wrist, and then feel the shafts of the metacarpals on the back of the hand. Identify the MCP joints at the knuckles and check the movements that occur at these joints – flexion, extension, abduction and adduction.*
  Identify the PIP and DIP joints and check the movements – flexion and extension only.
- *PALPATE the first metacarpal bone of the thumb, which moves independently of the other metacarpals.*

During many functional activities, the hand closes round an object to hold or move it. In **closing the hand**, the fingers are flexed and adducted; the thumb is in opposition (Fig. 6.10c). The hand also opens to release an object and set it down. In **opening the hand**, the fingers and the thumb are extended and abducted (Fig. 6.10a).

- *OPEN the hand. Notice how the fingers and thumb abduct as they extend in opening the hand. CLOSE the hand. Notice how the fingers and thumb adduct as they flex to close the hand.*

The muscles moving the hand will be described under three headings based on the functional use of the hand: (a) muscles that close the hand around an object to grasp it; (b) muscles that open the hand in preparation for gripping or to release an object; and (c) muscles that move an object in a precise way.

6.4.1 Muscles closing the hand

The muscles closing the hand lie in the anterior part of the forearm deep to the wrist flexors, and in the palm of the hand. 'Digitorum' (the Latin for fingers) is included in the names of the muscles moving the fingers, and 'pollicis' (the Latin for thumb) in those moving the thumb.

Forearm muscles

The forearm muscles that close the hand are: the *flexor digitorum superficialis*, the *flexor digitorum profundus* and the *flexor pollicis longus*.

The **flexor digitorum superficialis** originates at the medial side of the elbow with the wrist flexors, i.e. from the medial epicondyle of the humerus. The origin of the muscle continues diagonally across the bones below the elbow, attached to the coronoid process of the ulna and the anterior shaft of the radius (Fig. 6.11a).

The **flexor digitorum profundus** lies deep to the superficialis and takes origin from the anterior and medial shaft of the ulna (Fig. 6.11b).

The **flexor pollicis longus** also lies deep to the superficialis and is attached to the anterior shaft of the radius (Fig. 6.11b).

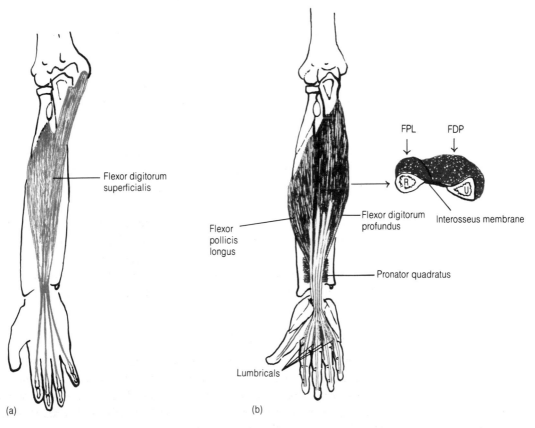

Fig. 6.11. Muscles seen in the anterior view of the right forearm and hand: (a) middle layer, flexor digitorum superficialis; (b) deep layer, flexor digitorum profundus and flexor pollicis longus.

The flexor digitorum profundus and flexor pollicis longus appear as one muscle in the deep layer on the anterior part of the forearm covering the radius, the ulna and the interosseus membrane in between them.

All three muscles pass down the anterior forearm to the wrist where the two muscles which insert into the fingers each divide into four tendons. Each of these tendons passes through the palm and over the palmar surface of each finger, where the flexor digitorum superficialis divides to insert into the sides of the middle phalanx. This allows the deeper flexor digitorum profundus tendon to pass on to insert into the distal phalanx. Figure 6.18 shows how these two muscles insert into each finger. The tendon of flexor pollicis longus turns laterally to reach the thumb and insert into the base of the distal phalanx.

The three muscles together flex all the joints of the fingers and the thumb. The tendons of the index, ring and little fingers diverge from the axis of the hand from wrist to finger tip. This means that as the fingers flex, they also adduct towards each other.

Muscles of the hand

Five *intrinsic muscles* of the hand also assist the forearm muscles in closing the hand, acting on the thumb and little finger.

The **flexor pollicis brevis** and **opponens pollicis** move the thumb and lie in the thenar eminence of the hand (Fig. 6.12a and b).

The **flexor digiti minimi** and **opponens digiti minimi** are comparable muscles in the hypothenar eminence below the little finger (Fig. 6.12a and b).

The **adductor pollicis** lies deep in the palm of the hand covered by the long flexor tendons and the flexor pollicis brevis (Fig. 6.12b).

A band of fibrous tissue, known as the flexor retinaculum crosses the palmar side of the carpal bones over the long flexor tendons. The thenar and hypothenar muscles originate from this retinaculum.

The flexor digiti minimi is inserted into the base of the proximal phalanx of the little finger, and the flexor pollicis brevis is attached to the proximal phalanx of the thumb. The opponens muscles are attached to the length of the shaft of the metacarpal bone of their corresponding little finger or thumb. During the opposition movement of the thumb, the shaft of the first meta-carpal is rotated about its axis by the pull of the opponens

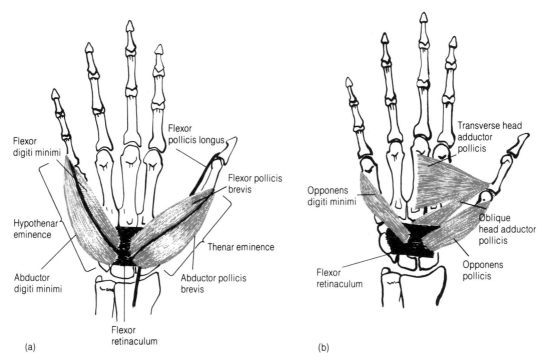

Fig. 6.12. Palmar view of the right hand: (a) flexor and abductor of the thumb and of the little finger; (b) opponens muscles and adductor pollicis.

pollicis. At the same time, the flexor draws the thumb across and towards the palm.

The opponens digiti minimi increases the bulk of the medial border of the hand in a cupping movement used to grasp a round knob, such as the gear lever of a car.

The adductor pollicis is attached along a wide origin in the centre of the palm on the shaft of the third metacarpal and has a second head from the capitate bone. This muscle forms the web of the thumb and inserts into the proximal phalanx of the thumb on the ulnar side (Fig. 6.12b). The adductor pollicis acts strongly to draw the thumb towards the hand in pinching movements between the thumb and index finger.

The connective tissues of the hand

The connective tissue in the *palm* of the *hand* plays an important role in the protection and binding of the muscles and tendons, so that smooth movement in the correct direction is achieved. Three particular sites are worthy of description: the *flexor retinaculum*, the *palmar aponeurosis* and the *flexor tendon sheaths*.

The **flexor retinaculum of the wrist**. The long finger flexors of the forearm enter the hand over the anterior side of the wrist. They are held in position by a band of fibrous tissue called the flexor retinaculum. This also provides a base for the attachment of some of the thenar and hypothenar muscles (Fig. 6.12).

- *LOOK at the skeleton of the hand and note how the carpal bones form a trough on the palmar side for the long flexor tendons. Look at the arrangement of the carpal bones and find four raised bony points on either side of this trough. These are: the pisiform and the hook of the hamate medially, and the tubercle of the scaphoid and crest of the trapezium laterally.*

The flexor retinaculum stretches across the carpal bones, converting the trough into a tunnel known as the *carpal tunnel* (Figure 6.13). Note: the exact position of the flexor retinaculum is across the base of the hand, i.e. under the heel of the hand, and not in the position of a bracelet around the wrist.

The **palmar aponeurosis**. The palmar aponeurosis is a triangular sheet of fibrous tissue covering all the long muscle tendons of the palm. The apex is joined to the flexor retinaculum at the wrist and receives the insertion of the palmaris longus (if this muscle is present), see Figure 6.5a. The sides of the triangle blend with the fascia covering the muscles of the thumb and

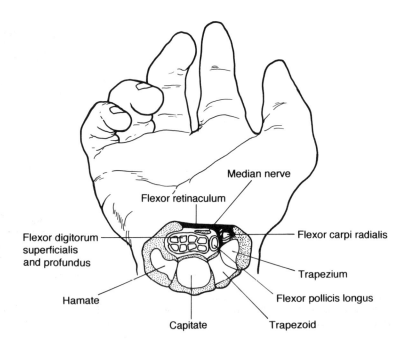

Median nerve

Flexor retinaculum

Flexor digitorum superficialis and profundus

Flexor carpi radialis

Trapezium

Hamate

Flexor pollicis longus

Capitate

Trapezoid

Fig. 6.13. Section through the carpus to show the carpal tunnel.

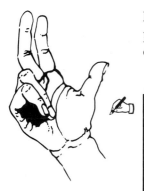

little finger, and the sheet ends at the base of the fingers. The palmar aponeurosis is anchored to the metacarpals and to the deep transverse palmar ligament.

Clinical note-pad 6B: Dupuytrens contracture

This condition occurs when there is shrinkage of the fibrous tissue in the palmar aponeurosis, usually on the ulnar side. The little and ring fingers are pulled down so that they curl into the palm of the hand (Fig. 6.14).

Fig. 6.14. Right hand with Dupuytren's contracture.

The **flexor tendon sheaths**. As the long flexor tendons pass through the carpal tunnel and up over the palmar surface of each finger, they are wrapped in a double layer of synovial membrane known as a tendon sheath (Fig. 6.15). Each tendon sheath is held in position on the palmar surface of the bones of the finger by fibrous bands forming tunnels. These fibrous bands are also joined to the palmar aponeurosis and are thin over the IP joints to allow flexibilty of the fingers.

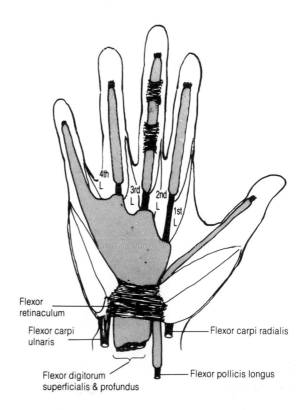

Fig. 6.15. Palmar view of the right hand showing tendon sheaths (shaded) of the long flexor tendons.

Clinical note-pad 6C: Tenosynovitis

Tenosynovitis is an inflammation of the synovial sheaths around the tendons of muscles, when there is swelling due to an accumulation of fluid. This may be due to overuse, for example in racquet games. The tendons passing through the carpal tunnel at the wrist are confined to a narrow space so that any increase in fluid compresses the median nerve. This condition sometimes occurs in pregnancy, in middle-aged women and in rheumatoid arthritis. See Chapter 7, clinical note pad 7D, carpal tunnel syndrome.

6.4.2 Muscles opening the hand

The muscles opening the hand lie in the posterior part of the forearm, and include one muscle in each of the thenar and hypothenar groups.

Forearm muscles involved in opening the fingers

The forearm muscles that open the fingers are the *extensor digitorum*, the *extensor indicis* and the *extensor digiti minimi*.

The **extensor digitorum** and the **extensor digiti minimi** originate with the wrist extensors from the lateral epicondyle of the humerus. The **extensor indicis**, a deep muscle, takes origin on the posterior border of the ulna. The tendons formed from these three muscles pass posteriorly over the wrist held down by a band of fibrous tissue, the extensor retinaculum. On the dorsal side of the hand, the extensor digitorum divides into four. The extensor indicis lies adjacent to the index finger tendon of the extensor digitorum and blends with it. The extensor digiti minimi lies medial to the other tendons and blends with the little finger tendon of extensor digitorum (Fig. 6.16). The tendons of the muscles insert into the dorsal surface of the fingers via a complex arrangement of fibrous tissue known as the dorsal extensor expansion. This will be described in more detail at the end of Section 6.4.3.

- *PALPATE the extensor tendons as they pass over the posterior side of the wrist and on to the back of the hand.*
- *OBSERVE how the long extensor tendons can be seen on the back of the hand when it is opened. Notice how the tendons are close together at the level of the wrist. The tendons of the index, ring and little fingers diverge away from the central axis of the hand to reach the fingers. The pull of the extensor tendons, therefore, abducts as well as extends these three fingers.*

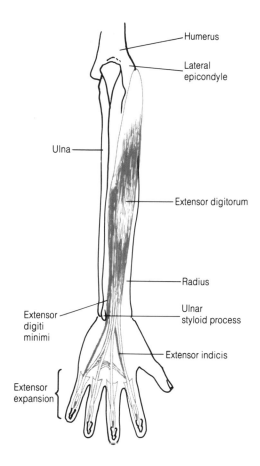

Humerus

Lateral epicondyle

Ulna

Extensor digitorum

Radius

Extensor digiti minimi

Ulnar styloid process

Extensor indicis

Extensor expansion

Fig. 6.16. Extensors of the fingers; posterior view of the right forearm and hand.

Forearm muscles involved in opening the thumb

Three forearm muscles act in separating the thumb when opening the hand, the *abductor pollicis longus*, the *extensor pollicis longus* and the *extensor pollicis brevis*.

The three muscles originate from the posterior shaft of the radius and ulna as follows: (a) the abductor pollicis longus from the upper shaft of the radius and ulna; (b) the extensor pollicis longus from the shaft of the ulna below; and (c) the extensor pollicis brevis from the shaft of the radius below.

All three muscles pass deep to the extensor digitorum and become superficial on the radial side of the wrist to reach the thumb (Fig. 6.17). At the base of the thumb they form the borders of the 'anatomical snuff box'. These long muscles of the thumb are called the 'deep outcropping muscles' of the forearm, since they begin deep in the posterior forearm and emerge near to the surface on the radial side of the wrist. Each muscle inserts into a different bone in the thumb: (a) the abductor

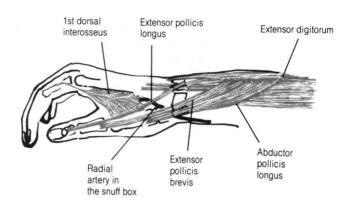

1st dorsal
interosseus

Extensor pollicis
longus

Extensor digitorum

Fig. 6.17. Radial side of the right wrist
and hand showing the muscles of the
'anatomical snuff box'.

Radial
artery in
the snuff box

Extensor
pollicis
brevis

Abductor
pollicis
longus

pollicis longus inserts into the first metacarpal; (b) the extensor
pollicis brevis inserts into the proximal phalanx; and (c) the
extensor pollicis longus inserts into the distal phalanx.

- *OBSERVE the 'anatomical snuff box' by extending the thumb with the
  wrist extended. A depression appears bounded by tendons below the
  thumb.*
- *PALPATE the abductor pollicis longus and extensor pollicis brevis
  lying together in the same boundary of the 'snuff box'. The other dorsal
  boundary is formed by the tendon of the extensor pollicis longus, which
  uses the dorsal tubercle of the radius to change direction at the wrist.*

Intrinsic muscles involved in opening the hand

Two intrinsic muscles of the hand assist the forearm muscles in
opening the hand, acting on the thumb and the little finger: (a)
the *abductor pollicis brevis* lies in the thenar eminence; and (b) the
abductor digiti minimi lies in the hypothenar eminence. Both these
muscles originate at the flexor retinaculum at the palmar side of
the base of the hand.

The **abductor pollicis brevis** is inserted into the base of the
proximal phalanx of the thumb on the lateral side (see Fig.
6.12a). Note: the thumb faces inwards at right angles to the
palm, so that when the abductor pollicis brevis contracts, it
draws the thumb away from the palm by movement at the base
of the first metacarpal (saddle joint of the thumb). Just as the
thumb reaches its fully abducted position, the opponens pollicis
pulls on the shaft of the first metacarpal, so turning the pad of
the thumb to face the pads of the fingers. In this way, the
precision grips of pinch and pincer take place between the two
digits (see Section 6.5.2).

The fibres of the **abductor digiti minimi** originate from the flexor retinaculum and pisiform bone, and insert into the base of the proximal phalanx of the little finger on the medial side (see Fig. 6.12a).

The action of opening the hand is important in releasing a grip and in placing an object on a surface. A young baby can grasp a toy in the hand, but drops it randomly. At a later stage, when coordination between opposing groups of muscles has developed, the child can then put the toy down precisely as the hand opens.

6.4.3 Precision movements

The fingers and thumb perform a variety of skilled movements: for example, alternate action of flexors and extensors at all the joints of the fingers is required to press the keys of a typewriter or a piano. When the fingers and thumb grip a pen or paint-brush, fine movements of flexion and extension of the distal joints carry the pen or brush over the paper.

Three sets of intrinsic muscles deep in the palm of the hand are important in precision movements: the *lumbricals*, the *dorsal interossei* and the *palmar interossei*.

The **lumbricals** are four small muscles which originate from the tendons of flexor digitorum profundus, the deepest long finger flexor in the palm (Fig. 6.18). Each muscle passes in front of the MCP joint of the corresponding finger, passes backwards on the radial side of this joint, and inserts into the dorsal surface of the finger on the radial side. The detail of the insertion will be considered later with the description of the dorsal extensor expansion of the fingers.

The actions of the lumbricals are flexion of the MCP joints and extension of the IP joints. They link the long flexor tendons in the palm to the long extensor insertion on the dorsal side of the fingers. In this way, they act as a bridge between the two, which balances the flexion and extension movements of the fingers. There is evidence that the lumbricals are active in all fine movements of the fingers.

The **interosseous muscles** lie in the spaces between the meta-carpal bones. There are two layers of interosseous muscles. The dorsal layer is the most superficial on the back of the hand. The palmar layer lies between the dorsal layer and the lumbricals.

- *PALPATE the dorsal interossei between the shafts of the metacarpals on the dorsal surface of the hand.*
- *MOVE the index finger into abduction (radial deviation) and palpate*

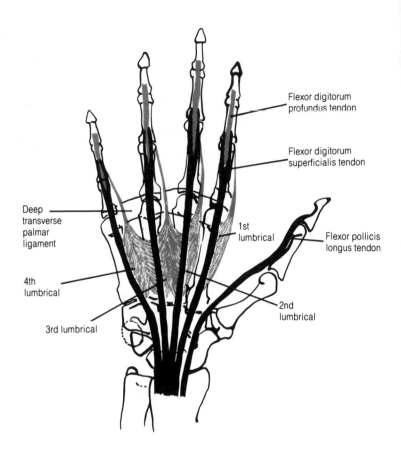

Flexor digitorum profundus tendon

Flexor digitorum superficialis tendon

Deep transverse palmar ligament

1st lumbrical

Flexor pollicis longus tendon

4th lumbrical

2nd lumbrical

3rd lumbrical

Fig. 6.18. Lumbrical muscles; position in a palmar view of the right hand.

the muscle on the radial side of the first metacarpal. This is the first dorsal interosseous muscle.

There are four **dorsal interossei** originating from the sides of adjacent shafts of metacarpals 1–5, deep to the extensor tendons. The position of these muscles is best understood from a diagram, see Figure 6.19a. Note: the two lateral (thumb side) dorsal interossei pass on the radial side of the MCP joints of the index and middle fingers; the medial two muscles pass on the ulnar side of the MCP joints of the middle and ring fingers. The tendons of all four muscles reach the dorsal surface of the fingers to blend with the outer bands of the extensor expansion of the index, middle and ring fingers, just beyond the level of the MCP joints (Fig. 6.20a).

Action of all four dorsal interossei will spread the fingers away from the central axis of the hand. The middle finger has two dorsal interosseous muscles, and therefore can abduct from the central axis to either side. The attachment of each tendon

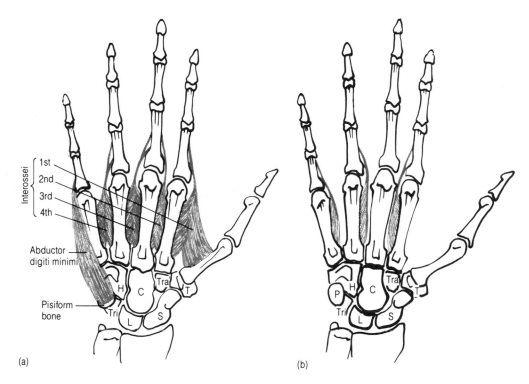

Interossei
1st
2nd
3rd
4th

Abductor
digiti minimi

Pisiform
bone

H C Tra T
Tri L S

(a)

P H C Tra T
Tri L S

(b)

Fig. 6.19. Interosseous muscles in a palmar view of the right hand: (a) dorsal interossei and abductor digiti minimi; (b) palmar interossei.

into the dorsal surface of the finger means that each muscle will also assist in extension of the DIP joints.

The dorsal interossei can be palpated between the shafts of the metacarpals. When these muscles are wasted, due to nerve damage, the skin sinks between the metacarpals and the back of the hand looks like a skeleton.

The three **palmar interossei** lie on the palmar side of the dorsal interossei. The position of these muscles can be seen in Figure 6.19b. Each is attached to one side of a metacarpal shaft, and is inserted into the outer band of the dorsal expansion of the same finger. From their attachments it can be seen how they will draw the fingers together in adduction when they contract.

One way to remember the actions of the two sets of interossei is by the initials: dorsal aBduct – DAB; palmar aDduct – PAD.

Both the dorsal and the palmar interossei cooperate with the lumbricals in flexion of the MCP joint and extension of the IP joints.

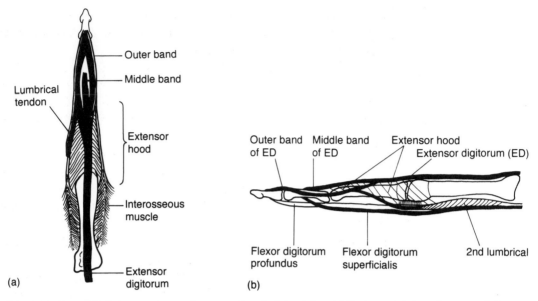

Fig. 6.20. Dorsal digital expansion and extensor hood of the right middle finger: (a) dorsal view; and (b) side view (second dorsal interosseus removed).

✍️ **Clinical note-pad 6D: Rheumatoid hand**

The fingers of the hand may be seen to be angled towards the ulnar side at the MCP joints. This ulnar drift deformity is due to subluxation of the proximal phalanx within the MCP joint capsule, particularly the index and middle fingers. The MCP joints are swollen and painful. It is important to maintain the strength of the first dorsal interosseous muscle to keep the fingers in alignment.

Dorsal (extensor) digital expansion of the fingers

The insertion of muscles on to the dorsal surface of the fingers is a complex system of fibrous bands known as the dorsal digital expansion. The extensor digitorum, the lumbricals and the interossei are inserted into it.

The tendon of extensor digitorum divides into three as it crosses the MCP joint. The middle band is inserted into the base of the middle phalanx, and the outer bands into the base of the distal phalanx (Fig. 6.20a). The outer bands receive the insertions of the lumbricals and the interossei. Fine transverse fibres spread out from the middle band to form a moveable extensor hood (Fig. 6.20b) over the proximal phalanx and the head of the metacarpal. The base of the hood extends to be attached to the deep transverse palmar ligament. This extensor hood prevents any bowstring of the extensor tendon.

Each lumbrical lies on the palmar side of the metacarpal at first, and then crosses the MCP joint to insert into the outer band of the dorsal expansion on the radial side. In this way the lumbricals can flex the MCP joint and extend the IP joints of each finger.

The interossei lie in parallel with the metacarpals and are held down by the extensor hood at the MCP joint. The interossei pull on the outer band of the dorsal expansion to produce abduction and adduction of the fingers. The attachment of the interossei to the dorsal digital expansion means that they also assist the lumbricals in flexion of the MCP joints and extension of the IP joints.

The functional significance of the dorsal digital expansion is to allow the complex movements of the fingers to occur. Activities such as writing involve simultaneous flexion of some joints and extension of others. A balance between flexor and extensor muscle activity is required to produce this. All the precision movements of the hand result from a variety of combinations of movements at the joints of the fingers and the thumb.

- *LOOK at the palmar side of a hand skeleton and your own hand. Work out how the lumbricals begin in the palm with the long flexor tendons, and end on the dorsal side of each finger, passing round the radial (thumb) side of the MCP joint.*
- *DRAW a line on the hand for the main axis through the middle finger and work out how the dorsal and palmar interossei are positioned around it.*
- *PALPATE the first dorsal interosseous muscle by abducting the index finger whilst the thumb is in abduction.*
- *LOOK at the dorsal side of the right middle finger and Figure 6.20a. Locate the position of the dorsal digital expansion and the insertion of extensor digitorum by three bands. A lumbrical is inserted into the outer band on the radial side. A dorsal interosseus muscle is inserted into the outer band on each side.*
- *LOOK at the side view of the right middle finger and Figure 6.20b. Work out where the tendons of extensor digitorum, flexor digitorum superficialis and flexor digitorum profundus each insert in the finger.*

Clinical note-pad 6E: Finger deformity

In rheumatoid arthritis

(1) Swan neck deformity. Hyperextension of the PIP joint and flexion of the DIP joint caused by rupture of the tendon of flexor digitorum profundus and the pull of the lumbricals on the outer bands of the extensor expansion.

(2) Trigger finger. A flexor tendon may become trapped at the entrance to its sheath. The cause may be thickening of the tendon sheath, or the swelling and/or nodules around the tendons. The finger lies in flexion and it has to be extended passively by the other hand when it straightens with a snap. The ring and middle fingers are most commonly affected.

Trauma to the finger

(1) Mallet finger due to injury to the outer bands of the extensor expansion proximal to the DIP joint by a ball travelling at speed which hits the tip of the finger. Active extension of the DIP is absent but passive movement is normal.

(2) Button hole deformity is caused by lesion to the middle band of the extensor expansion by a direct cut or burn. The PIP remains flexed by the outer bands of the extensor expansion being drawn forwards until they lie anterior to the fulcrum of the joint and there is no extensor to act upon the joint to extend it.

Repetitive strain injury (RSI)

Also known as cumulative trauma disorder (CTD), this is caused by overuse of the fingers in work such as poultry processing and keyboard operation. The synovial tendon sheaths become thickened and painful. The most usually affected tendons are abductor pollicis longus and extensor pollicis longus and brevis.

6.5 Types of grip

The hand is used in a variety of ways to grasp and hold handles, tools, levers and so on. The different types of grip made by the hand in daily activities involve particular movements at the various joints of the hand, and the combination of activity in muscle groups in the forearm and hand. The ability to grip various objects is an important part of the assessment of the damaged hand.

- *OBSERVE the different ways that people use their hands to grip objects over a whole day, while dressing, cooking, eating, travelling, working and during leisure.*

The type of grip selected depends upon the shape of the object to be grasped, what we want to do with it and the texture of its surface. Naming all the different types of grip is a difficult task when the hand is used in such a wide variety of ways, and individuals approach each method of grasp according to their own style of working.

There are two main types of grip: (a) power grips; and (b) precision grips.

6.5.1 Power grips

In the power grips all the fingers are flexed around an object. The thumb is curled round in the opposite direction to press against, or meet the fingers around the object. All the muscles that close the hand are active. Both the thenar and hypothenar muscles keep the hand in contact with the object grasped.

The hypothenar muscles are important to stabilise the medial side of the palm against a handle, and the muscles of the fingers and the thumb grip the object firmly. The wrist extensors are active to give a stable base for the gripping action, they increase the tension in the long finger flexors and prevent them from acting on the wrist as well. As the hand grips harder, the wrist extensors increase their activity.

The power grips bring the maximum area of sensory surface of the fingers, thumb and palm into contact with the object being grasped, so that feedback from the receptors of the hand ensures that exact pressure and control is being exerted on the handle or tool.

The power grip is the most primitive grasping movement. One of the primary reflexes of the newborn baby is finger flexion in response to touching the palm. By 6 months, the whole hand can form a palmar grasp with the thumb in opposition. Exertion of power by the finger flexors requires the additional group action of the wrist extensors and elbow stability which does not develop until later. By the fifth year the child can grip strongly with each hand individually.

The unique feature of the power grip is to hold an object firmly so that it can be moved by the more proximal joints of the upper limb, such as the shoulder, elbow or radioulnar joints. For example, the hand grasps a door handle, but it is the elbow and shoulder muscles that press it down, and the muscles acting on the radioulnar joints that turn the knob. The hand moulds itself to the shape of the object grasped in the power grip before the power is exerted to move it.

(1) The **cylinder grip** is used for handles that lie at right angles to the forearm, such as a racquet, a jug handle or the hand brake of a car (Fig. 6.21a). The skin of the palmar surface of the fingers and the palm curves round the handle, and the thumb lies in opposition over the finger tips.

Where a tool or object is being used in line with the forearm, such as a hammer, screwdriver or trowel, the fingers flex around the handle in a graded way with maximum degrees of flexion in the little finger and least in the index finger. The thumb either lies over the finger tips or lies along the handle of the tool being grasped. The wrist is ulnar deviated and the maximum area of skin of the palm, thenar and hypothenar eminences is in contact with the handle of the tool. This is a grip giving considerable control, together with powerful manipulation of the tool (Fig. 6.21a).

(2) The **ball grip** encompasses circular knobs, balls and the top of mugs or jam jars (Fig. 6.21b). The fingers and thumb adduct onto the object and sometimes the palm of the hand is not involved.

(3) The **hook grip** is used for carrying a suitcase, bucket or shopping bag by the side of the body with a straight elbow and wrist. Only the flexed fingers are used in this grip, the thumb is not involved (Fig. 6.21c). Following a median nerve lesion (see

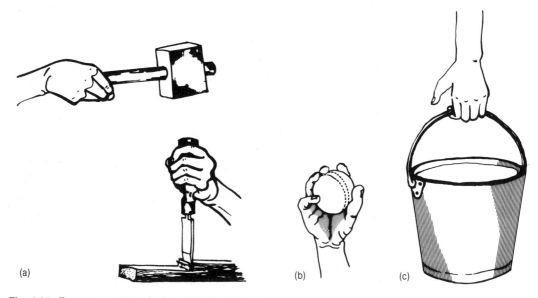

(a) (b) (c)

Fig. 6.21. Power grips: (a) cylinder; (b) ball; (c) hook.

Chapter 7) the thumb cannot be opposed and the hook grip is the only power grip possible.

6.5.2 Precision grips

The hand in the precision grip holds an object between the tips of the thumb and one, two or three fingers, e.g. holding a pencil or small tool. The intrinsic muscles of the hand are now involved, in cooperation with the long flexors and extensors of the digits. The hand is positioned by the wrist and forearm, and the gripping is performed by the muscles acting on the joints of the fingers and thumb.

The precision grip is a more advanced manipulative movement than the power grip, appearing around 9 months of age in child development. Complex integration of the flexor – extensor mechanism of the fingers is essential for grasping a small object and moving it precisely.

The digits have serially arranged joints to perform these manipulative movements. The thumb has three: the first (CMC) carpometacarpal joint; the (MCP) metacarpophalangeal joint; and the interphalangeal (IP) joint. Each finger also has three: the metacarpophalangeal (MCP) joint; the proximal interphalangeal (PIP) joint; and the distal interphalangeal (DIP) joint. It is the variety of movements at all these joints that combine to execute the different precision grips. The lumbrical and interosseus muscles form the balancing forces between the long finger flexors and extensors, and the intrinsic muscles of the thumb bring the pad of the thumb into opposition.

(1) The **plate grip**. The MCP joints of the fingers are flexed with the IP joints extended; the thumb is opposed across the palmar surface of the fingers. The grip is used when holding a plate or other object that needs to be kept horizontal (Fig. 6.22a). An alternative name is the lumbrical grip.

(2) The **pinch grip**. The MCP and PIP joints of the index finger are flexed and the finger meets the opposed thumb. The DIP is pushed into extension in the finger and thumb. The pinch grip may include the middle finger (Fig. 6.22b). This is also known as the pad to pad grip.

(3) The **key grip**. The extended thumb is held on the radial side of the index finger (Fig. 6.22c). This is also known as the lateral grip.

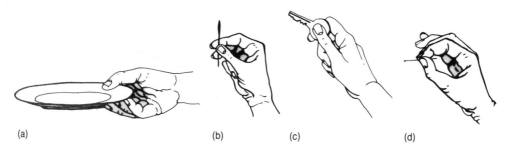

Fig. 6.22. Precision grips: (a) plate; (b) pinch; (c) key; (d) pincer.

(4) The **pincer grip**. All the joints of the index finger are flexed and the finger tip is brought into contact with the tip of the abducted thumb (Fig. 6.22d). The grip may be called the tip to tip grip.

Manipulative movements

The bilateral activity in the two hands working together is an important feature of many manipulative tasks. The two hands may be performing similar movements, as in rolling pastry or pressing the keys of a keyboard. At other times, one hand may provide stability while the other hand makes precise movements, for example in stirring the contents of a saucepan, unscrewing the top of a jar or sewing. The coordination of activity in the two hands is under the control of the nervous system. The hand is represented by large areas in both the somatosensory and the primary motor cortex of the brain. Together with the motor centres of the brain stem and the cerebellum, there is the capacity to develop highly skilled movements in the two hands. For example, complex coordinated activity is required to play many musical instruments (Fig. 6.23).

6.6 Summary of the muscles of the forearm and the intrinsic muscles of the hand

The muscles of the forearm and hand have been described in three functional groups. For revision purposes, the muscles will now be grouped in their anatomical position with notes on common points of origin to assist the learning of the attachments of the individual muscles.

The **forearm muscles** lie in the following positions:

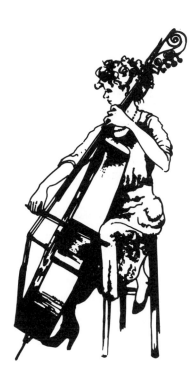

Fig. 6.23. Highly skilled bilateral movements of the hands.

Anterior

(1) Superficial layer: pronator teres, flexor carpi radialis, palmaris longus, flexor carpi ulnaris (common flexor origin is the medial epicondyle of the humerus).

(2) Middle layer: flexor digitorum superficialis.

(3) Deep layer: flexor digitorum profundus, flexor pollicis longus, pronator quadratus.

Posterior

(1) Superficial layer: brachioradialis, extensor carpi radialis longus and brevis, extensor digitorum, extensor digiti minimi, extensor carpi ulnaris, anconeus (common extensor origin is the lateral side of the elbow).

(2) Deep layer: supinator, abductor pollicis longus, extensor pollicis longus and brevis, extensor indicis (origins from the posterior surface of the radius and ulna).

The 12 posterior muscles can be divided into the following.

(1) Three act on elbow and radio-ulnar joints: brachioradialis, supinator and anconeus.

(2) Three act to extend the wrist: extensor carpi ulnaris, extensor carpi radialis longus and brevis.

(3) Three act to extend the fingers: extensor digitorum, extensor indicis and extensor digiti minimi.

(4) Three act on the thumb: extensor pollicis longus and brevis, abductor pollicis longus.

The **intrinsic muscles of the hand** are arranged as follows.

Palmar view

(1) Thenar muscles – bulge of muscles found below the thumb: flexor pollicis brevis, abductor pollicis brevis and opponens pollicis (some include adductor pollicis).

(2) Hypothenar muscles – bulge found below the little finger: flexor digiti minimi, abductor digiti minimi and opponens digiti minimi.

The six thenar and hypothenar muscles all originate on the flexor retinaculum at the base of the hand. The three thenar muscles are the mirror image of the three hypothenar muscles and *vice versa*. The opponens muscles of the two eminences are deep as they are inserted into the metacarpal shafts.

Deep muscles of the palm of the hand

(1) Lumbricals, palmar interossei, dorsal interossei, adductor pollicis.

At the end of this chapter, you should be able to:

(1) List the functions of the hand.

(2) Describe the structure and movements of the joints of the forearm (radioulnar), the wrist (radiocarpal and midcarpal), the fingers and the thumb. Discuss their importance in the use of the hand in daily living.

(3) Describe the position, attachments and actions of the muscles that:
   (a) pronate and supinate the forearm;
   (b) move the wrist in flexion, extension, abduction (radial deviation) and adduction (ulnar deviation);
   (c) open and close the hand; and
   (d) move the thumb and fingers in manipulative and expressive activity.

(4) Describe and give examples of power and precision grips.

7 / The Nerves of the Upper Limb

7.1 Introduction

The lower spinal nerves in the neck (C5, C6, C7, C8, T1) provide the nerve supply to the whole of the upper limb. Movement in the limb as a whole depends on activity in these five spinal nerves which form the roots of the *brachial plexus*. The nerves branch and join in a complex manner as they pass over the first rib and under the clavicle to reach the axilla.

Five terminal branches of the plexus are formed in the axilla. The movements of the upper limb activated by each of the nerves can be summarised as follows.

(1) **Axillary nerve**: shoulder movement.

(2) **Radial nerve**: extensors of the elbow, wrist and fingers.

(3) **Musculocutaneous nerve**: flexors of the elbow.

(4) **Median nerve**: flexors of wrist and fingers, grip of thumb.

(5) **Ulnar nerve**: fine movements of the fingers.

Injury to the brachial plexus in the neck can have a widespread effect on upper limb movements.

In the embryo, as the upper limb grows out from the side of the trunk, the nerve from the central segment, C7, grows down towards the end of the limb (Fig. 7.1a). The spinal nerves from segments C5 and 6 join to form the upper trunk of the plexus and supply the lateral border of the limb. C8 and T1 unite to form the lower trunk and its branches supply the medial border of the limb. The dermatomes lie in order down the lateral side of the limb, across the hand and up the medial side (Fig. 7.1b).

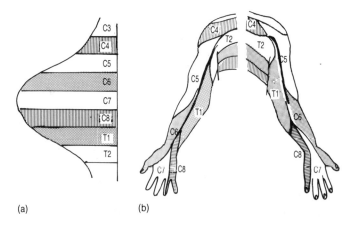

Fig. 7.1. Distribution of spinal segments C5 to T1 to the skin of the upper limb: (a) limb bud in the embryo; (b) anterior and posterior views of dermatomes in the adult.

(a)   (b)

176

In general, the nerves supplying the muscles of the shoulder originate from the upper segments (C5 and 6), and those concerned with movements of the fingers are derived from the lower segments (C8 and T1).

7.2 The brachial plexus (Fig. 7.2)

The *roots* of the brachial plexus are the anterior primary rami of the spinal nerves C5, 6, 7, 8 and T1.

The three *trunks*, formed by joining of the upper two and lower two roots pass downwards and laterally between two muscles of the neck – the scalenus anterior and medius. The trunks meet the axillary artery and continue with it behind the clavicle. Each trunk then divides into anterior and posterior *divisions* – the posterior divisions forming the nerves to the posterior muscles of the limb, and the anterior divisions forming the nerves to the anterior muscles. The six divisions formed in this way continue through the axilla, then combine to form three cords.

The three *cords* lie just behind the pectoralis minor muscle (Fig. 5.10) and take their name from their relationship with the axillary artery. The three *cords* are formed in the following way: Three posterior divisions combine to form the posterior cord. Two anterior divisions from the upper and middle trunks form the lateral cord. One anterior division of the lower trunk becomes the medial cord.

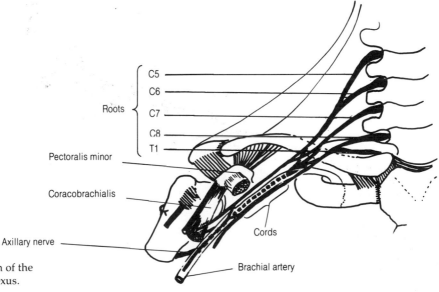

Fig. 7.2. Position of the right brachial plexus.

The cords lie in the axilla close to the axillary artery, which forms the blood supply to the upper limb. At the lower part of the axilla, the cords split into the named nerves which enter the arm.

The **posterior cord** represents the *extensor* nerve of the upper limb.

The **medial** and **lateral cords** represent the *flexor* nerves of the limb.

- *LOOK at the articulated skeleton to identify the exact position of the brachial plexus, starting at the cervical vertebrae, passing over the first rib under the clavicle, to the axillary region below the shoulder joint.*
- *STUDY the plan of the brachial plexus shown in Figure 7.3 to see the arrangement of the roots, trunks, divisions and cords.*
- *IDENTIFY: (a) the branches leaving the plexus which supply most of the muscles of the shoulder region; and (b) the terminal branches that enter the arm.*

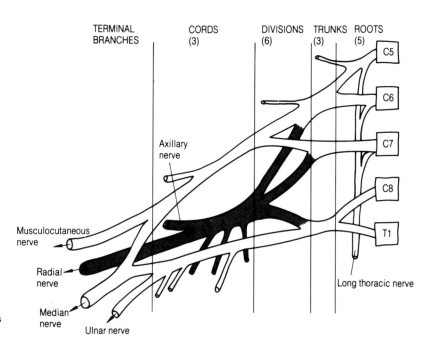

Fig. 7.3. Plan of the brachial plexus and its main branches.

> ### Clinical note-pad 7A: Brachial plexus lesions
>
> The brachial plexus may be damaged in a variety of ways.
>
> (1) At birth.
>
> (2) By traction injuries to the neck.
>
> (3) By traction on the outstretched hand.
>
> (4) Through compression in the axilla. For example in 'Saturday night palsy' when a person goes to sleep in an armchair with the arms hanging over the edge of the chair. Compression from a tight haversack can give a similar effect to that of ulnar nerve damage (see clinical note-pad 7E).
>
> The resulting loss of function is variable. The upper roots C5 and 6 may be damaged in 1, 2 or 3, when there is loss of function in the abductors and flexors of the shoulder, and flexors and extensors of the elbow. The arm cannot be lifted from the side, and hangs in a position of adduction, medial rotation, pronation and finger flexion – waiter's tip position, known as Erb's paralysis.
>
> Damage to the lower roots produces weakness of the intrinsic muscles of the hand, especially on the medial side, which is the ulnar or 'power' side. This is known as Klumpke's paralysis.

7.3 Terminal branches of the brachial plexus

Five terminal branches are formed from the three cords in the axilla and enter the arm. One of the branches can be considered as two parts, one from each of the lateral and medial cords. Then each of the cords has two terminal branches.

The **posterior cord** forms the *radial* and *axillary nerves*.

The **medial cord** forms the *ulnar* and medial half of the *median nerve*.

The **lateral cord** forms the *musculocutaneous* and lateral half of the *median nerve*.

● *Trace from the roots to the formation of the five nerves in Figure 7.3.*

Note: the ulnar nerve originates from the lower roots of the plexus. The radial nerve has fibres from all the roots.

7.3.1 Shoulder movement – the axillary nerve

The **axillary** nerve, a branch of the posterior cord, is important in all movements that lift the arm from the side, since it supplies the deltoid muscle and teres minor (Fig. 7.4). From the posterior

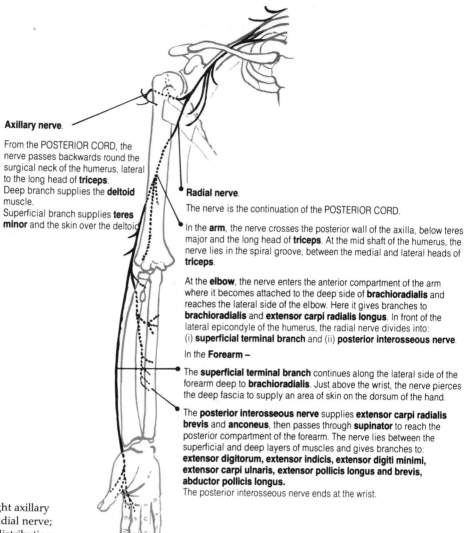

Axillary nerve.

From the POSTERIOR CORD, the nerve passes backwards round the surgical neck of the humerus, lateral to the long head of **triceps**.
Deep branch supplies the **deltoid** muscle.
Superficial branch supplies **teres minor** and the skin over the deltoid

Radial nerve.
The nerve is the continuation of the POSTERIOR CORD.

In the **arm**, the nerve crosses the posterior wall of the axilla, below teres major and the long head of **triceps**. At the mid shaft of the humerus, the nerve lies in the spiral groove, between the medial and lateral heads of **triceps**.

At the **elbow**, the nerve enters the anterior compartment of the arm where it becomes attached to the deep side of **brachioradialis** and reaches the lateral side of the elbow. Here it gives branches to **brachioradialis** and **extensor carpi radialis longus**. In front of the lateral epicondyle of the humerus, the radial nerve divides into:
(i) **superficial terminal branch** and (ii) **posterior interosseous nerve**.

In the **Forearm** –

The **superficial terminal branch** continues along the lateral side of the forearm deep to **brachioradialis**. Just above the wrist, the nerve pierces the deep fascia to supply an area of skin on the dorsum of the hand.

The **posterior interosseous nerve** supplies **extensor carpi radialis brevis** and **anconeus**, then passes through **supinator** to reach the posterior compartment of the forearm. The nerve lies between the superficial and deep layers of muscles and gives branches to: **extensor digitorum, extensor indicis, extensor digiti minimi, extensor carpi ulnaris, extensor pollicis longus and brevis, abductor pollicis longus**.
The posterior interosseous nerve ends at the wrist.

Fig. 7.4. Right axillary nerve and radial nerve; course and distribution, anterior view.

cord, the axillary nerve branches backwards under the capsule of the shoulder joint, and winds round the surgical neck of the humerus to supply the whole of the deltoid muscle. A branch to teres minor continues as a cutaneous nerve supplying the skin over the deltoid muscle.

The other muscles moving the shoulder are mainly supplied by branches of the roots, the upper trunk and the three cords (see Section 7.4).

Clinical note-pad 7B: Axillary nerve lesion

Fracture of the neck of the humerus or subluxation of the shoulder joint may damage the axillary nerve. The resulting loss of function is the inability to make movements that lift the arm away from the body.

7.3.2 Extensor nerve of the upper limb – the radial nerve

The radial nerve is the largest branch of the brachial plexus, formed as the continuation of the posterior cord (Fig. 7.4). In the arm, the radial nerve supplies the whole of the triceps muscle. The nerve is essential for extension movement of the elbow, since the triceps is the only muscle capable of this movement with any power (see Chapter 5).

In front of the lateral epicondyle of the humerus at the elbow, the nerve divides into two.

The *superficial terminal branch* continues along the lateral side of the forearm under the brachioradialis. Just above the wrist, the nerve pierces the deep fascia to supply a variable area of skin over the dorsal surface of the hand on the thumb side (Fig. 7.5).

The *posterior interosseous nerve* supplies the extensor muscles in the forearm, ending at the wrist, where it supplies all the joints of the wrist.

Note: the radial nerve as a whole supplies all the *extensor muscles* of the upper limb, but does not supply the intrinsic muscles of the hand that insert into the dorsal digital expansion of the fingers.

Extension of the wrist is important in maintaining the functional position of the hand (Fig. 7.6a) for all movements of the fingers and thumb.

Fig. 7.5. The right hand. Areas of skin supplied by the radial, median and ulnar nerves: (a) palmar; (b) dorsal.

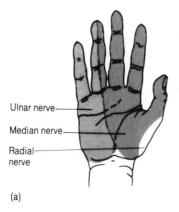
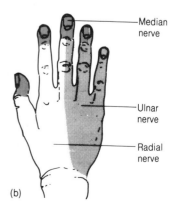

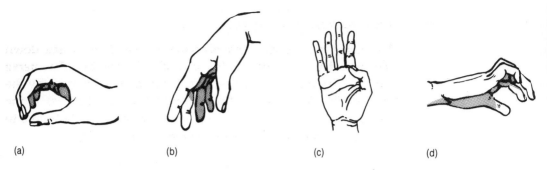

(a)   (b)   (c)   (d)

Fig. 7.6. Positions of the right hand: (a) functional position of the normal hand; and after damage to (b) the radial nerve – 'wrist drop'; (c) the median nerve – 'ape hand'; (d) the ulnar nerve – 'claw hand'.

Clinical note-pad 7C: Radial nerve lesion

Injuries to the radial nerve most commonly occur as a complication of the fracture of the **midshaft of humerus** where the radial nerve lies in the radial groove (Fig. 7.4). This injury results in 'wrist drop' (Fig. 7.6b); the hand cannot be lifted against gravity and the power grip is weak. There is weakness which leads to inability to reach up to a high shelf or to push against a resistance, e.g. a door.

Injury at the **elbow**, which may occur as a complication of supracondylar fracture of the humerus, gives weakness of extension of the fingers and the thumb, particularly at the MCP joints.

Injury at the **wrist**, due to laceration or burns, only results in a small area of sensory loss on the dorsum of the hand over the first dorsal interosseus muscle.

- *WATCH the hand and forearm of a partner doing daily activities such as making a cup of tea and eating with a knife and fork. Note the position of the wrist during the movements. If the wrist could not be held in extension, the hand would drop under its own weight and the weight of any object held in it.*

7.3.3 Flexor nerves of the upper limb – the musculocutaneous and median nerves

There are two terminal branches of the lateral cord of the brachial plexus that are important for flexion movements of the upper limb. The *musculocutaneous nerve* supplies the elbow flexors; and the *median nerve* supplies the wrist, fingers and thumb flexors, working in cooperation with the ulnar nerve.

The musculocutaneous nerve

The nerve pierces the coracobrachialis, and then passes down the arm between the biceps and the brachialis. The nerve supplies these three muscles, which can be remembered by the initials BBC. At the elbow, the nerve becomes cutaneous at the lateral side of the tendon of the biceps, to become the nerve to the skin on the lateral side of the forearm (Fig. 7.7).

The median nerve

This is formed from the lateral and medial cords of the brachial plexus. The course and distribution of the median nerve can be seen in Figure 7.8. There are no branches of the median nerve

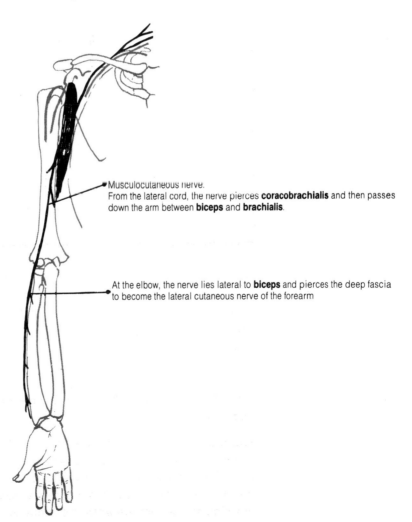

Musculocutaneous nerve.
From the lateral cord, the nerve pierces **coracobrachialis** and then passes down the arm between **biceps** and **brachialis**.

At the elbow, the nerve lies lateral to **biceps** and pierces the deep fascia to become the lateral cutaneous nerve of the forearm

Fig. 7.7. Right musculocutaneous nerve; course and distribution, anterior view.

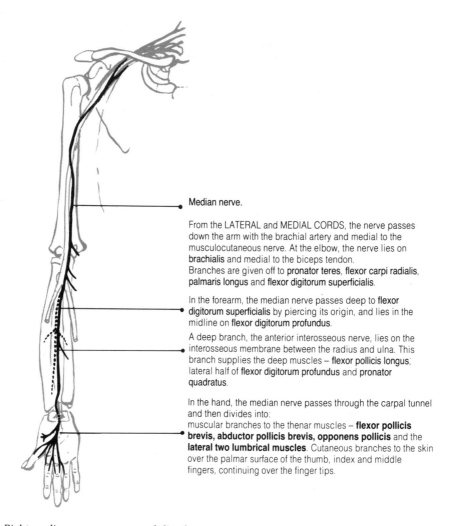

Median nerve.

From the LATERAL and MEDIAL CORDS, the nerve passes down the arm with the brachial artery and medial to the musculocutaneous nerve. At the elbow, the nerve lies on **brachialis** and medial to the biceps tendon.
Branches are given off to **pronator teres, flexor carpi radialis, palmaris longus** and **flexor digitorum superficialis.**

In the forearm, the median nerve passes deep to **flexor digitorum superficialis** by piercing its origin, and lies in the midline on **flexor digitorum profundus.**

A deep branch, the anterior interosseous nerve, lies on the interosseous membrane between the radius and ulna. This branch supplies the deep muscles – **flexor pollicis longus**; lateral half of **flexor digitorum profundus** and **pronator quadratus.**

In the hand, the median nerve passes through the carpal tunnel and then divides into:
muscular branches to the thenar muscles – **flexor pollicis brevis, abductor pollicis brevis, opponens pollicis** and the **lateral two lumbrical muscles**. Cutaneous branches to the skin over the palmar surface of the thumb, index and middle fingers, continuing over the finger tips.

Fig. 7.8. Right median nerve; course and distribution, anterior view.

in the arm; it is a nerve of the forearm and hand only. A communicating branch with the musculocutaneous nerve in the arm is present in some individuals.

At the *elbow*, the median nerve lies anteriorly and medial to the tendon of the biceps.

In the *forearm*, branches are given off to four of the muscles attached to the medial epicondyle of the humerus. A deep branch is given off, the *anterior interosseus nerve*, which lies on the interosseous membrane between the radius and ulna, and supplies the three muscles of the deep layer.

Note: the median nerve supplies all the flexors in the forearm except flexor carpi ulnaris and the medial half of flexor digitorum profundus (to the ring and little fingers).

The median nerve enters the *hand* in the midline, passing underneath the flexor retinaculum, i.e. through the carpal tunnel and lying on top of the synovial sheath containing the eight long finger flexors (see Chapter 6, Fig. 6.15). In the hand there are two main branches: (a) to the three thenar muscles and first two lumbricals; and (b) a cutaneous branch to the skin over the palmar surface of the thumb, index and middle fingers, continuing over the finger tips to the dorsal side (Fig. 7.5).

Clinical note-pad 7D: Median nerve lesion

The appearance of the hand in median nerve lesions is often called ape or monkey hand. The thenar eminence is wasted and the thumb is drawn backwards in line with the fingers, due to unopposed action of the extensor pollicis longus (Fig. 7.6c). The loss of function of the lateral two lumbricals leads to flattening of the lateral side of the palm; the MCP joints are drawn into extension and the IP joints into slight flexion.

The most usual site of damage is at the **wrist**. Then the thumb is unable to oppose, and this, together with the loss of sensation from the finger tips, makes many gripping movements difficult. If the nerve is damaged at the **elbow**, there is added loss of finger flexion, particularly the index and middle fingers, which also affects gripping. It is the precision grips that are most affected by median nerve damage.

In carpal tunnel syndrome, the median nerve is compressed in the carpal tunnel at the wrist by increase in pressure from the swelling of flexor tendon sheaths or carpal joints. It can be very painful, and the loss of sensation and muscle weakness leads to clumsiness and 'dropping things'.

- *PULL your THUMB back and to the side of the palm of your dominant hand by winding a bandage round the wrist and round the thumb. Now try to use your hand in everyday activities to experience the problems when the thumb cannot be opposed to the fingers.*
- *WEAR a thin plastic glove with the ring and little fingers cut away on your dominant hand during hand activities. You will then experience the effects of loss of skin sensation in median nerve injury.*

7.3.4 Fine movements of the fingers – the ulnar (and median) nerve

The *ulnar nerve*, is a continuation of the medial cord of the brachial plexus. Figure 7.9 shows the course and distribution of the ulnar nerve.

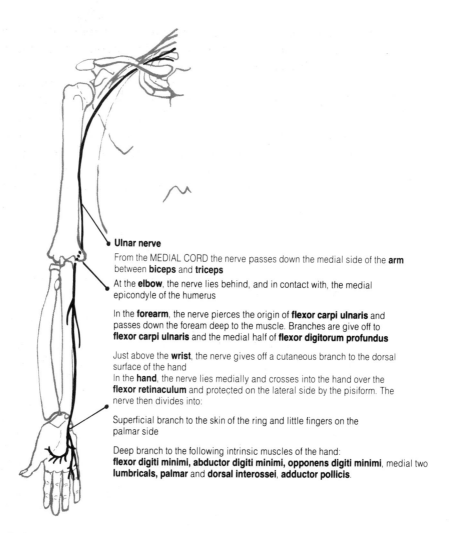

Ulnar nerve

From the MEDIAL CORD the nerve passes down the medial side of the **arm** between **biceps** and **triceps**

At the **elbow**, the nerve lies behind, and in contact with, the medial epicondyle of the humerus

In the **forearm**, the nerve pierces the origin of **flexor carpi ulnaris** and passes down the foream deep to the muscle. Branches are give off to **flexor carpi ulnaris** and the medial half of **flexor digitorum profundus**

Just above the **wrist**, the nerve gives off a cutaneous branch to the dorsal surface of the hand
In the **hand**, the nerve lies medially and crosses into the hand over the **flexor retinaculum** and protected on the lateral side by the pisiform. The nerve then divides into:

Superficial branch to the skin of the ring and little fingers on the palmar side

Deep branch to the following intrinsic muscles of the hand:
flexor digiti minimi, abductor digiti minimi, opponens digiti minimi, medial two **lumbricals, palmar** and **dorsal interossei, adductor pollicis**.

Fig. 7.9. Right ulnar nerve; course and distribution, anterior view.

There are no branches of the ulnar nerve in the arm. The course of the nerve in the forearm and hand is apparent when the inside of the elbow is bumped. 'Banging the funny bone' gives a tingling sensation down the inside of the forearm and on to the little finger.

In the *forearm*, the ulnar nerve supplies the one and a half muscles not supplied by the median nerve.

At the *wrist*, the nerve lies medially and passes over the flexor retinaculum. Two cutaneous nerves are given off at, or above, the wrist to supply the skin over the palmar and dorsal sides of the hand medially, and the ring and little fingers (Fig. 7.5).

The terminal branches in the *hand* supply all the intrinsic muscles not supplied by the median nerve, which includes all the muscles moving the ring and little fingers.

The ulnar nerve is important for keyboard operators, musicians and all those who need fine coordinated movements of the fingers. The grips particularly dependent on the ulnar nerve are the *power grip* for stabilising the medial side of the hand, and the *span grip* when the fingers must be separated to spread over a large object. Because of the importance of sensory feedback in all movements of the hand, both power and precision, the median and the ulnar nerves are codependent in all hand function.

Clinical note-pad 7E: Ulnar nerve lesion

The ulnar nerve is most frequently damaged when the hand is put through glass, as when falling through a window. The ulnar nerve is in a vulnerable position when the hand is put out as the body falls. The appearance of the hand in ulnar nerve lesion is known as 'claw hand' (Fig. 7.6d). The ring and little fingers curl in a flexion deformity, with hyperextension at the MCP joints, due to paralysis of the medial two lumbricals. Loss of the dorsal interossei means that the fingers cannot be separated. The web between the thumb and index finger, formed by the adductor pollicis and the first dorsal interosseous muscle, is wasted. The loss of thumb opposition in median nerve damage can sometimes be compensated for by use of the adductor pollicis, if the ulnar nerve is intact.

The ulnar and median nerves may be damaged together in severe laceration of the wrist. The result is impairment of total hand function, with loss of all grips.

- *REVISE the intrinsic muscles of the hand from Chapter 6.*
- *LIST all the muscles and their nerve supply.*

7.4 Outline of the direct branches from the brachial plexus

The five terminal branches of the brachial plexus supply all the muscles moving the elbow, forearm, wrist and hand. The deltoid and teres minor are supplied by the axillary nerve, but the other muscles moving the shoulder region receive branches direct from the plexus.

Return to Figure 7.3 to identify the branches direct from the plexus.

(1) Branches from the **roots** of the plexus are:
 (a) C5 supplies the levator scapulae, the rhomboids and the subclavius; and
 (b) C5, C6 and C7 form the *long thoracic nerve* to the serratus anterior on the floor of the axilla.

(2) One branch from **upper trunk** C5 and C6:
The *suprascapular nerve* leaves the upper trunk and passes over the upper border of the scapula at the suprascapular notch to reach the supraspinous fossa. The two posterior rotator cuff muscles, the supraspinatus and infraspinatus, are supplied by this branch.

(3) Branches from the **cords**:
 (a) The **posterior cord** has three branches that supply the muscles of the posterior wall of the axilla – the subscapularis, the teres major and the latissimus dorsi.
 (b) The **lateral cord** gives a branch to the muscle of the anterior wall of the axilla – the pectoralis major.
 (c) The **medial cord** has three branches. Two form separate cutaneous nerves to the skin on the medial side of the arm and forearm. The third branch supplies the pectoralis minor and the lower fibres of the pectoralis major.

The trapezius is the only muscle attached to the scapula that is not supplied by a branch of the brachial plexus. The spinal root of the *spinal accessory nerve* (cranial nerve XI) branches to the anterior of the trapezius.

At the end of this chapter, you should be able to:

(1) Outline the position and arrangement of the roots, trunks, divisions and cords of the brachial plexus.

(2) Describe the course, distribution and functional importance of the *five* terminal branches of the brachial plexus: the axillary, radial, musculocutaneous, median, ulnar and radial nerves.

(3) Outline the effects of injury to the nerves listed in (2).

8 / Support and Propulsion: The Lower Limb

8.1 Functions of the lower limb

The lower limbs are the supporting pillars when we stand. A pillar must have strength and must not collapse under the weight above. The bones, joints and muscles together convert the lower limb into a stable support. The pillar is divided into segments, the thigh, leg and foot. The segments are linked by joints, the hip, knee, ankle and joints of the foot, which can adjust to the changes that occur in the line of weight through the limbs as the head and trunk move above. The muscles around the joints counteract the effects of gravity and any external forces that disturb the balance of the body.

Daily activities such as getting out of bed, sitting down on a chair, getting up from a chair, using the toilet, all involve the lower limb. Weakness of muscles or loss of joint mobility make these transfer activities difficult and the upper limb then has to compensate. (This is discussed in Chapter 5.)

The sole of the foot is the contact area of the lower limb with the ground, and plays an important role in sensing the texture and friction properties of the supporting surface. Feedback from receptors in the skin and muscles of the sole of the foot is essential for an economical pattern of locomotion. The absence of this sensory information results in an abnormal gait.

The overall functions of the lower limb, in summary, are as follows.

(1) Support in standing.

(2) Swing and support in locomotion.

(3) Transfer of the body from lying to sitting, to standing.

(4) Provision of sensory information from supporting surfaces.

The muscles of the lower limb are as active in stabilising the joints and converting the limb into a lively pillar of support, as they are in producing movement of the limb. The attachments of the muscles are often anchored in sheets of dense fibrous tissue. An example of this fibrous tissue is the fascia on the lateral side of the thigh, known as the iliotibial tract, which passes over the hip and the knee. Two muscles keep the hip and knee extended by producing tension in the iliotibial tract. Other muscles are attached to bony points and make precise movements, e.g. the calf muscles pull on the heel to raise the foot on to the toes.

Locomotor movements require one limb to support the body weight while the other limb swings forward. In walking, running and climbing stairs, the lower limb has to keep its function as a support and also propel the body forwards or upwards. As we walk, the alternation of swing and support means that the limb as a whole must combine strength with mobility, and change its role every second. The lower limb acts as a unit. This is different from the upper limb, where the shoulder is concerned with mobility, and the elbow and wrist with stability for movements of the hand.

In this chapter, the muscles of the lower limb will be described in relation to three functions in locomotion: (a) support in standing upright; (b) swing, when one limb is free while the opposite limb is in support; and (c) propulsion to move the body forwards and/or upwards.

8.2 Movements of the lower limb

The joints of the lower limb combine to give stability for the support of the body weight, and adequate range of movement for the limb as a whole. These joints are the hip, the knee, the ankle and two main joints in the foot, the subtalar and mid-tarsal joints.

The *hip joint* is a stable ball and socket joint, whose articulating surfaces fit closely, and the capsule is strengthened by ligaments on all sides. The *knee* is a modified hinge joint allowing movement in the sagittal plane with some rotation in full flexion and at the end of extension. The *ankle* is a true hinge joint, with collateral ligaments and no lateral or rotatory movement. The joints of the foot allow the sole to turn inwards and outward, by movement at the joints between the bones of the foot – the *subtalar* and *mid-tarsal joints* in particular.

- *LOOK at the movements of the major joints of the lower limb, and contrast them with the upper limb joints. Note any difference in the range of movement between the hip and the shoulder, the knee and the elbow, the ankle and the wrist, the toes and the fingers.*

8.2.1 The hip joint

The hip joint, like the glenohumeral joint at the shoulder, is a ball and socket type, but there the similarities end. The shoulder joint is designed for mobility, but the hip joint has to fulfil two functions, that of mobility and stability. The socket of the hip joint is formed by the acetabulum, a name which means 'little vinegar cup'. The acetabulum lies at the side of the pelvis and is

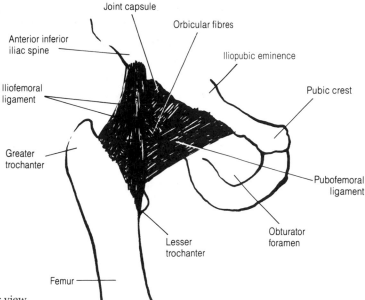

Joint capsule

Orbicular fibres

Anterior inferior
iliac spine

Iliopubic eminence

Iliofemoral
ligament

Pubic crest

Greater
trochanter

Pubofemoral
ligament

Lesser
trochanter

Obturator
foramen

Femur

Fig. 8.1. Right hip joint, anterior view.

a deep, outwards facing cup surrounded by a rim of fibrocartilage, known as a labrum. The head of the femur forms the ball which is two-thirds of a sphere. When the ball is in the socket, the labrum curves inwards beyond the equator of the head of the femur to grip it and help to hold it in place.

The hip joint has a strong capsule that includes most of the femoral neck. The capsule is further strengthened by very strong ligaments anteriorly, and by small half rotator cuff muscles posteriorly. The iliofemoral ligament is the strongest in the body, it is 'Y' shaped, passing across the front of the joint (Fig. 8.1). This ligament limits the range of extension of the hip and therefore can be used to support the trunk on the lower limb, see Section 8.3.1. Stability is also assisted by circular fibres within the capsule, called the orbicular fibres, which give the capsule a 'waist', so increasing the suction effect of the cup on the head of the femur (Fig. 8.1).

The *movements* of the hip joint are: flexion, extension, abduction, adduction, and medial and lateral rotation.

> ### Clinical note-pad 8A: Fracture of the neck of the femur
>
> This is usually due to a fall, particularly in the elderly, when osteoporosis has weakened the bone by withdrawal of calcium. This fracture can interrupt the main blood supply to the head of the femur and the bone fails to unite. The fracture is usually reduced by inserting a dynamic screw, or by replacement of the head with an artificial one (arthroplasty).
>
> Hip arthroplasty is also used in osteoarthritis.

8.2.2 The knee joint

The rounded condyles of the femur articulate with the shallow saucer shaped condyles of the tibia. Note that the fibula is not included in the joint. A fibrocartilaginous semicircular disc, known as a meniscus, lies on each of the tibial condyles (Fig. 8.2a). The menisci have four important functions within the knee: (a) to increase congruence between the femur and the tibia; (b) to act as shock absorbers as the body weight falls on to the tibial plateau; (c) to assist in weight bearing across the joint; and (d) to aid lubrication by the circulation of synovial fluid within the knee joint.

The knee joint has strong collateral ligaments, and an oblique ligament that passes posteriorly across the joint. The medial collateral ligament is a broad band whose posterior margin is attached to the medial meniscus. The lateral collateral ligament is a round cord which is mobile and not attached to the capsule or the lateral meniscus. Anteriorly, the knee joint is strengthened by the tendon of the quadriceps muscle (see Section 8.5) as it passes over the patella to be inserted into the anterior tubercle of the tibia (Fig. 8.2b).

- *FEEL the front of the knee joint and locate the patella. Three fingers breadth below the lower border of the patella you will feel a large lump. This is the anterior tubercle of the tibia where the quadriceps is inserted.*

Within the knee joint, there are two further very important ligaments. These are attached to the centre of the tibial plateau and pass upwards to attach within the intercondylar notch of the femur (Appendix 1). They appear to cross one another and so they are called the cruciate ligaments (Fig. 8.2a). The position of the cruciate ligaments in the centre of the joint means that they prevent the femur rolling off the tibia. The cruciate ligaments also form a fulcrum for the 'locking action' of the knee

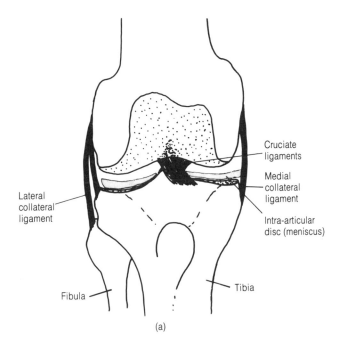

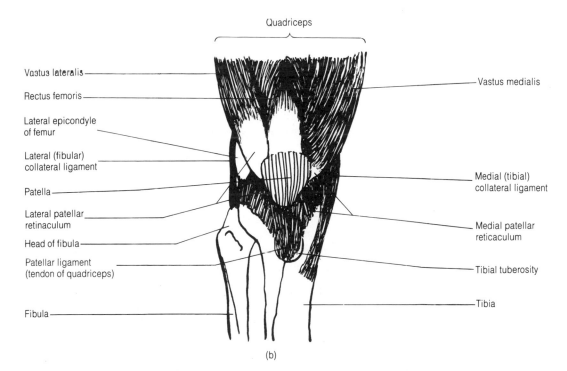

Fig. 8.2. Right knee joint, anterior view: (a) capsule and muscle removed; (b) showing the patella and quadriceps tendon.

which occurs when the femur rotates slightly medially at the end of full extension.

- *STAND upright and extend the knees as far as possible in 'standing to attention'. Note how the femur rotates medially at the end of the movement.*

   SIT and extend the knee with the leg off the ground. Note how the tibia rotates laterally at the end of the movement turning the toes to point laterally. Both these movements demonstrate the 'locking action' of the knee.

The *movements* of the knee joint are flexion and extension with some rotation in full flexion and at the end of extension.

Clinical note-pad 8B: Meniscal and ligament injuries of the knee

Twisting injuries of the knee occur in sport, particularly football. The following damage may occur.

   The medial meniscus tears and splits in its length. The torn portion sometimes becomes displaced and lodged between the femur and the tibia.

   The medial ligament is most commonly torn, and in severe cases the anterior cruciate ligament is involved as the tibia rotates laterally. Less commonly, the lateral ligament is torn, and the posterior cruciate ligament tears when the tibia is forced backwards in relation to the femur.

   There may be spontaneous healing of the collateral ligaments, but torn cruciates are more serious.

8.2.3 The ankle joint

The articular surfaces of the ankle joint are the upper surface of the talus bone of the foot and the inferior surface of the tibia. The weight bearing surfaces are the curved trochlear of the talus and the reciprocal shallow notch of the tibia. Stabilising surfaces are the medial malleolus of the tibia and the lateral malleolus of the fibula, which provide a firm grip on the sides of the talus, creating a bony mortice and tenon joint.

   The medial collateral ligament (also known as the deltoid ligament) is very strong and fan shaped (Fig. 8.3a). Its attachment to the navicular bone of the foot makes it an important support mechanism for the medial arch of the foot (see Section 8.6.3). The lateral ligament has three bands binding the lower end of the fibula to the talus and the calcaneum (Fig. 8.3b).

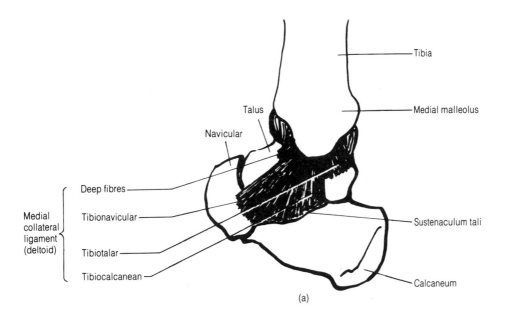

(a)

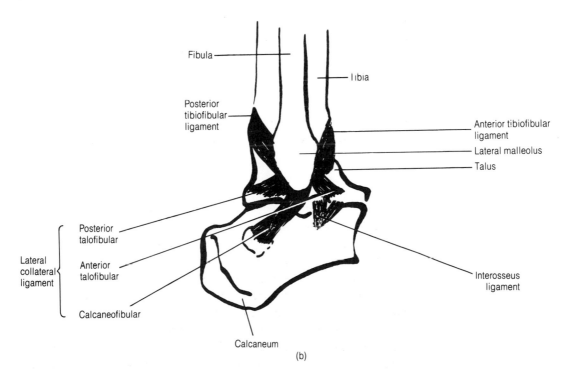

(b)

Fig. 8.3. Right ankle joint: (a) medial aspect; (b) lateral aspect.

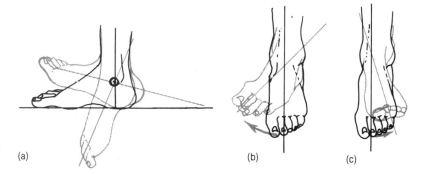

Fig. 8.4. Movements at the ankle and foot: (a) dorsiflexion and plantar flexion; (b) inversion; (c) eversion.

The ankle joint is a true hinge joint and the *movements* are in the sagittal plane only, known as dorsiflexion and plantar flexion. The neutral position of the ankle joint is the position of the foot in the normal standing position, when the foot makes a right angle with the leg. In *dorsiflexion* the foot is drawn upwards towards the leg. In *plantar flexion* the movement is in the opposite direction from the neutral position (Fig. 8.4a).

- *SIT with the foot off the ground. Start with the foot at right angles to the leg. MOVE the ankle through dorsiflexion (toes up), and then plantar flexion (toes down).*
- *STAND upright and lift the body up onto the toes. Note how this is a plantar flexion movement at the ankle.*

Clinical note-pad 8C: Ankle injuries

In injury to the ankle, the foot is usually twisted and turns inwards, which tears the calcaneofibular component of the lateral ligament (Fig. 8.3b). More severe injury causes a fracture of the fibula (Pott's fracture) when the lateral malleolus is pushed off the talus. In some cases both malleoli are fractured.

8.2.4 Joints of the foot

A concave facet on the undersurface of the talus articulates with a convex surface on the upper surface of the calcaneum to form the *subtalar joint*. Strong ligaments unite the bones, particularly an interosseous ligament which acts as a fulcrum for movements of the foot on the leg.

The *mid-tarsal joint* is formed by the articulation between the talus and the navicular, together with that between the calcaneum and the cuboid, extending from one side of the foot to the other. These two articulations combine in the movements of the foot.

The *movements* of the foot are known as inversion and eversion (Fig. 8.4b and c). In inversion, the foot turns so that the sole faces inwards, the medial border is raised and the lateral border is depressed. In eversion, the opposite movement occurs and the sole faces outwards. Most of the movement occurs at the mid-tarsal joint. Some adduction accompanies inversion, and some abduction accompanies eversion. It is easy to notice these movements of the foot in dancing and gymnastics, but inversion and eversion are very important when putting the foot down on sloping ground or on an irregular surface (see Section 8.6.2).

- *REMEMBER how difficult it is to walk on loose shingle, a rocky hillside or down the aisle of a moving train.*

8.3 Support

8.3.1 Double support and change to single support

There is a remarkable economy of muscle activity involved in standing upright on two legs. The joints of the lower limb are in a close packed position when standing, and stability depends largely on the tension of the ligaments around the joints. Two particular structures are important.

(1) The anterior ligament of the hip joint, the *iliofemoral ligament* (Fig. 8.1), is important in resisting the tendency for the trunk to fall backwards on the lower limbs when the line of the body weight falls behind the hip joint. Little activity is required in the hip flexors and extensors. The paraplegic with paralysed hip muscles learns to place the hips well in front of the line of gravity and relies entirely on the tension in the iliofemoral ligament for stability at the hips in standing (Fig. 8.5a).

(2) The **iliotibial tract** (also known as the fascia lata) is a band of dense fascia which extends across the hip and knee on the lateral side of the thigh. In standing, the tension in a small muscle, known as the *tensor fascia lata*, which originates on the anterior superior spine of the ilium and inserts into the iliotibial tract, keeps the hip and knee extended, with the help of the *gluteus maximus*, the large superficial muscle of the buttock (Fig. 8.5b).

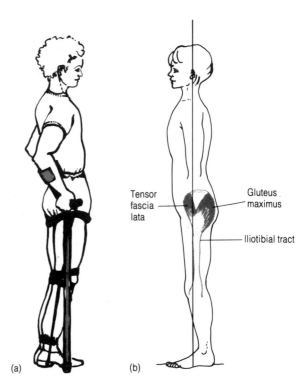

Fig. 8.5. Upright standing viewed from the side: (a) paraplegic standing; (b) iliotibial tract in double support.

The line of body weight lies in front of the ankle joints, so that some activity in the calf muscles is needed to keep balance over the foot base.

(The gluteus maximus and the calf muscles will be described in detail in Section 8.5.)

We rarely stand to attention like the guardsmen on parade, but adopt changing positions of 'slack standing' with the knees slightly flexed and the weight shifting from one leg to the other.

- *WATCH people standing at a bus stop, queueing for tickets at a station, or talking in groups. Note the variety of lower limb positions. Shop assistants, teachers, nurses and surgeons spend long periods of time standing. The constant shifting of position reduces fatigue in any one muscle group, and also aids the return of blood to the heart by the pumping action of leg muscles.*

The change from standing on two legs to standing on one, is the first stage in beginning to propel the body forwards. When one leg is lifted from the ground, muscles around the hip of the supporting leg are active to: (a) move the body weight over the

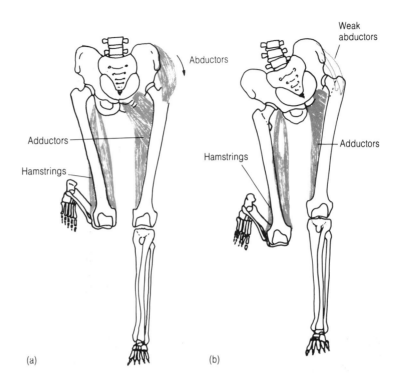

Fig. 8.6. Single support: (a) action of the hip abductors and adductors to keep the pelvis level; (b) Trendelenburg's sign.

supporting leg; and (b) prevent the pelvis from dropping on the unsupported side.

The **adductor** group of muscles on the inside of the thigh contract to shift the pelvis over the supporting side. At the same time, the tendency for the pelvis to drop is counteracted by activity in the **abductors** of the hip in the supporting leg. Figure 8.6a shows the position of the abductors and adductors in the supporting leg. You should be able to see how contraction of the abductors will pull on the pelvis and keep it level. Further tilt of the pelvis gives added clearance for the raised foot.

8.3.2 Muscles of the hip in single support

Abductors of the hip

The abductors of the hip are the *gluteus medius* and *gluteus minimus*.

These two fan shaped muscles lie deep to the gluteus maximus, the largest muscle of the buttock. Gluteus medius and minimus originate from the outer surface of the ilium, and both muscles insert into the greater trochanter of the femur (Fig. 8.7).

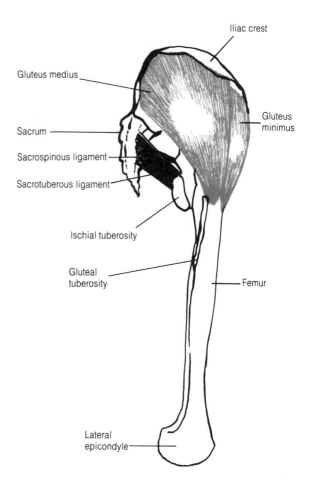

Fig. 8.7. Gluteus medius and minimus, seen in the lateral view of the right pelvis and femur.

When the leg is not acting as a support, the abductors lift the leg sideways.

- *STAND some distance from a long mirror, and take a few steps slowly. Note: if the right leg is off the ground, the right side of the pelvis is unsupported and could drop to the right, and so the left abductors must contract. For the next step, the opposite abductor muscles contract. (There is also a muscle of the trunk involved, quadratus lumborum, and this will be described in Chapter 10.)*

The changes in hip position with each step can be seen if you walk behind someone wearing tight jeans. Notice how the sway varies in different people, at different speeds of walking, and with mood.

Clinical note-pad 8D: Trendelenburg's sign

Problems of the hip, e.g. congenital dislocation, fracture of the neck of the femur, or paralysis of hip abductors, produce an abnormal pattern of walking. The hip drops to the opposite side when weight is taken on the affected hip; this is known as *Trendelenburg's sign* (Fig. 8.6b).

Adductors of the hip

These are a group of five muscles lying on the inner side of the thigh (Fig. 8.8). In the various positions of the hip joint, the individual muscles of the adductor group can act as flexors, extensors and rotators. Strong adduction of the thigh is not very significant to everyday activities except when riding a bicycle or

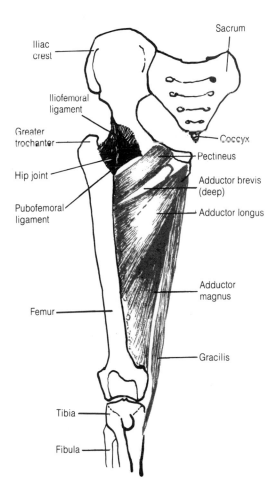

Fig. 8.8. Adductor group of muscles, seen in the anterior view of the right pelvis and thigh.

a horse, when contraction of the adductors keeps you on the saddle. When standing on an unstable platform, the adductors act with the abductors to keep the body weight over the feet.

The names of the adductors of the hip are *adductor magnus, adductor longus, adductor brevis, pectineus* and *gracilis*. The group of adductors originates from the anterior surface of the body of the pubis extending medially on to the superior and inferior ramus. Adductor magnus is the most posterior muscle of the group, and its origin extends back to the ischial tuberosity. From the small area of origin, the muscles fan out to insert into the full length of the posterior shaft of the femur. The posterior fibres of adductor magnus pass vertically down to the adductor tubercle, just above the medial side of the knee. Gracilis is a strap muscle lying medially in the group and ends below the knee.

The shift of the body weight over the supporting leg demands more stability at the knee. The large muscle on the front of the thigh, quadriceps femoris, acts to keep the knee joint extended. The quadriceps muscle will be described in more detail in Section 8.4 (Fig. 8.14).

The muscles around the ankle are important to keep the lateral balance when the body weight is supported on one foot. It is the muscles that turn the foot inwards and outward (known as invertors and evertors respectively) that provide this stability. These muscles will be described in Section 8.5.

- *WATCH a partner in bare feet stand on one leg. Notice any changes in the level of the pelvis, and the side to side movement of the foot taking place just below the ankle joint.*

During walking, the relative amount of time spent in single support at each step depends on the speed of walking. At slow speeds, the swinging leg is only off the ground for a short time, and most of the cycle is spent in double support. As the speed increases, single support occupies a relatively longer time, so that patients with hip problems, weak quadriceps and inability to balance, can only walk at slow speeds.

8.4 Swing

8.4.1 Leg swing in daily activities

Leg swing can occur when one leg is free to move while the opposite leg is supporting the body weight. The movements of the free leg swing the limb to place the foot forwards, upwards or to the side.

- *STAND on one leg and swing the free leg in all directions. Think about the daily activities that use these movements.*

  How does the leg swing in: (a) walking; (b) climbing stairs; (c) stepping into the bath; (d) getting into a car; and (e) getting on to a bicycle?

8.4.2 Muscles of the hip, knee and ankle in leg swing

The muscles involved in swinging the leg forwards are found in: (a) the *hip* (flexors combined with abductors and rotators); (b) the *knee* (flexors); and (c) the *ankle* (dorsiflexors – to raise the toes clear of the ground).

Hip flexors

The main muscles that flex the hip are the *iliacus* and *psoas*, usually grouped together and called *iliopsoas*, assisted by the sartorius, the rectus femoris and the tensor fascia lata. The *iliopsoas* originates in the abdomen. The fibres of psoas are attached to the transverse processes, bodies and discs of the lumbar vertebrae. Iliacus takes origin from the inner surface of the ilium on the iliac fossa. The two muscles leave the abdomen together, passing under the inguinal ligament, over the front of the hip joint and insert into the lesser trochanter of the femur (Fig. 8.9).

- *SIT with the trunk slightly forwards. Place the hand at the waist between the lower ribs and iliac crest, with the fingers across the lower back. Raise the foot off the ground and feel the activity in psoas just lateral to the vertebral column. The bulk of the muscle you are feeling lies posteriorly, but remember its tendon passes over the **anterior** side of the hip joint to reach the femur.*

The iliopsoas is active in *walking, climbing stairs* and *sitting up*.

In **walking** the iliopsoas is used to start the leg swinging forwards. On level ground the leg then moves like a pendulum to complete the swing phase. Greater activity in the hip flexors is needed in walking up hill and running. Figures 8.10a and b show the hip flexion during swing.

In **climbing stairs** the iliopsoas lifts the leg and puts the foot

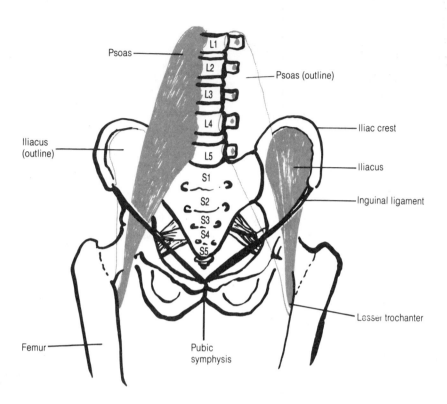

Fig. 8.9. Iliacus and psoas, seen in the anterior view of the pelvis and hip joints.

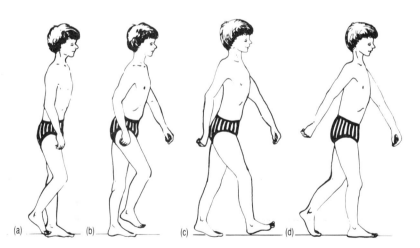

Fig. 8.10. Walking: (a) start of swing phase; (b) swing phase; (c) heel strike; (d) propulsion and support phase.

on the step above. Figures 8.11a shows the flexion in the left hip.

In **sitting** and preparing for standing, the iliopsoas is used to pull the trunk forwards, i.e. the femur is fixed (Fig. 8.11c). As the trunk leans forwards, the centre of gravity of the trunk moves over the feet before standing upright (Fig. 8.11d).

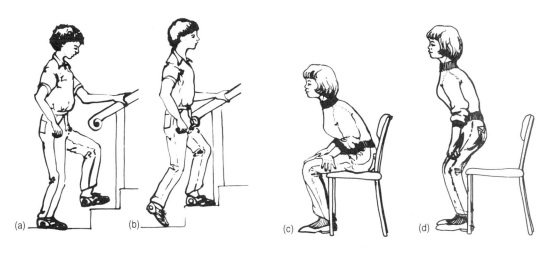

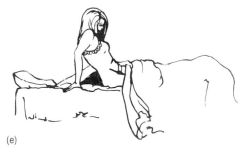

Fig. 8.11. Movements of the lower limb in climbing stairs, stand up from sitting and sit up from lying: (a) lift leg on to step; (b) lift body weight on to the step; (c) lean forwards; (d) stand up; (e) sit up from lying.

In **sitting up** from lying (Fig. 8.11e), the iliopsoas acts by pulling on the ilium of the pelvis and the lower vertebrae. The abdominal muscles (described in Chapter 10) start the movement, and iliopsoas is active at the end of the movement to pull the trunk upright.

Hip rotators and abductors

Many muscles around the hip have rotatory actions. The particular active muscles vary with the position of the femur in relation to the pelvis. The swinging leg in **walking** is rotated laterally to keep the foot pointing forwards. In **standing**, the hip rotators control the position and stability of the pelvis, particularly when the body is being rocked from side to side on a train or a bus. In **sitting** and **turning over in lying**, the same muscles control the movements of the pelvis on the flexed thigh.

There are six small *lateral rotator muscles* arranged close to the hip joint, in a similar way to the rotator cuff muscles of the shoulder. The six muscles lie across the posterior side of the hip joint deep to the gluteus maximus. The names of the muscles are: piriformis, obturator internus, gamellus superior, gamellus inferior, quadratus femoris and obturator externus. Detailed attachments of these muscles can be found in standard anatomy textbooks.

Sartorius is a long thin strap like muscle that crosses the anterior thigh (Fig. 8.12). When the hip and the knee are flexed, the lateral rotation action at the hip produced by sartorius is important. The overall actions of sartorius put the limb into the cross legged position, adopted by the early tailors (hence the name). The same movement is used to draw up the lower limbs in swimming and in Yoga.

The abductors of the hip, *gluteus medius* and *gluteus minimus*, are involved in **swinging** the leg **to the side**. Walking in daily living includes considerable side stepping to avoid obstacles. In sitting, the hip abductors are used to swing the thigh from one chair to another, or from a car seat to prepare to stand.

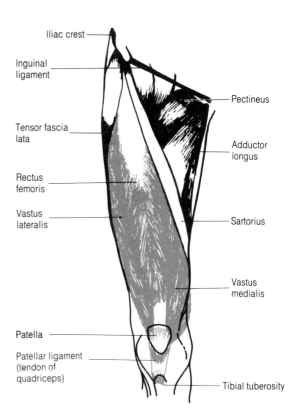

Iliac crest

Inguinal ligament

Pectineus

Tensor fascia lata

Adductor longus

Rectus femoris

Vastus lateralis

Sartorius

Vastus medialis

Patella

Patellar ligament (tendon of quadriceps)

Tibial tuberosity

Fig. 8.12. Quadriceps femoris and sartorius, seen in the anterior view of the right thigh.

Knee flexors

When the lower limb swings, the knee flexes to lift the foot clear of the ground. Look at Figure 8.10b to see the knee flexion during swing. The muscles active in flexion of the knee are the *hamstring* group at the back of the thigh, and the medial part of adductor magnus.

The three hamstring muscles are the *biceps femoris*, the *semimembranosus*, and the *semitendinosus*.

- *FEEL the tendons of the hamstrings in the fold of the knee in the sitting position. Two tendons lie medially (semimembranosus and semi-tendinosus), and one tendon can be felt laterally (biceps femoris).*

All three hamstrings originate on the ischial tuberosity of the pelvis (Fig. 8.13). Biceps femoris also has a short head of origin from the linea aspera of the femur and, passing laterally to the knee, both heads are inserted into the head of the fibula. The semimembranosus begins as a flat tendon which forms a third of its length, and the muscle fibres insert by a thick tendon behind the medial condyle of the tibia. The semitendinosus begins as muscle fibres and becomes tendinous two-thirds of the way down the thigh, to insert into the tibia on the medial side below the knee.

All the hamstrings flex the knee to lift the leg towards the thigh. When the trunk leans forwards, the ischial tuberosities (origin of the hamstrings) are carried upwards and backwards in relation to the hip and the muscles can be felt stretching in the thigh. Contraction of the hamstrings then extends the hip, and the trunk is raised to the upright position. The action of the hamstrings in extension of the hip will be discussed again in Section 8.5.

Ankle dorsiflexors

The weight of the foot in the swinging leg will tend to pull the toes downwards, and so drag the toes on the ground. To counteract this dropping of the foot, the muscles passing over the front of the ankle on to the dorsal surface of the foot contract. Look at the ankle movement during swing in Figures 8.10a and b. Dorsiflexion of the ankle joint lifts the toes clear of the ground during the swing.

The individual muscles in the group of dorsiflexors are

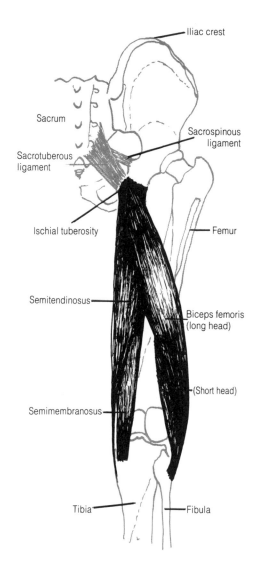

Fig. 8.13. The hamstring group of muscles seen in the posterior view of the right pelvis and thigh.

the *tibialis anterior*, the *extensor hallucis longus*, and the *extensor digitorum longus*.

- *PALPATE the bulge of muscles below the knee and lateral to the shin. Lift the toes upwards by dorsiflexing the ankle and feel the group in action. Tibialis anterior is the most superficial muscle that can be felt.*
- *OBSERVE the three tendons passing over the front of the ankle, tibialis anterior medially adjacent to the medial malleolus, then extensor hallucis longus going to the big toe, and extensor digitorum longus laterally. Check with Figure 8.14.*

The *tibialis anterior* is attached to the anterolateral shaft of the

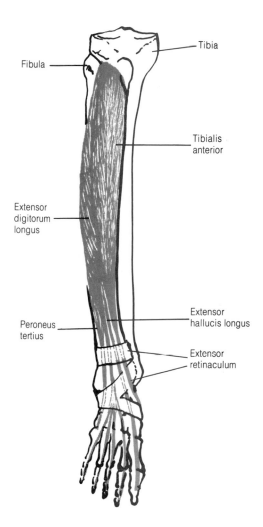

Fig. 8.14. The anterior tibial group of muscles, seen in the anterior view of the right leg and foot.

tibia and inserts on the medial side of the foot into the medial cuneiform and the base of the first metatarsal.

The *extensor hallucis longus* originates on the shaft of the fibula and inserts into the distal phalanx of the big toe.

The *extensor digitorum longus* has fibres attached to the shafts of the tibia and fibula and the interosseous membrane in between. The common tendon passes over the front of the ankle and divides into four, each inserting via an extensor expansion to the toes, in a similar way to the extensors of the fingers. A fourth tendon is sometimes present, which is the tendon of *peroneus tertius*, inserting into the base of the fifth metatarsal.

Two transverse bands of fascia over the anterior side of the leg above the ankle hold the tendons of the dorsiflexors in position during movements of the ankle (Fig. 8.14).

8.5 Propulsion

So far we have considered movements of the lower limb in support and swing. Next we shall look at the muscles which exert force against the ground to move the body forwards and upwards.

Muscle groups used in propulsion movements are found in: (a) the *hip* (extensors); (b) the *knee* (extensors); (c) the *ankle* (plantar flexors); and (d) the *toes* (flexors).

Hip extensors

The main extensor of the hip in propulsion movements is the *gluteus maximus* (Fig. 8.15). The most superficial muscle of the gluteal group, the gluteus maximus is the largest muscle in the body. The gluteus maximus can be seen when lying prone or standing upright, forming the curve of the buttocks. Strong contractions can be felt in climbing stairs, running and jumping.

The extensive origin of the gluteus maximus spreads from the posterior corner of the iliac crest across the posterior side of the sacrum and coccyx with some fibres attached to the fascia of

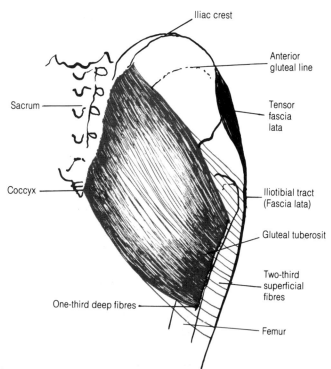

Fig. 8.15. Gluteus maximus, seen in the posterior view of the right hip.

the lower back (thoracolumbar fascia) and to sacrotuberous ligament of the pelvis. All the fibres pass downwards and laterally
over the posterior side of the hip joint. The main insertion of
the muscle is into the iliotibial tract, with the remaining fibres
passing deeply to attach to the gluteal tuberosity on the posterior
shaft of the femur.

The extensor action of the gluteus maximus is used in the
following activities.

(1) **Walking** up hill requires strong action of the gluteus maximus
to propel the body onwards.

(2) In **climbing stairs** the gluteus maximus is important in the
supporting leg during swing, and in the stepping leg when the
body is lifted up on to the step (Fig. 8.11b). In going down
stairs, the gluteus maximus works eccentrically in the trailing
leg.

(3) **Standing up** from sitting requires strong hip extension (Fig.
8.11d), together with knee extension. The gluteus maximus
works eccentrically in sitting down from standing.

The *hamstring* muscles also extend the hip, working with the
gluteus maximus, for propulsion forwards in walking. The activity begins at heel strike and continues as the supporting hip
moves over the foot (Fig. 8.10c and d).

Knee extensors

The muscles active in extension of the knee are the *quadriceps
femoris* group. Four muscles on the anterior of the thigh form
this group. The individual muscles are: (a) the *rectus femoris*, the
most superficial in the midline; (b) the *vastus medialis* on the
medial side; (c) the *vastus lateralis* on the lateral side; and (d)
the *vastus intermedius* which lies deep to the rectus femoris.
These muscles can be clearly seen in athletes and footballers
when the vasti in particular become enlarged in response to
weight training.

● *SIT on a chair and put your hands on the top of your thighs. Now stand
up slowly and feel the quadriceps in action. Pause in standing and feel
the tension is less. Then sit down slowly to feel the quadriceps in action
again. The muscle is working concentrically to extend the knee and lift
the body upwards; then working eccentrically against gravity as the
knee flexes and the body lowers to the seat of the chair again.*

The quadriceps group can be seen in anterior view in Figure 8.12, with the exception of the vastus intermedius which lies deep to the rectus femoris.

The *rectus femoris* is the only part of the quadriceps that passes over the hip joint. This muscle is attached by two heads, one from the anterior inferior iliac spine, and the other from just above the acetabulum.

The three vastus muscles surround the shaft of the femur:

The *vastus medialis* begins posteriorly on the spiral line and down the medial side of the linea aspera. The fibres wrap round medially to approach the knee.

The *vastus lateralis* is attached posteriorly to the lateral side of the linea aspera and wraps round the lateral side of the femoral shaft.

The *vastus intermedius* originates on the anterior and lateral shaft of the femur.

Figure 8.16 shows how the muscles of the quadriceps group extend around three sides of the femur.

All four muscles meet at the patella on the front of the knee, and insert by a common quadriceps tendon, the ligamentum patellae, to the anterior tubercle of the tibia. The ligamentum patellae provides extra stability for the knee joint on the anterior side where the capsule is absent. The lower horizontal fibres of

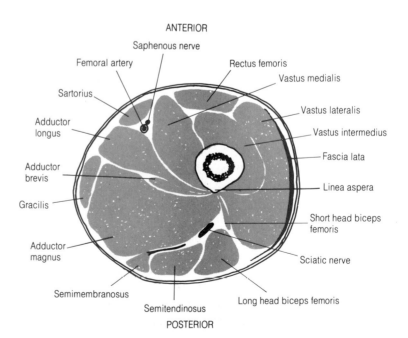

Fig. 8.16. Transverse section through the right thigh at the level of the upper third.

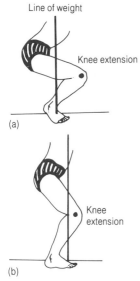

Line of weight

Knee extension

(a)

Knee extension

(b)

Fig. 8.17. Rise from a squat: (a) low position; (b) higher position. Note the change in the line of weight relative to the knee joint.

the vastus medialis prevent lateral displacement of the patella at the end of knee extension.

The quadriceps group is a powerful extensor of the knee, while the rectus femoris alone has a weak flexor action on the hip. Acting with the gluteus maximus, the quadriceps raise the body from sitting and squatting. When the knees are flexed at an angle less than a right angle, the quadriceps has to develop a force of 4–5 times body weight to hold the position. The knees are under great stress when the body is raised from a low squat position since the line of body weight is some distance from the knee joint (Fig. 8.17) (see also Chapter 2).

When the knee is injured, or after a period of bed rest, the quadriceps wastes very rapidly. The strength of this muscle is restored by knee extension exercises, at first lifting the weight of the leg alone and then by adding weights to the leg. Equipment operated by knee extension pressing a foot pedal or plate, e.g. treadle lathe or sewing machine, can also be used.

Ankle plantar flexors

When the heel is raised from the ground, the body is lifted up or forwards in a 'push off' movement (Fig. 8.10d). The calf muscles, attached by the Achilles' tendon to the heel, are active in this movement.

- *STAND on your toes and feel the calf muscles contracting. The muscles are also working eccentrically when you lower your heels to the ground.*

When the calf muscles are weak, the 'push off' in the trailing leg in walking is lost, and the body weight is transferred by trunk flexion; the thrust in jumping is also reduced.

The active muscles in plantar flexion of the ankle, which lie in the calf, are the *gastrocnemius* and the *soleus* (Fig. 8.18a).

The *gastrocnemius* is attached by two heads to the posterior surface of the femur, one above each femoral condyle.

The *soleus* attaches below the knee, across the soleal line on the posterior shaft of the tibia, and to the head and shaft of the fibula.

Both muscles join to form the very strong Achilles' tendon attached to the posterior surface of the calcaneum. The length of the calcaneum behind the axis of the ankle joint gives good leverage to the calf muscles.

There is a small muscle, the *plantaris*, lying between the gastrocnemius and the soleus. The short belly of this muscle

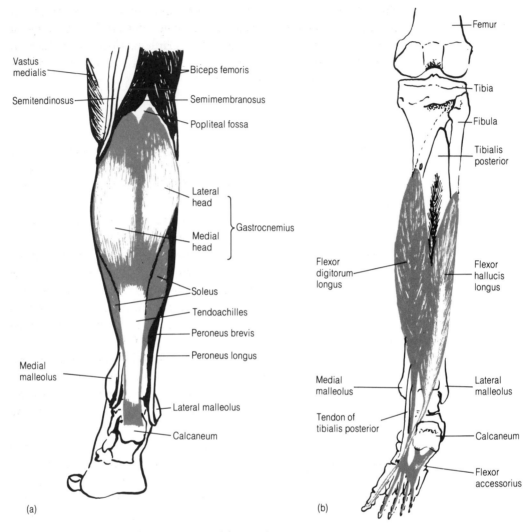

Fig. 8.18. Posterior view of the right leg and foot to show: (a) gastrocnemius and soleus (superficial); (b) the flexor muscles of the toes (deep).

originates above the lateral condyle of the femur, near to the lateral head of the gastrocnemius, and becomes a thin tendon just below the knee joint. The tendon passes down the length of the calf to insert on to the calcaneum in the Achilles' tendon.

Another small muscle, the *popliteus*, is found at the back of the knee joint, deep to the gastrocnemius. It is attached to the triangular area above the soleal line of the tibia, and passes upwards to the lateral condyle of the femur.

Deep to the gastrocnemius and soleus are three muscles whose tendons pass round the medial side of the ankle to enter the sole of the foot. They assist the calf muscles in propulsion at the ankle, and are known as the deep plantar flexors. One of these muscles (tibialis posterior) will be described with the foot in Section 8.6. The other two muscles are flexors of the toes as well as plantar flexors of the ankle.

Flexors of the toes

In the propulsion movements, it is important to keep the toes firmly on the ground while the body moves above. At the end of the movement, some thrust is added by flexion of the toes, particularly the great toe in running.

The muscles involved in flexion of the toes are the *flexor hallucis longus* and the *flexor digitorum longus* (Fig. 8.18b).

The *flexor hallucis longus* is attached to the posterior shaft of the fibula below the soleus. The tendon crosses the lower end of the tibia to pass through a groove on the back of the talus, and under the sustentaculum tali of the calcaneum, to continue along the sole of the foot on the medial side to insert on the distal phalanx of the great toe.

The *flexor digitorum longus* also arises below the soleus on the posterior shaft of the tibia, and passes round the medial side of the ankle with the flexor hallucis longus. In the sole of the foot, the tendon divides into four to insert on the distal phalanx of the four lesser toes.

The tendons of both these muscles are held in position at the ankle by the flexor retinaculum, a band of fibrous tissue from the medial malleolus to the medial tubercle of the calcaneum. In the sole of the foot the tendons are enclosed in synovial sheaths, similar to the flexors of the fingers in the hand.

> ### Clinical note-pad 8E: Avulsion of the Achilles' tendon
>
> The Achilles' tendon may sustain spontaneous avulsion (severing) with a feeling of being struck just above the heel and inability to tiptoe. This occurs in tennis players and athletes who rely on thrust at the ankle, and sometimes in middle age when the tendon is degenerate.

8.6 The foot

8.6.1 Functions and movements of the foot

The foot is a relatively small area that makes contact between the body weight and the ground. The surface of the ground may be rough, smooth, hard, soft, level or sloping, and the sole of the foot has to be able to accommodate all these. The weight of the body above compresses the parts of the foot in different directions as the body moves.

The muscles acting on the foot originate in the leg and pass around the ankle to insert into the bones of the foot. Like the hand, the foot also has intrinsic muscles that begin and end in the foot. The arrangement of the intrinsic muscles of the foot is similar to those in the hand. Children with malformation of the upper limb may develop the muscles of the foot to take over the manipulative functions of the hand.

The most important function of all the muscles of the foot is to resist deformation of the foot by the ground, or any obstacle in contact with the foot. When the foot is off the ground (e.g. in the swing phase in walking) the muscles act to change the position of the foot in relation to the leg. For most of the time, however, the feet are in contact with the ground, supporting the body weight in standing, and providing momentum for moving the body around. When the foot is firmly planted on the ground, the extrinsic muscles can move the leg on the foot, e.g. the dorsiflexors of the ankle pull the body forwards on to the leading leg in walking. The muscles are then acting in the opposite direction to pull the proximal attachments in the leg towards the foot.

Dorsiflexion and plantar flexion movements at the ankle (see Fig. 8.4a) have already been described in Sections 8.4.2 and 8.5 respectively. *Inversion* and *eversion* movements of the foot occur independently in the joints of the foot (Fig. 8.4b and c).

Inversion is the movement which turns the sole of the foot inwards when the foot is off the ground, or shifts the weight to the lateral side of the foot when weight bearing.

Eversion turns the sole of the foot outwards with the foot off the ground, or shifts the weight towards the medial side of the foot in weight bearing.

The muscles involved in **inversion** are *tibialis anterior* and *tibialis posterior*; while those producing **eversion** are *peroneus longus* and *peroneus brevis*.

Invertors

The **tibialis anterior** is one of the dorsiflexors already described in Section 8.4. Its tendon inserts on the medial side of the foot into the medial cuneiform and base of the first metatarsal, so that it lifts the medial border of the foot.

The **tibialis posterior** is the deepest muscle of the calf, originating on the posterior shaft of the tibia and fibula. The tendon of this muscle passes round the medial malleolus at the ankle and it inserts on the plantar surface of the navicular and adjacent tarsal bones (Fig. 8.19a). Note the relationship between the tendons of the tibialis anterior and posterior on the medial side of the foot (Fig. 8.19b).

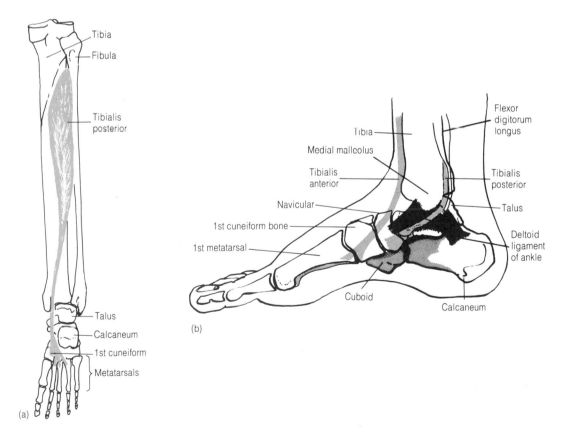

Fig. 8.19. (a) Posterior view of the right leg and the sole of the foot to show the tibialis posterior. (b) Medial aspect of the right ankle showing the insertions of the tibialis anterior and the tibialis posterior.

Evertors

The **peroneus longus** and **brevis** are attached to the lateral shaft of the fibula and their tendons pass round the lateral malleolus at the ankle. At the base of the fifth metatarsal, the peroneus brevis tendon ends, and the peroneus longus turns under, crossing the sole of the foot in a groove on the cuboid bone, to reach the medial cuneiform and base of the first metatarsal (Fig. 8.20).

When the evertors are weak, lateral stability of the ankle is lost, and the lateral ligament of the ankle is often torn.

When the foot is in contact with an uneven surface, the movements of inversion and eversion, together with the actions of the intrinsic muscles of the foot, allow the foot to adjust to

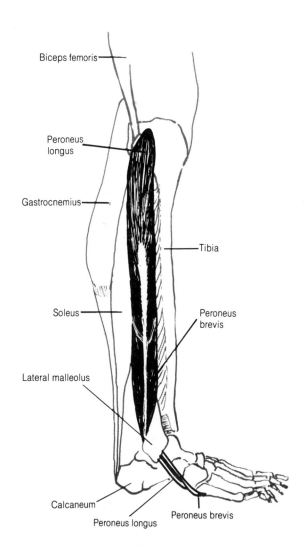

Fig. 8.20. Peroneus longus and brevis seen in the lateral view of the right leg and foot.

the ground and stabilise the ankle. Shoes reduce the amount of adaptation required, but the foot and shoe still have to accommodate sloping ground and avoid slipping on wet or icy surfaces.

8.6.2 The arches of the foot

The complex mechanism of the foot has resilience and spring to respond and adapt to the stress and strain of the body weight above.

- *REVISE the bones of the foot. Place an articulated skeleton of the foot on a flat surface. Note which bones are in contact with the table, and which bones are wholly or partly raised above the surface.*
- *STAND the feet in a tray of water soluble paint, then make foot prints on a sheet of lining paper laid out on the floor: (a) sitting on a chair, i.e. non-weight-bearing; (b) standing upright; and (c) walking several steps. Note the variation in pattern of footprint in (a), (b) and (c). Compare your foot prints with those of other students and note any individual differences.*

From (a) to (c) above there will be an increase in the area of foot in contact with the ground. In all the prints, the heel and ball of the foot will be seen. The lateral border of the foot will be present when the foot is bearing weight. The medial border of the foot remains absent, except when there is abnormal flattening of the foot.

Looking at the bones of the foot and the foot prints, it can be seen that the foot is arched in different directions. A longitudinal arch from the heel to the ball of the foot is easy to recognise. The foot is also arched transversely across the distal row of tarsals and the metatarsals (Fig. 8.21).

Ligaments bind the bones of the foot together and provide the main factors supporting the arches in standing. During movement, it is the muscles of the leg acting as slings from above, and the intrinsic muscles of the foot acting as bow strings across the base of the arches, that maintain the arches. The height of the arches varies during different phases of locomotor movements, particularly the medial part of the longitudinal arch.

Bony compartments of the arches

(1) **Medial longitudinal arch**. This arch is formed by the calcaneum, talus, navicular, three cuneiforms and metatarsals 1, 2 and 3.

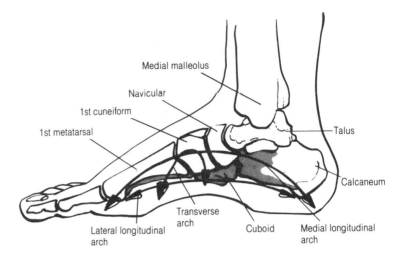

Fig. 8.21. Medial view of the right ankle to show the arches of the foot.

The highest part of the arch is the talus, which sits on the calcaneum supported by a shelf on the medial side known as the sustentaculum tali.

(2) **Lateral longitudinal arch**. This arch also begins at the calcaneum and extends along the lateral side of the foot to the cuboid and metatarsals 4 and 5. There is considerable stress on this arch during running when the body weight is transferred along the lateral border of the foot and on to the big toe. The shoes of a marathon runner, which are often worn down on the outer border, show how high this stress can be.

(3) **Transverse arch**. The foot is most arched in the transverse direction across the distal row of tarsals – the three cuneiforms and the cuboid. The metatarsals are also arched transversely; the region of the heads of the metatarsals is sometimes called the anterior arch. When the foot is stressed from above in standing, the anterior arch is flattened as the weight is taken by the heads of the metatarsals.

Ligaments bonding the arches

(1) **Spring ligament**. A tough fibrous band extends from the sustentaculum tali of the calcaneum to the navicular, and supports the head of the talus. This ligament is very elastic and responds to compression of the medial longitudinal arch (Fig. 8.22a).

(2) **Long** and **short plantar ligaments**. These two ligaments bind the bones of the lateral longitudinal arch. The long plantar ligament stretches from the calcaneum to the ridge on the cuboid and the

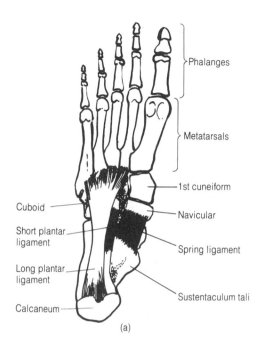

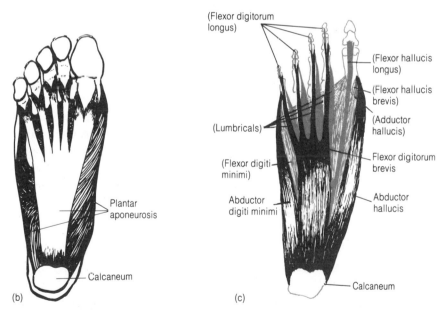

Fig. 8.22. The plantar surface of the right foot: (a) plantar ligaments; (b) plantar aponeurosis; (c) three muscles of the first layer (muscles of the second and third layers named in brackets).

bases of the middle metatarsals. Deep to this, the short plantar ligament is attached to the anterior end of the calcaneum and to the cuboid (Fig. 8.22a).

(3) **Plantar aponeurosis (Fig. 8.22b)**. A thick sheet of dense fibrous tissue is attached to the tuberosities of the calcaneum, and passes forwards over the muscles of the sole, to blend with the ligaments joining the heads of the metatarsals (deep transverse metatarsal ligaments). There are five main bands in the plantar aponeurosis, and each band blends with a fibrous sheath round a flexor tendon to a toe. The plantar aponeurosis tightens when the heel of the trailing leg is lifted off the ground in walking. This raises the longitudinal arch.

Muscles supporting the arches

(1) **Muscles of the leg**. The tibialis anterior inserts on the dorsal surface of the medial cuneiform and base of the first metatarsal, while the tendon of tibialis posterior unites the plantar surfaces of the medial tarsal bones. These two muscles therefore support the medial longitudinal arch, and the tendon of the flexor hallucis longus acts as a bow string for it. Further support for the longitudinal arch is provided by the tendons of flexor digitorum longus lying along the plantar surface of the foot.

The peroneus longus has a tendon that crosses the foot from the cuboid and the base of metatarsal 5 laterally, to insert on the plantar surface of the medial cuneiform and base of metatarsal 1 medially. Crossing the foot in this way, the peroneus longus is the chief support for the transverse arch. The tendon of the peroneus longus resists any compression of the outer side of the foot and protects the lateral ligament of the ankle.

(2) **Intrinsic muscles of the foot**. Three muscles of the first layer of the foot originate on the calcaneum and insert into the toes. Like the plantar aponeurosis, these muscles (abductor hallucis, flexor digitorum brevis and abductor digiti minimi) join the proximal and distal ends of the longitudinal arches (Fig. 8.22c). The muscles function by responding to depression of these arches by the weight above.

The transverse head of the adductor hallucis, in the third layer of the foot, crosses the anterior end of the transverse arch, from the heads of metatarsals 3, 4 and 5 to the proximal phalanx of the big toe. This muscle is the main support for the anterior arch.

The interosseous muscles of the foot are arranged around the second metatarsal, which forms the axis of the foot. (The axis of the hand is the third metacarpal.) Activity in the interossei and the flexors draws the metatarsals towards the axis of the foot and maintains the transverse arch.

- *PLACE the foot flat on the ground while sitting in a chair. Try to pull up the centre of the foot (flexion) with the toes kept flat on the ground. Notice how the foot arches both longitudinally by some flexion at the tarso-metatarsal joints, and transversely as the shafts of the metatarsals move towards the axis of the foot.*

The maintenance of the flexibility of the foot is important for mobility, especially in dancers and gymnasts who need to balance the body on the whole, or part of, one foot. The bony arches respond to the compression of the foot by the body weight. In the supporting foot in walking and running, the body weight is transmitted from the heel to the big toe at each step. The big toe takes most of the weight in standing, and provides the thrust in driving the body forwards in walking and running. Long distance runners commonly experience pain in the big toe as a result of the stress on it.

> **Clinical note-pad 8F: Flat foot, hallux valgus**
>
> Flat foot is the collapse of the medial arch so that the medial border of the foot almost touches the ground. Predisposing factors are muscle weakness or joint erosion, e.g. rheumatoid arthritis.
>
> Hallux valgus is the most common deformity of the foot. The first metatarsal deviates medially away from the second metatarsal, and the big toe slants laterally towards the second toe. The head of the metatarsal develops a protective bursa where the shoe rubs. There is some evidence for shoes with inadequate support in standing contributing to the condition. It does not occur in people who have never worn shoes.

8.7 Summary of the lower limb muscles

(1) *Muscles around the hip*: gluteus maximus, medius and minimus, tensor fascia lata, iliacus and psoas (ilio-psoas), six lateral rotators.

(2) *Anterior thigh*: quadriceps femoris, sartorius.

(3) *Medial thigh*: adductor magnus, longus and brevis, pectineus, gracilis.

(4) *Posterior thigh*: hamstrings – biceps femoris, semitendinosus, semimembranosus.

(5) *Anterior leg*: tibialis anterior, extensor hallucis longus, extensor digitorum longus.

(6) *Posterior leg*: gastrocnemius, soleus (plantaris and popliteus), flexor hallucis longus, flexor digitorum longus, tibialis posterior.

(7) *Lateral leg*: peroneus longus and brevis.

(8) *Sole of the foot*:
first layer – abductor hallucis, flexor digitorum brevis, abductor digiti minimi;
second layer – lumbricals, flexor digitorum accessorius;
third layer – flexor hallucis brevis, flexor digiti minimi brevis, adductor hallucis;
fourth layer – interossei, three plantar and four dorsal.

At the end of this chapter, you should be able to:

(1) Discuss the functions of the lower limb.

(2) Describe the structure and movements of the hip, knee and ankle joints in relation to lower limb function.

(3) Describe the changes from standing with double support to single support, including the names and position of the muscles involved.

(4) Describe the muscle action at the hip, knee and ankle in: (a) swinging the lower limb; and (b) propelling the body forwards and upwards, with special reference to walking, climbing stairs and standing up from sitting.

(5) Outline the functions of the foot.

(6) Distinguish between the movements of the ankle (dorsiflexion and plantar flexion) and the movements of the joints of the foot (inversion and eversion). Name the muscles producing these movements.

(7) Outline the importance of the arches of the foot and list the factors maintaining them.

9 / The Nerves of the Lower Limb and some Observations of Gait

9.1 Introduction

The nerves of the lower limb are formed from the lumbar and sacral spinal nerves. Movement in the limb as a whole depends on activity in spinal nerves from the first lumbar down to the fourth sacral nerves. The spinal roots branch and join in the abdomen and pelvis before forming the peripheral nerves in the limb. The first four lumbar nerves form the **lumbar plexus** which lies embedded in the psoas muscle in the posterior abdominal wall. A second plexus is formed from the fifth lumbar to the fourth sacral spinal nerves. These roots of the **sacral plexus** are part of the cauda equina (see Fig. 4.4) and enter the pelvis through the anterior foramina of the sacrum.

The **terminal branches** of the lumbar plexus and sacral plexus which supply the large muscle groups of the lower limb are: (a) the *femoral nerve* – to the anterior muscles of the thigh; (b) the *obturator nerve* – to the medial muscles of the thigh; (c) the *gluteal nerves* – to the muscles of the buttock; and (d) the *sciatic nerve* – to the posterior muscles of the thigh (this branches to form the *tibial* and *common peroneal nerve* – to all the muscles below the knee.

The lumbar and sacral plexi are less vulnerable to injury than the brachial plexus. The femoral, sciatic and common peroneal nerves may be damaged by trauma, and the obturator nerve may be compressed by any rise in pressure in the pelvis due to enlargement of pelvic organs. Injury to the back may compress the roots of the lumbar nerves, particularly L4 and L5.

In development, the lower limb bud grows out from the side of the embryo. The nerve from the central segment, S1, grows down the limb, to end along the outer side of the foot (see Fig. 4.5) in the same way that the middle segments of the brachial plexus supply the hand. Later in development, the lower limb rotates medially as it extends, so that the dermatomes of the upper segments (L2, L3, L4, L5) lie along the front of the limb, and those of the lower segments (S2, S3) lie on the back of the leg. The rotation also means that the anterior and posterior divisions of the spinal nerves forming the plexi do not pass to the corresponding side of the lower limb.

(1) **Lumbar plexus**: (a) posterior divisions – anterior muscles of thigh; (b) anterior divisions – medial muscles of thigh.

(2) **Sacral plexus**: (a) posterior divisions – muscles of the buttock, anterior and lateral muscles of the leg; (b) anterior divisions – posterior muscles of the thigh, leg and sole of foot.

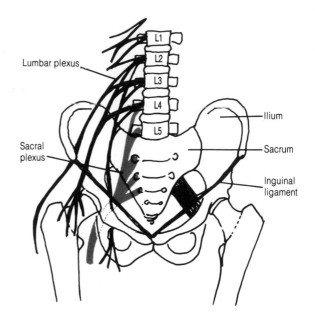

Fig. 9.1. Lumbar and sacral plexi; position and relations.

Figure 9.1 shows the position of the lumbar and sacral plexi in relation to the lumbar spine, the sacrum and the hip. The course of the muscular branches will be described, the cutaneous branches will be mentioned in outline only.

9.2 The lumbar plexus: position and formation

The lumbar plexus is formed by the anterior primary (ventral) rami of the upper four lumbar nerves. The psoas muscle lies alongside the lumbar vertebrae in the posterior abdominal wall, so that the lumbar plexus lies in this muscle and the branches of the plexus emerge from it. Most of the fibres of L4 join the lumbar plexus, but the remainder join L5 to form the *lumbosacral trunk* which is part of the sacral plexus.

Branches direct from the plexus supply the psoas, iliacus and quadratus lumborum.

Figure 9.2 shows the five roots of the lumbar plexus and the formation of the main terminal branches.

9.3 Terminal branches of the lumbar plexus

There are three important nerves that are formed from the lumbar plexus: the *femoral*, the *lateral cutaneous*, and the *obturator nerves*. Each nerve passes through the pelvis to enter the thigh: (a) the *femoral nerve* passes anteriorly to supply the quadriceps

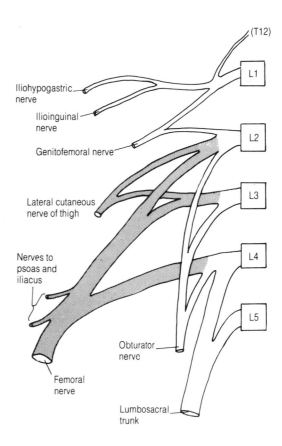

Fig. 9.2. Lumbar plexus; roots and main terminal branches.

and sartorius; (b) the *lateral cutaneous nerve* passes laterally to the skin on the lateral side of the thigh; and (c) the *obturator nerve* passes medially to supply the adductor group of muscles.

Figure 9.1 shows the way that the three nerves leave the pelvis.

- *LOOK at Figures 9.3 and 9.4 to follow the course and distribution of the femoral, lateral cutaneous and obturator nerves.*

The femoral nerve

This is the largest nerve of the lumbar plexus. It lies in the psoas muscle in the pelvis, and then emerges from the lateral border of the muscle to lie between the psoas and iliacus, leaving the pelvis anteriorly under the inguinal ligament. In the thigh, the femoral nerve branches to supply the quadriceps group of muscles. The saphenous nerve, a branch of the femoral nerve in the thigh becomes cutaneous at the medial side of the knee and continues on to the medial side of the ankle (Fig. 9.3).

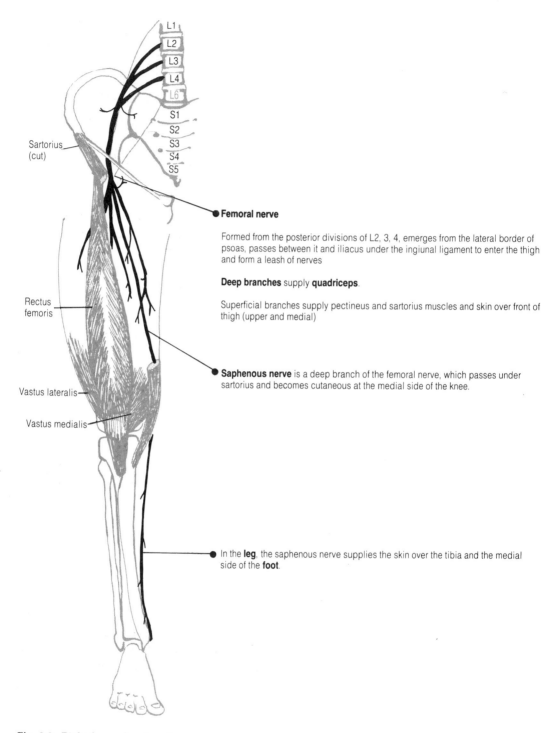

Femoral nerve

Formed from the posterior divisions of L2, 3, 4, emerges from the lateral border of psoas, passes between it and iliacus under the inguinal ligament to enter the thigh and form a leash of nerves

Deep branches supply **quadriceps**.

Superficial branches supply pectineus and sartorius muscles and skin over front of thigh (upper and medial)

Saphenous nerve is a deep branch of the femoral nerve, which passes under sartorius and becomes cutaneous at the medial side of the knee.

In the **leg**, the saphenous nerve supplies the skin over the tibia and the medial side of the **foot**.

Fig. 9.3. Right femoral and saphenous nerve.

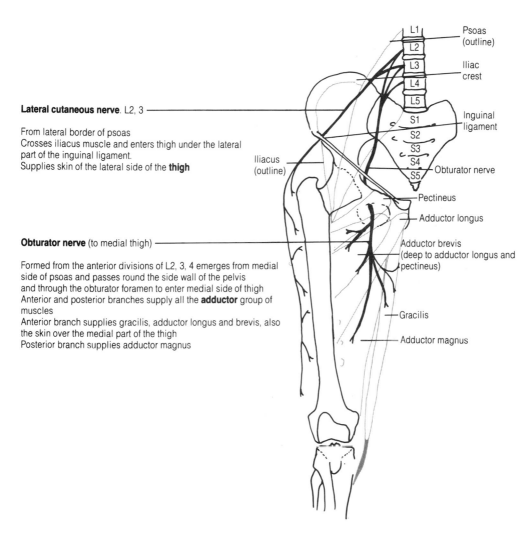

Lateral cutaneous nerve. L2, 3

From lateral border of psoas
Crosses iliacus muscle and enters thigh under the lateral
part of the inguinal ligament.
Supplies skin of the lateral side of the **thigh**

Iliacus
(outline)

L1
L2
L3
L4
L5
S1
S2
S3
S4
S5

Psoas
(outline)

Iliac
crest

Inguinal
ligament

Obturator nerve

Pectineus

Adductor longus

Adductor brevis
(deep to adductor longus and
pectineus)

Gracilis

Adductor magnus

Obturator nerve (to medial thigh)

Formed from the anterior divisions of L2, 3, 4 emerges from medial
side of psoas and passes round the side wall of the pelvis
and through the obturator foramen to enter medial side of thigh
Anterior and posterior branches supply all the **adductor** group of
muscles
Anterior branch supplies gracilis, adductor longus and brevis, also
the skin over the medial part of the thigh
Posterior branch supplies adductor magnus

Fig. 9.4. Right obturator and lateral cutaneous nerve.

The lateral cutaneous nerve

This nerve emerges from the lateral side of the psoas muscle and
crosses the iliacus obliquely to the anterior superior spine of the
ilium. The nerve passes under the lateral end of the inguinal
ligament and becomes cutaneous in the lateral thigh. Pressure
on the nerve in the area of the iliac spine causes loss of sensation
on the lateral side of the thigh (Fig. 9.4).

The obturator nerve

This leaves the medial side of the psoas muscle at the brim of the pelvis and passes through the obturator foramen of the hip bone to reach the medial side of the thigh. In the medial compartment of the thigh, the obturator nerve supplies all the adductor group of muscles.

The functional importance of the femoral and obturator nerves

The femoral and obturator nerves are both important in walking. The quadriceps, supplied by the femoral nerve, stabilises the knee during support, and propels the body upwards when walking uphill and climbing stairs. The adductors, supplied by the obturator nerve, are active in the supporting leg when the other leg is off the ground. If the adductors are weak due to damage of the obturator nerve, the leg swings outward instead of forwards in the swing phase in walking.

Other nerves of the lumbar plexus

Three other cutaneous nerves are formed from the first two nerves of the lumbar plexus. The first lumbar nerve divides into two, the **iliohypogastric** and the **ilioinguinal** nerves, which supply the skin of the buttock and groin respectively. A third cutaneous nerve, the **genitofemoral**, is formed from L1 and L2, and supplies a small area of skin on the upper front part of the thigh (Fig. 9.2).

9.4 The sacral plexus: position and formation

The sacral plexus is formed in the pelvis from the joining of the anterior primary (ventral) rami of the lumbosacral trunk (L4, L5), the first three and part of the fourth sacral nerves. The landmark to find the position of the sacral plexus in the pelvis is the *piriformis*, one of the six lateral rotator muscles of the hip. (The piriformis is attached to the anterior aspect of the second, third and fourth segments of the sacrum, and passes out of the pelvis into the thigh through the greater sciatic notch of the pelvis to attach to the apex of the greater trochanter of the femur. Figure 9.6 shows a posterior view of the piriformis muscle.) The main part of the plexus passes backwards with piriformis to enter the posterior compartment of the thigh. Figure 9.1 shows the emerging sacral nerves lying on the anterior surface of the sacrum. Figure 9.5 shows the roots of the sacral plexus and the main terminal branches.

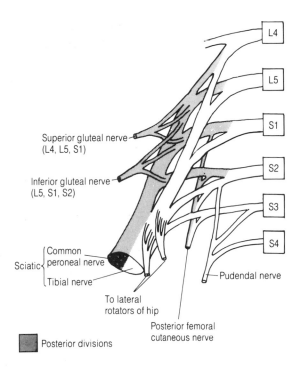

Fig. 9.5. Sacral plexus; roots and main terminal branches.

- *LOOK at an articulated skeleton and identify the greater sciatic notch of the pelvis, which is converted into the greater sciatic foramen by the sacrospinous ligament joining the sacrum to the ischial spine.*
- *LOOK at the anterior surface of the sacrum to see how spinal nerves originating inside the pelvis from the sacral foramina reach the back of the thigh by passing through the greater sciatic foramen. (Remember how the femoral nerve passed anteriorly under the inguinal ligament, and the obturator nerve passed medially through the obturator foramen.)*

You should now understand the three directions of exit of nerves to the thigh. Return to Figure 8.14 and identify each nerve in a transverse section of the thigh.

9.5 Terminal branches of the sacral plexus

9.5.1 Branches to the posterior thigh, leg and foot muscles

The three main nerves from the sacral plexus important for movement of the lower limb are: the *superior gluteal nerve* which passes above piriformis to supply the gluteus medius, gluteus minimus and tensor fascia lata; the *inferior gluteal nerve* which passes below piriformis to supply the gluteus maximus; and, most importantly, the *sciatic nerve* which emerges below

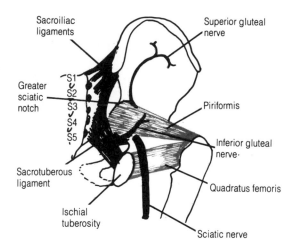

Fig. 9.6. Posterior view of the right pelvis and hip to show nerves emerging through the greater sciatic foramen.

piriformis to supply the hamstrings, and branches to all the muscles below the knee.

Figure 9.6 shows the three nerves emerging through the greater sciatic notch and branching to supply the muscle groups.

The sciatic nerve

This is the largest in the body, about the same size as the thumb or 2 cm in diameter. The posterior divisions of L4, L5, S1 and S2 form the common peroneal component of the sciatic nerve. The anterior divisions of L4, L5, S1, S2 and S3 form the tibial component of the sciatic nerve (Fig. 9.5). These two components lie together in the thigh until they divide above the knee. Branches high in the thigh supply the hamstring group of muscles. Only the nerve to the short head of the biceps comes from the common peroneal division, all other branches to the hamstrings are from the tibial component. The sciatic nerve also supplies the fibres of adductor magnus that originate from the ischium. Trauma to the sciatic nerve in the middle of the thigh does not usually affect the hamstrings since the branches to these muscles begin high in the thigh.

Figures 9.7a and b show the course and distribution of the sciatic nerve. The *branches* of the sciatic nerve are as follows.

(1) The **tibial nerve** (Fig. 9.7a). This is the nerve of the posterior muscles of the calf, supplying all the plantar flexors – gastrocnemius, soleus, flexor hallucis longus, flexor digitorum longus and tibialis posterior. The tibial nerve lies in the popliteal fossa at the back of the knee and continues on down the leg

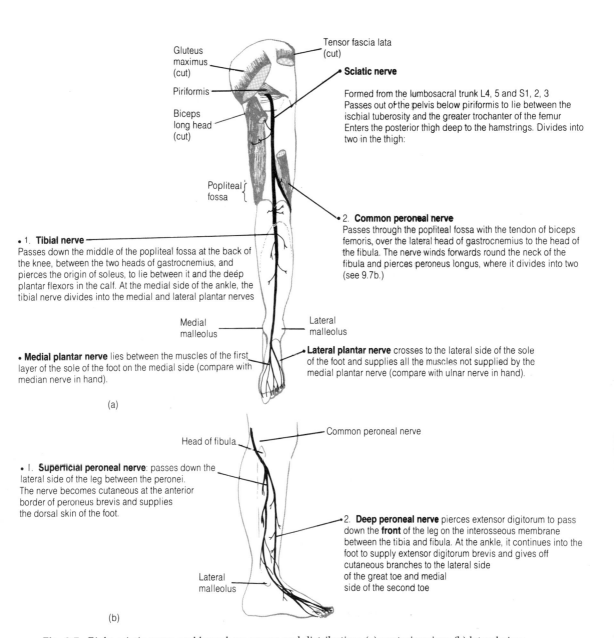

Gluteus maximus (cut)

Piriformis

Biceps long head (cut)

Popliteal fossa

Tensor fascia lata (cut)

Sciatic nerve

Formed from the lumbosacral trunk L4, 5 and S1, 2, 3
Passes out of the pelvis below piriformis to lie between the ischial tuberosity and the greater trochanter of the femur
Enters the posterior thigh deep to the hamstrings. Divides into two in the thigh:

2. Common peroneal nerve
Passes through the popliteal fossa with the tendon of biceps femoris, over the lateral head of gastrocnemius to the head of the fibula. The nerve winds forwards round the neck of the fibula and pierces peroneus longus, where it divides into two (see 9.7b.)

1. Tibial nerve
Passes down the middle of the popliteal fossa at the back of the knee, between the two heads of gastrocnemius, and pierces the origin of soleus, to lie between it and the deep plantar flexors in the calf. At the medial side of the ankle, the tibial nerve divides into the medial and lateral plantar nerves

Medial malleolus

Lateral malleolus

Medial plantar nerve lies between the muscles of the first layer of the sole of the foot on the medial side (compare with median nerve in hand).

Lateral plantar nerve crosses to the lateral side of the sole of the foot and supplies all the muscles not supplied by the medial plantar nerve (compare with ulnar nerve in hand).

(a)

Head of fibula

Common peroneal nerve

1. Superficial peroneal nerve: passes down the lateral side of the leg between the peronei. The nerve becomes cutaneous at the anterior border of peroneus brevis and supplies the dorsal skin of the foot.

2. Deep peroneal nerve pierces extensor digitorum to pass down the **front** of the leg on the interosseous membrane between the tibia and fibula. At the ankle, it continues into the foot to supply extensor digitorum brevis and gives off cutaneous branches to the lateral side of the great toe and medial side of the second toe

Lateral malleolus

(b)

Fig. 9.7. Right sciatic nerve and branches; course and distribution: (a) posterior view; (b) lateral view.

between the muscles of the calf. The *sural nerve* is a cutaneous branch of the tibial nerve in the calf that supplies the skin on the lateral side of the leg and foot (Fig. 9.8a). A branch of the tibial nerve at the ankle supplies the skin of the heel.

At the medial side of the ankle, the tibial nerve divides into two nerves that supply the muscles of the sole of the foot. (a) The **medial plantar nerve** supplies the abductor hallucis, flexor

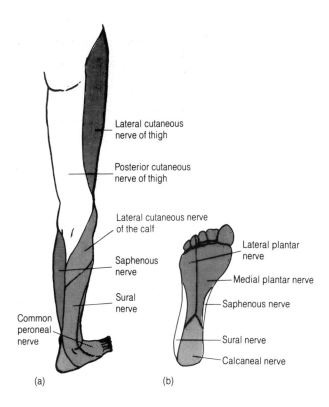

Fig. 9.8. Cutaneous nerve supply to the right lower limb: (a) posterior view; (b) sole of foot.

(a)

(b)

hallucis brevis, flexor digitorum brevis and the first lumbrical. (b) The **lateral plantar nerve** supplies the lateral three lumbricals, all the interossei, abductor digiti minimi, flexor digiti minimi and adductor hallucis.

(2) The **common peroneal nerve** (Fig. 9.7a and b). This is the lateral part of the sciatic nerve that forms in the upper part of the popliteal fossa. It travels with the biceps femoris to the head of the fibula where it passes around the neck into the peroneus longus. There it divides into the superficial and deep peroneal nerves. (a) The **superficial peroneal nerve** supplies the evertors, peroneus longus and brevis. This nerve lies deep to peroneus longus in the leg and continues over the front of the ankle to supply the skin of the dorsum of the foot. (b) The **deep peroneal nerve** supplies the dorsiflexors, the tibialis anterior, extensor hallucis longus, the extensor digitorum longus and peroneus tertius. This nerve ends on the dorsum of the foot where it supplies the extensor digitorum brevis and the skin over the first and second toes.

> **Clinical note-pad 9A: Peroneal nerve lesion**
>
> The common peroneal nerve is vulnerable to damage at the lateral side of the knee, where it is subcutaneous as it winds round the neck of the fibula. The result is loss of dorsiflexion and eversion of the ankle producing 'foot drop' when the leg is lifted off the ground.
>
> Fracture of the shaft of the fibula, common in skiing and skating falls, may injure the superficial peroneal nerve. The foot then tends to go into inversion, and the ankle loses stability.

● *Revise the muscle groups involved in the support and swing phases of walking described in Chapter 8. Now add the nerve supply to each of the groups of muscles. You should now be able to work out how the activation of the muscles used in walking depends on the following:*

(1) *The superior and inferior gluteal nerves, and the femoral nerve keep the pelvis level and stabilise the hip and knee in support. The sciatic and deep peroneal nerves flex the knee and dorsiflex the ankle respectively during swing.*

(2) *The tibial nerve initiates 'push off' by plantar flexing the ankle.*

(3) *The superficial peroneal nerve stabilises the ankle and protects its lateral ligament, particularly on rough ground.*

9.5.2 Pudendal nerve

The pudendal nerve (S2, S3, S4) (Fig. 9.5) passes out of the greater sciatic foramen medial to the sciatic nerve, and then turns below the ischial spine to supply the muscles of the pelvic floor.

9.5.3 Cutaneous nerves of the sacral plexus

Posterior femoral cutaneous nerve

Branches of the posterior femoral cutaneous nerve (S1, S2, S3) (Fig. 9.5) supply the skin over the posterior side from the buttock to the upper calf.

Sural nerve

The sural nerve is a branch of the tibial nerve at the back of the knee which supplies the skin of the lateral side of the lower calf and the lateral side of the foot. A branch of the tibial nerve at the ankle supplies the skin of the heel.

9.5.4 Summary of the cutaneous supply in the foot

The nerve supply to the skin of the sole of the foot is important for sensory information about the contact of the foot with the ground during standing and walking, and the distribution of the body weight over the feet. The major part of the skin of the sole of the foot is supplied by the medial and lateral plantar nerves. The heel receives the calcaneal nerve, a branch of the tibial nerve. The lateral border of the foot is supplied by the sural nerve (Fig. 9.8b).

The dorsal surface of the foot is largely supplied by branches of the superficial peroneal nerve, except a triangular area over the first and second toes which receives branches of the deep peroneal nerve. The saphenous nerve, a branch of the femoral nerve in the thigh, becomes the cutaneous nerve to the medial side of the lower leg and continues to the medial dorsal surface of the foot.

9.6 Some observations of gait

Walking is a pattern and sequence of movements performed by the lower limbs to propel the upright body in one direction, usually forwards. To keep the balance of the body, the head and trunk constantly adjust their position, so that the centre of gravity remains over the foot base. In fast walking and in running, the forward propulsion is aided by swinging the arms, but the upper limbs only play a minor role in walking at average speeds. The timing and coordination of all the active muscles is controlled by the central nervous system.

- *WATCH people walking to the shops, to the station and in the park; alone and in groups. Notice the variety of walking speed, length of stride, rate of stepping, position of the head and body, and amount of arm swing.*

Each person seems to have his or her own way of walking, which varies with mood, time of day and many other factors. If you try to 'walk in step' with someone else, it is always difficult, especially if you are not the same height. All the measurable parameters of gait, such as stride length and step frequency are related to stature. Tall people take long strides and make fewer steps per minute compared with short people walking at the same speed. Other features of gait are not easy to measure, but can be observed by the experienced eye of the therapist and athletics coach. The walking pattern should be stable, rhythmic and coordinated. The ability to change direction and speed, and to accommodate changing surfaces on the ground, are all part of the demands of normal walking. Knowledge of the features of walking patterns makes it easier to observe deviations from the normal in those who have difficulty in walking.

9.6.1 The walking cycle

The cycle of movements in walking is usually divided into: (a) the support or stance phase; and (b) the swing phase. In Chapter 8 the lower limb actions in support and swing have been considered. Figure 9.9 shows the stages in swing and support during walking. The changes occurring during support and swing will be considered in more detail here.

Support phase

When the heel of the leading leg is lowered to the ground at 'heel strike' the support phase begins (Fig. 9.9c). The leading leg is now preparing to receive the body weight transferred from the trailing leg: contraction of the quadriceps and hamstrings stabilises the hip and the knee; the ankle is dorsiflexed at heel strike, and then plantar flexes (by eccentric action of the anterior tibial muscles) to place the whole foot flat on the ground.

The 'mid stance' phase is when the leading leg has become a support for the body weight.

At the end of the support phase, the heel is raised in plantar

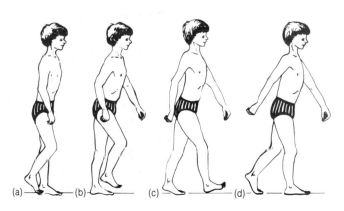

Fig. 9.9. Walking cycle: (a) start of swing; (b) swing phase; (c) heel strike; (d) propulsion and support.

(a) (b) (c) (d)

flexion at 'push off' to transfer the weight forwards to the opposite leg (Fig. 9.9d).

During support the hip and knee extensors stabilise the leg; the hip abductors and adductors stabilise the pelvis.

- *WATCH a partner walking slowly and notice the changes in the pattern of movements of the leg from heel strike to push off in the supporting leg at each step.*

Swing phase

After push off, the trailing leg is lifted from the ground and starts the forwards swing (Fig. 9.9a). The hip flexors start the swing and, in walking at slow speeds on level ground, the limb then swings like a pendulum. During the swing the knee flexes and the ankle dorsiflexes to lift the toes clear of the ground (Fig. 9.9b).

The swinging leg carries the pelvis forwards on that side. To counteract this rotation of the pelvis, the femur is rotated laterally by the hip rotators. In this way, the toes are kept pointing forwards. At the same time the trunk is carried forwards on the side of the swinging leg, so the trunk rotators are active to keep the shoulders facing forwards and the eyes looking ahead. At the end of the swing, the hip extensors halt the thigh, the knee extends and the heel is placed on the ground.

- *WATCH a partner walking and observe the changes in the pattern of the swinging leg at each step. The leg accelerates, swings and then decelerates at each step.*

When one leg is in the swing phase the other leg is in the support phase. At most natural speeds of walking, there is a 'double support phase' in between when both feet are on the ground. With an increase in the speed of walking, there is a decrease in the time of double support. In running, double support disappears altogether.

9.6.2 Abnormal gait

An abnormal pattern of walking may have mechanical or neurological origin. Only one side of the body may be affected or both sides. Walking demands the ability to perform the swing and support movements of the lower limb, at the same time as maintaining the balance of the body. Coordination of the bilateral movements of the lower limbs, trunk and arms is essential. The postural reflexes, largely based on the brain stem, control the balance reactions, such as the trunk moving laterally over the supporting leg at each step.

Some possible causes of abnormal gait

(1) **Mechanical**
   (a) Inability of skeletal structures to bear the body weight. For example, fracture or osteoporosis of bone, pain in lower limb joints.
   (b) Weakness of muscles.
   c) Restricted range of movement at joints.

(2) **Neurological**
   (a) Abnormal muscle tone – hypotonia, spasticity or rigidity.
   (b) Presence of abnormal movement synergy in the lower limb.
   (c) Disturbance of postural reflexes.
   (d) Absence of sensory feedback from the sole of the foot and from proprioceptors in muscles and joints.
   (e) Loss of body image when one side is ignored and the affected side is 'left behind'.
   (f) Perceptual problems leading to difficulty in judging distances and depths and therefore where to put limbs.

Apparently minor problems such as a painful toe or ill fitting shoes can produce marked changes in gait. Also, one particular feature of abnormal gait may occur for a variety of reasons. For example, the forefoot may drop during the swing and the toes drag on the ground due to damage to the common peroneal nerve, or general weakness of lower limb muscles, or increased tone in the plantar flexors. It is therefore important to *observe* the particular features in each individual (Fig. 9.10), including any abnormal movements of body segments and also the ability to: (a) balance; (b) coordinate the two sides of the body; (c) maintain walking rhythm; and (d) change direction and speed of walking as required.

Some types of abnormal gait

(1) **Shuffling gait**. The feet make short shuffling steps with rigidity in hip and knee extensors. There is little movement of the trunks and arms (Parkinson gait).

(2) **High stepping gait**. During the swing phase, the foot is lifted

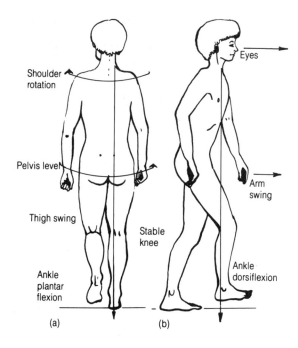

Fig. 9.10. Observation of gait.

(a)   (b)

high off the ground. This is due to loss of sensory information from the skin of the sole of the foot and from the proprioceptors in the muscles of the limb, known as *sensory ataxia*. If this gait is unchanged when the eyes are closed, then the cerebellum is involved and it is known as *cerebellar ataxia*.

(3) **Spastic gait** (with hypertonia). The lower limb shows extensor synergy with overactive adductors, extensors and invertors. The thigh swings across the body during the swing (called *scissors gait*). There is difficulty in putting the heel down at the beginning of the support phase.

(4) **Hemiplegic gait** (with hypotonia). The pelvis is lifted on the affected side by 'hip hitching', and the thigh swings out to that side due to weak adductors. The foot drops during the swing, and the toes or lateral border of the foot are placed on the ground first.

(5) **Waddling gait**. General weakness in the supporting muscles means that the pelvis tilts with every step and the trunk is thrown from side to side.

At the end of this chapter, you should be able to:

(1) Outline the position and arrangement of the lumbar plexus.

(2) Describe the course and distribution of the main branches of the lumbar plexus: femoral, lateral cutaneous and obturator nerves. Explain their function for muscle action at the hip and knee during standing and walking.

(3) Outline the position and arrangement of the sacral plexus.

(4) Describe the course and distribution of the main branches of the sacral plexus: superior gluteal, inferior gluteal, sciatic, tibial and common peroneal nerves. Deduce the functional importance of each nerve by revision of the muscles of the lower limb from Chapter 8.

(5) Explain the role of the branches of the common peroneal nerve (superficial and deep peroneal nerves) for movement and stability of the ankle.

(6) Summarise the nerve supply to the skin of the sole of the foot.

(7) Describe the swing and support phases of the walking cycle. List the main features of abnormal gait patterns.

10 / Posture and Breathing: The Trunk

10.1 Functions of the trunk

The trunk is the central axis of the body. The limbs use the trunk as a base on which to move. When the body is upright, the trunk supports the head and maintains the erect posture with minimal effort.

The trunk consists of the *thorax, abdomen and pelvis*, three cavities stacked one above the other (Fig. 10.1). Any change in the pressure inside one of the cavities affects the adjacent ones. The vertebral column links the three boxes posteriorly. The thoracic cavity extends from the clavicle and first rib above to the muscular diaphragm below. The abdominal cavity has the dome of the diaphragm as the roof. The blade of the iliac bone of the pelvis lies in the abdomen and the cavity leads down into the pelvis below. The pelvic cavity is a bowl formed by the sacrum and the two inferior bones (pubis and ischium), with a muscular floor. It is important to consider the three parts of the trunk as a functional unit, as changes in one part affect the other two.

The joints and muscles of the trunk combine to form a stable system when standing upright. The muscles act like guy ropes

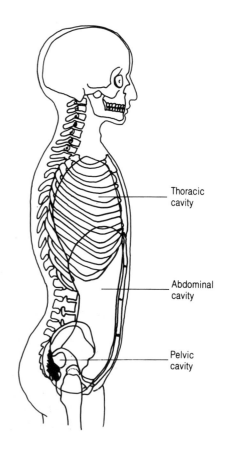

Thoracic cavity

Abdominal cavity

Pelvic cavity

Fig. 10.1. Side view of the trunk. Outlines of the thoracic, abdominal and pelvic cavities.

keeping the balance when external forces act on the trunk. If a group of muscles becomes weak, the trunk changes its position, just as a tent will lean to one side if a guy rope is loosened.

The trunk has a protective function for the lungs, heart, digestive tract, kidneys and pelvic organs (bladder, rectum and reproductive organs). The spinal cord is also protected by being enclosed by the bones of the vertebral column, with pairs of spinal nerves emerging between adjacent vertebrae to be distributed to all parts of the body.

Ventilation of the lungs is the result of movements of the thorax, the anterior abdominal wall and the muscular diaphragm. The muscle action of the anterior abdominal wall exerts its effect either on the diaphragm above to expel air, or on the pelvic cavity below to expel urine or faeces.

Lifting, carrying, pushing and pulling heavy loads all involve the trunk, which counteracts the forces on the limbs, and adjusts the line of weight over the foot base. Carrying a heavy load of shopping in one hand requires muscle activity on the opposite side of the trunk to balance the weight. Activity in the anterior abdominal muscles is important to reduce the load on the back in lifting loads from the front.

To summarise, the overall functions of the trunk are:

(1) To maintain the upright posture.

(2) To protect organs.

(3) To aid ventilation of the lungs.

(4) To adapt to changes in internal pressures when lifting loads.

(5) To expel urine, faeces and the foetus at birth.

Most of the movements of the trunk are performed by large muscles arranged in sheets around the axial skeleton. The position of the muscles and direction of the fibres determine the ways in which each contributes to trunk movement.

10.2 Upright posture

The bones and ligaments of the *vertebral column* form a stable balanced support that requires little muscle activity when standing still. Any slight sway is counteracted by the tension in the strong longitudinal ligaments joining the individual vertebrae. Each bone of the vertebral column articulates with the one above and the one below by a cartilaginous joint (intervertebral disc) between the bodies, and by four synovial joints between the articular processes. The position of the articular processes is shown in Appendix 1.

At birth, the vertebral column has a primary curve, concave forwards. As the baby learns to support the weight of the head and trunk in sitting and then standing, two secondary curves develop in the neck and lower back. From 2 years onwards, the vertebral column has four curves as follows: seven cervical vertebrae, convex forwards, secondary; twelve thoracic vertebrae, concave forwards, primary; five lumbar vertebrae, convex forwards, secondary; five sacral vertebrae, concave forwards, primary (fused); and three coccygeal vertebrae. The four curves provide an ideal way of combining support with flexibility and resilience (Fig. 10.2).

● *OBSERVE a partner standing upright. Look first from the side to imagine a line from the ear through the vertebral column to the hip and knee, ending just in front of the ankle. Move the trunk until the position looks balanced. Notice the curves of the back. Refer to an articulated skeleton to see the curves more easily. Next, look at your partner from the front to see if the shoulders and hips are level, i.e. no lateral curves.*

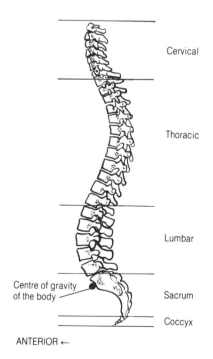

Cervical

Thoracic

Lumbar

Centre of gravity
of the body

Sacrum

Coccyx

Fig. 10.2. Vertebral column viewed from the side. Cervical, thoracic, lumbar and sacral curves.

ANTERIOR ←

- *WATCH a person sitting at a keyboard and notice the shape of the back in relation to the shape of the back of the chair. Try raising and lowering the keyboard to see the effect on the working posture.*
- *LOOK at elderly people sitting in easy chairs. Think where a cushion should be placed to support the lumbar curve of the back.*

If an abnormal posture is adopted over long periods of time, a balanced position is progressively lost and muscle activity must be used to a greater extent. Examples of abnormal posture are: **kyphosis**, standing with rounded shoulders; **lordosis**, standing with a hollow back; and **scoliosis**; lateral curvature to the spine, and tilting of the shoulders.

Shoes with high heels throw the body weight forwards and the vertebral column adapts by increasing the lumbar curvature (lordosis). Problems with breathing may develop in scoliosis due to the effect on the shape of the thorax. Poor working posture increases the possibility of low back pain, even in the young. In the elderly, degenerative changes in the vertebrae and discs due to disease or ageing, coupled with the loss of the need and motivation to move about during the day, give general loss of mobility, and deformity develops which may become permanent.

10.3 Movements of the trunk

When the trunk moves in different directions, the movement at the synovial joints between adjacent vertebrae is small, but the result of combined movement of vertebrae at all levels results in a considerable range of movement. During movement of the vertebral bodies, the fibrocartilaginous discs are compressed on one side (see Fig. 1.7b). The collagen fibres in the intervertebral discs are arranged in concentric layers, the annulus fibrosus. The semi-fluid central mass of the disc is the nucleus pulposus.

Clinical note-pad 10A: Prolapsed intervertebral disc

A movement that involves a sudden compression of the intervertebral disc may result in tearing of the annulus fibrosus, and this allows the nucleus pulposus to protrude and press on the spinal cord or the roots of a spinal nerve. Severe pain then radiates down the path of the affected nerve.

The movements of the trunk, seen in Figure 10.3, are described as follows.

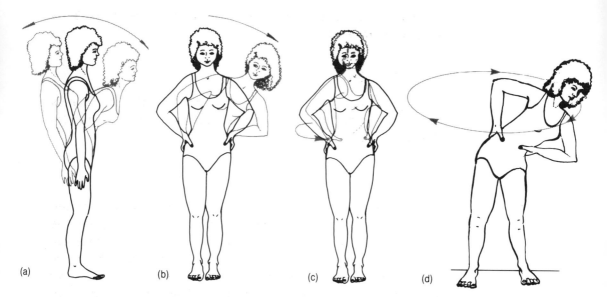

Fig. 10.3. Movements of the trunk: (a) flexion (forwards) and extension (backwards); (b) lateral flexion; (c) rotation; (d) circumduction.

Flexion: bend forwards, or sit up from lying, the ribs move towards the pelvis.

Extension: straighten the back and bend backwards; the ribs move away from the pelvis.

Lateral flexion: bend to the side, e.g. pick up a basket or case; the ribs move towards the pelvis on one side only.

Rotation: the trunk twists, the head and shoulders are turned so that the eyes can look to the side or behind, either to the right or left.

The 'trunk rolling' exercise shown in Figure 10.3d is a combination of all these movements.

The range of the individual movements varies in different parts of the vertebral column, depending on the thickness of the intervertebral discs, the direction of the articular facets of the synovial joints, and the length and angulation of the spines. The regions with secondary curves have the greatest mobility.

Movements of the cervical region are important for the eyes to scan a large area. Reversing a car becomes difficult when there is loss of mobility in the neck. The lumbar region has the greatest range for flexion and extension movements. The extreme bending movements of the acrobat and gymnast are made by continual exercises to stretch the intervertebral ligaments and increase the separation of the lumbar vertebrae. Conversely, the fusion of the lumbar vertebrae in some pathological changes of the spine will reduce the overall mobility of the trunk by a significant amount.

10.3.1 Muscles moving the trunk

Two systems of muscles collectively perform all the movements of the trunk: (a) the deep posterior muscles of the back; and (b) the abdominal muscles.

Deep posterior muscles of the back

The posterior aspect of the vertebral column, from the sacrum to the skull, provides a long line of bony processes for the attachment of muscle fibres. Some of these muscles fibres are long, extending from the sacrum to the thorax, while others are short and only span one, two or three vertebrae. The vertical fibres pull the column into extension, those arranged obliquely can rotate one vertebra on the next, and the lateral fibres which are attached to the angles of the ribs can assist lateral flexion.

The largest muscle in this group of deep back muscles is the **erector spinae** (also known as *sacrospinalis*) which originates from the sacrum by a thick broad tendon. In the lumbar region, this muscle is thick and can be palpated in the lower back. Continuing upwards, the muscle is in three bands in the thoracic region, attached to the spines, transverse processes and ribs. The uppermost fibres in the cervical region end on the base of the skull.

The muscles connecting the trunk to the upper limb, for example the latissimus dorsi and trapezius (described in Chapter 5), are separated from the deep muscles of the back by a layer of deep fascia.

Figure 10.4 follows the line of the erector spinae on the right hand side of the vertebral column. Note how the muscle starts at the sacrum and climbs up the back to the head. Deep to the erector spinae another group of muscles is found (Fig. 10.4, left hand side of vertebral column). Most of the fibres in this deeper group lie obliquely from the transverse process of one vertebra to the spine of the vertebra above, or they may span three or four vertebrae. The parts found in the thorax and neck are known as **semispinalis**.

In movements of the trunk, the erector spinae acts strongly to raise the body from flexion to an upright position.

The erector spinae is important in stabilising the bones of the vertebral column, and plays a role in lifting and carrying loads.

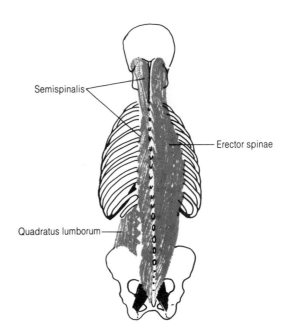

Fig. 10.4. Posterior view of the trunk to show the erector spinae on the right, the semispinalis and quadratus lumborum on the left.

Lifting from a starting position of bending forwards with straight legs is shown in Figure 10.5a. From this position, the erector spinae compresses the lumbar discs as it extends the back to raise the load of the trunk, the arms and the child. The line of weight is some distance from the fulcrum in the lower back, so that the load arm is long. The erector spinae, acting on a short lever arm, must develop considerable effort

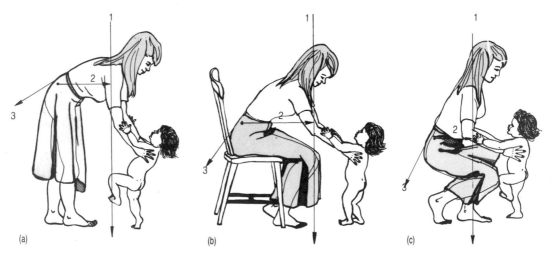

Fig. 10.5. Lifting: (a) straight legs; (b) sitting; (c) bent knees. 1 = line of weight, 2 = load arm, 3 = effort force.

force to overcome the moment of force of the trunk and the weight of the child. In lifting from the sitting position (Fig. 10.5b), the line of weight is even further from the fulcrum and the compression load on the discs is therefore much greater as the erector spinae extends the spine. People in wheelchairs should avoid lifting heavy loads, since the stress on the back will be greater than the same load lifted by someone who can stand close to the load. Lifting from a starting position with bent knees, and with the load as close to the body as possible (Fig. 10.5c) reduces the stress on the back by allowing the hip and knee extensors to contribute most of the power for the lift, and by shortening the lever arm of the trunk plus load.

It should now be clear how bending the knees as well as the back before lifting puts less stress on the back.

Abdominal muscles

The **anterior abdominal wall** consists of flat sheets of muscle forming a four-way corset or girdle between the ribs and the pelvis. The individual muscles are: (a) the *rectus abdominis*, which is a vertical panel down the centre of the abdomen; (b) the *external* and *internal obliques*, which form diagonal sheets of muscle at the side of the trunk; and (c) the *transversus abdominis*, which is a large horizontal band of muscle lying deep to the oblique muscles.

Figure 10.6a shows the direction of the fibres of the abdominal muscles seen from the side. The fibres of the two oblique muscles and transversus abdominis blend into an aponeurosis (dense fibrous tissue) towards the midline, connecting with those from the opposite side to form a sheath round the rectus abdominis.

The **rectus abdominis** (Fig. 10.6b) is a strap like muscle extending from the lower end of the sternum and the costal cartilages of the 5th, 6th and 7th ribs to the pubis below. The muscles fibres are usually interrupted at three intervals by transverse bands of fibrous tissue, known as tendinous intersections. The four bulges of muscle fibres in between can be seen in men who have done weight training.

The rectus abdominis flexes the trunk by pulling the sternum towards the pelvis, so acting strongly in sitting up from lying. When the body is lifted off the ground, as in running and jumping, the rectus abdominis supports the front of the pelvis.

Fibres of the **two oblique abdominal muscles** lie at right angles to each other. The **external oblique** is attached to the

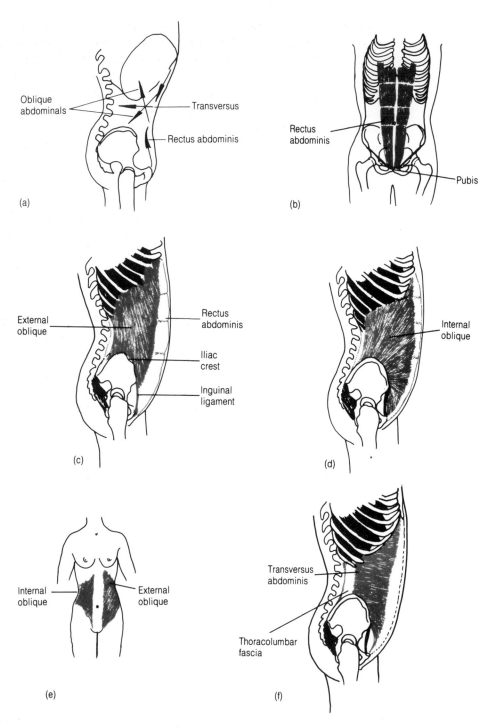

Fig. 10.6. Muscles of the anterior abdominal wall: (a) side view of the trunk to show the direction of the muscle fibres; (b) rectus abdominis, anterior view; (c) right external oblique abdominal, side view; (d) right internal oblique abdominal, side view; (e) oblique abdominals working together; (f) right transversus abdominis.

outer surfaces of the lower eight ribs. The posterior fibres pass vertically to insert on the posterior part of the iliac crest of the pelvis. All the other fibres lie in a direction downwards and forwards, i.e. like hands in a side pocket, to attach to the wide central aponeurosis (Fig. 10.6c). The lower margin of the muscle and aponeurosis is thickened to form the inguinal ligament, which extends from the anterior superior iliac spine to the pubic crest (see Chapter 8, Fig. 8.12). The inguinal ligament acts as a retinaculum forming the division between the trunk and the thigh. The **internal oblique** is attached to the fascia of the lower back (thoracolumbar fascia), the anterior iliac crest (deep to the external oblique), and the inguinal ligament. The muscle fibres pass upwards and inwards, to attach to the lower ribs, and become a wide aponeurosis as far as the midline (Fig. 10.6d). The aponeuroses of the right and left obliques meet in the midline at the linea alba, a strip of fascia from the lower end of the sternum to the pubic symphysis.

The various ways in which the two layers of oblique abdominal muscles work in combination to produce movements of the trunk will now be considered.

Flexion of the trunk involves the external and internal obliques on *both sides together*.

Lateral flexion involves the external and internal oblique on *one side only*.

Rotation of the trunk involves the external oblique on *one side* working with the internal oblique on the *opposite side*. The trunk then rotates towards the side of the internal oblique (Fig. 10.6e).

In standing and sitting, the oblique abdominals work with the neck muscles in turning to look to the side and behind. In walking, the pelvis is carried forwards on the side of the leading leg and the trunk rotates to keep the eyes looking forwards. The amount of rotation increases with the stride length.

● *LIE down supine and feel the abdominal muscles working in:*

(1) *Sitting up from lying.*

(2) *Lifting the head from lying. Feel the rectus abdominis working statically to fix the thorax so that the neck muscles can act on the head.*

(3) *Sitting up from lying while turning the trunk to the left at the same time. Think which abdominal muscles are working.*

The reasons why it is difficult to sit up from lying if the

abdominal muscles cannot function, for example after abdominal surgery, with fractured ribs, or in the late stages of pregnancy, should now be clear. In these instances sitting up can be performed by turning on to one side and pushing up with the opposite arm to raise the trunk. The legs can then be swung round to the sitting position.

The **transversus abdominis** is the deepest abdominal muscle originating from the inner aspect of the costal margin, the thoracolumbar fascia, iliac crest and inguinal ligament. From this extensive posterior origin, the fibres pass transversely round the abdomen to form a central aponeurosis anteriorly. The muscles from each side meet in the midline at the linea alba. Figure 10.6f shows the right transversus viewed from the side.

The transversus has no action in moving the trunk. The tension in transversus supports the abdominal organs and contraction increases the pressure inside the abdomen. This rise in pressure aids the expulsion of air from the lungs in breathing.

All the muscles of the **anterior abdominal wall** support and protect the organs of the abdomen and pelvis. A blow to the abdomen produces reflex contraction of the anterior abdominal wall and a temporary cessation of breathing.

When lifting loads with the back, contraction of the abdominal muscles can be used to reduce the pressure on the intervertebral discs of the lumbar region. The rise in intra-abdominal pressure during the lift is then distributed upwards and downwards, and this relieves the pressure on the lumbar vertebrae set up by the back muscles. Weight lifters learn to use the abdominal muscles to reduce the stress on the back. A sudden or unexpected demand for lifting can produce back strain, and even simple everyday tasks, like making a bed, can cause back injury. Some of the lifting tasks used in the care of the disabled have been replaced by the use of hoists, but it is still important to be aware that contraction of the abdominal muscles can relieve stress on the back when lifting a patient.

In straining movements to expel contents of the pelvic organs, for example urine and faeces, the muscles of the anterior abdominal wall contract to raise the pressure inside the abdomen and pelvis.

The function of the muscles in breathing will be discussed in Section 10.4.4.

The **posterior abdominal wall** between the twelfth rib and the posterior part of the iliac crest is formed by the *quadratus lumborum* (Fig. 10.4). This muscle lies lateral to the psoas and deep to the origin of the transversus abdominis.

Contraction of the quadratus lumborum on one side only, assists lateral flexion of the trunk. Acting in reverse, the muscle can lift the pelvic brim on the same side, which is important in single support, see Chapter 8, Section 8.3.2. When both sides contract, the lumbar vertebrae and the pelvis are stabilised for strong activity of the upper trunk and upper limb.

10.3.2 Muscles moving the head and neck

The two main functions of the muscles of the head and neck are to support the head so that it is held upright on the trunk, and to turn the head in all directions so that the eyes can focus over a wide field of vision.

Two of the muscles supporting the head on the trunk are the upper fibres of the trapezius (described in Chapter 5) and the upper part of the erector spinae (Section 10.3.1). Lying in between these two muscles at the back of the neck is another pair of muscles, the *splenius capitis* and *splenius cervicis* (Fig. 10.7).

Holding down the deep muscles of the neck in this region, the splenius capitis has been called the 'bandage muscle'. The splenius muscles are attached to the lower part of the ligament in the midline of the neck (ligamentum nuchae), and the spines of the upper four thoracic vertebrae. Passing upwards and laterally, the capitis is inserted on the base of the skull, to the mastoid process of the temporal bone and adjacent occipital bone. The splenius cervicis inserts on to the transverse processes of the cervical vertebrae 1 to 4. Working statically, the splenius

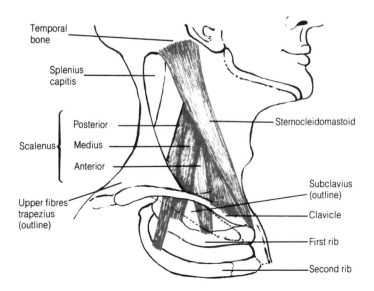

Fig. 10.7. Right side view of the neck to show the sternomastoid, and the scalenus anterior, medius and posterior.

muscles prevent the head from falling forwards. Both sides working together pull the head backwards in extension. If one side only contracts, the head is rotated to turn the face to the same side.

The most superficial muscle on the front of the neck, clearly visible in action, is the *sternocleidomatoid*, often shortened to sternomastoid (Fig. 10.7). This strap-like muscle crosses the neck diagonally, and combines with other muscles to perform all the movements of the head. Its name indicates the attachments of this muscle. From the upper end of the sternum and the medial end of the clavicle, the sternocleidomastoid crosses upwards and outwards to end on the mastoid process of the temporal bone of the skull, extending medially to meet the upper fibres of the trapezius.

Both sides of the sternomastoid working together draw the head forwards and act strongly to lift the head up when lying supine. One side contracting produces lateral flexion and rotation to the opposite side. These movements are important in looking from side to side to scan the visual field. The sternomastoid and the splenius muscles combine to produce most of the turning movements of the head. When the head is tilted backwards beyond the vertical, the sternomastoid can act as a neck extensor.

A group of three muscles in the lateral part of the neck are the **scalenes**; scalenus anterior, medius and posterior (Fig. 10.7). Attached centrally to the transverse processes of the cervical vertebrae, the scalenes pass downwards and laterally to the first and second ribs. These muscles are an important landmark in the location of the brachial plexus, which passes between the scalenus anterior and scalenus medius in its course towards the first rib.

The scalenes flex the cervical spine if both sides contract; or if one side only is active, produce lateral flexion. The muscles are also used to fix the first two ribs in deep inspiration prior to a powerful or long exhalation, as when singing or playing a wind instrument.

- *LIE SUPINE and lift the head. Feel the sternomastoid and scalenes in action.*
  Turn the head to the right and feel the left sternomastoid in action.

10.4 Movements of the thorax and abdomen in breathing

The action of the muscles moving the ribs, and the muscle dividing the thorax and abdomen (the diaphragm), combine to change the size of the thoracic cavity and to ventilate the lungs. The abdominal muscles are also involved in breathing, since their activity affects the position of the diaphragm.

The two lungs fill the thoracic cavity, apart from the space occupied by the heart and major blood vessels. Shaped like two cones, the base of each lung sits on the diaphragm and the apex of each lies above the clavicle. Each lung is surrounded by a narrow airtight space called the pleural cavity. The pleural membranes which form this cavity are attached to the outer surface of the lungs and the inner wall of the thorax. The cavity between the membranes is a completely enclosed space in which the pressure is lower than the pressure of the air outside the thorax. As the thorax expands due to muscle contraction, the lowered pressure in the pleural cavity causes the lungs to be expanded also. The two layers of pleura remain in contact like the sides of a new plastic bag when you try to separate them. When the lungs expand, the air pressure within the air sacs is reduced and atmospheric air is drawn in through the nose and trachea to equalise the pressure inside the lungs. Relaxation of the muscles reduces the size of the thorax to the resting volume and the pressure in the air sacs rises, therefore air passes out into the atmosphere.

The exact amount of air entering and leaving the lungs at any one time depends on the amount of movement of the thorax. Other factors that influence the volume of air breathed are the elasticity and inertia of the lung tissue, and the resistance offered by the airways in the lungs.

The increase in overall size of the thorax by muscle action is essential for the inspiration of air into the lungs. In quiet breathing, expiration is passive. The relaxation of the muscles active in inspiration allows the thorax to return to the resting size. The extra air ventilated by the lungs in deep breathing is the result of additional muscle activity during inspiration, and expiration involves active muscle contraction.

Clinical note-pad 10B: Pneumothorax

If the pleural membranes are punctured by a stab wound, or as a result of infection, then air can enter the pleural cavity and the pressure rises. This reduces tension on the elasticity of the lung and it collapses. Once the pleural membrane heals, the excess air is slowly absorbed into the blood stream and the lung reinflates. This process can be used clinically to allow lung tissue to rest and repair.

10.4.1 Movements of the ribs in quiet breathing

The 12 ribs articulate with the thoracic vertebrae posteriorly. The first seven ribs articulate directly with the sternum in front, while the 8th, 9th and 10th ribs are linked indirectly to the sternum by their costal cartilages. The 11th and 12th ribs, which are small and free anteriorly, play little part in breathing.

- *LOOK at the position of the ribs on an articulated skeleton. Posteriorly, identify the position of two synovial joints, one between the head of the rib and the body of the vertebra, one between the tubercle of the rib and the transverse process. Anteriorly, the first to seventh ribs join with the sternum by the costal cartilages.*

    Note two things about the general direction of ribs 2 to 7: (a) the anterior end is lower than the vertebral articulations; and (b) when viewed from the side, the central part of each rib is lower than both the anterior and the posterior ends.

Movement at the joints of ribs 2 to 7 occurs around two axes simultaneously. Figure 10.8 shows the two axes – AA' and BB'.

One axis (A–A') passes through the neck of each rib. When the rib moves about this axis, the sternum is raised upwards and forwards to increase the anterior to posterior diameter of the thorax.

The other axis (B–B') passes through the angle of the ribs posteriorly and the sternocostal joints anteriorly. Movement about this axis lifts the middle of the rib upwards and outwards to increase the transverse diameter of the thorax.

The eighth, ninth and tenth ribs have no sternocostal joints and therefore only move about one axis (A–A').

Fig. 10.8. Movement of a rib in side view and plan view. A–A' axis through the neck of the rib, B–B' axis through the vertebral and sternal ends of the rib.

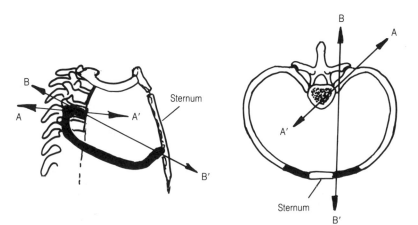

- *PLACE your hands on the thorax of a partner, first at the sides over the lower rib cage. Ask your partner to breathe in deeply and watch how your hands move further apart, i.e. the thorax becomes wider.*

  Next, stand at the side and place one hand flat on the sternum, the other hand flat on the thoracic vertebrae. Again ask your partner to breathe in deeply, and notice how the hand on the sternum moves forwards and upwards.

  These two movements occur together each time the ribs move.

Muscles acting on the ribs

The *external* and *internal intercostal muscles*, which form two layers in the space between adjacent ribs, move the ribs in quiet breathing.

The fibres of the **external intercostal muscles** pass obliquely from the lower border of one rib to the upper border of the rib below. At the anterior end of each intercostal space, the muscle is replaced by membrane. The posterior fibres pass downwards and laterally, and the more anterior fibres lie downwards and medially, i.e. in the same direction as the external oblique abdominal muscles. The first rib does not move in quiet breathing. Figure 10.9 shows the position of the external intercostal muscles in the spaces between ribs 1 to 6.

Contraction of the external intercostals lifts the ribs about the two axes described. The thorax increases in size by expanding in a forwards and sideways direction and air is drawn into the lungs.

The **internal intercostal muscles** lie deep to the external intercostals, and their fibres are at right angles, downwards and backwards from one rib to the one below. The muscle fibres are

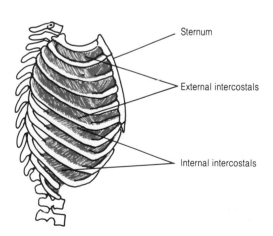

Sternum

External intercostals

Internal intercostals

Fig. 10.9. Side view of the thorax to show the intercostal muscles. Internal intercostal muscles (shown in the lower 6 spaces) lie deep to the external intercostals (shown in the upper 5 spaces).

replaced by membrane at the posterior end of the intercostal space, between the angle and head of each rib. Figure 10.10 shows the position of the internal intercostal muscles in the spaces between ribs 6 to 10. There is conflicting evidence about the action of the internal intercostals. It has been shown that the anterior fibres between the costal cartilages are active in inspiration. Other studies have shown activity during speech, which is expiratory. The contribution of the internal intercostals to rib movements probably depends on which fibres are active, and on the level of inflation of the lungs.

Relaxation of the intercostal muscles lowers the ribs to their resting position, and air leaves the lungs. Expiration in quiet breathing is therefore passive.

10.4.2 Movements of the ribs in deep breathing

The muscles in the neck which elevate the shoulder girdle and upper ribs allow the thorax to expand further in inspiration.

The main muscles that are recruited to increase the depth of inspiration are the *sternomastoid*, the *scalenes* (Fig. 10.7) and the *pectoralis minor*.

When the upper attachments of the sternomastoid and the scalenes are fixed, these two muscles will pull the clavicle and first two ribs upwards.

The pectoralis minor is a small muscle attached to the coracoid process of the scapula, and its fibres pass downwards to the third, fourth and fifth ribs (see Chapter 5, Fig. 5.10). If the scapula is fixed, this muscle will also lift the upper ribs.

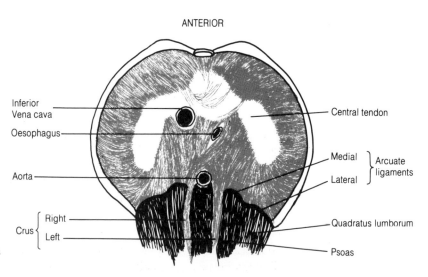

Fig. 10.10. Diaphragm viewed from below.

- *WATCH the neck of a person breathing deeply to see the activity in neck muscles.*

In deep expiration, the *latissimus dorsi* (Fig. 5.6a), which wraps round the rib cage from the lower back to the shoulder, can compress the ribs further if the humerus is fixed. The abdominal muscles are also involved (see Section 10.4.4) when expiration becomes active instead of passive.

Clinical note-pad 10C: Asthma and COAD

Asthma occurs in children and adults. There are attacks of breathing difficulty in response to certain protein substances, such as pollen or animal protein, which release allergens within the body. The muscular walls of the narrow airways in the lungs constrict. Inspiration which is initiated by muscle activity can take place, but passive expiration becomes difficult. Expiratory muscles have to be used to try to force the air out of the lungs.

Chronic obstructive airways disease (COAD) occurs in the elderly. There is a chronic inflammation of the lining of the airways (chronic bronchitis) and the air sacs become distended (emphysema). The thorax and the lungs become less elastic. The muscles of the neck and shoulders, normally used in deep inspiration, are used for quiet breathing, and diaphragmatic breathing becomes more important.

10.4.3 Movements of the diaphragm

The diaphragm is a dome shaped muscle which forms the floor of the thoracic cavity. At rest, the fibres of the peripheral part of the dome are almost vertical. Converging inwards, the muscle fibres end in a central tendon, a strong flat aponeurosis shaped like a trefoil or clover leaf. The central tendon is nearer to the front of the thorax than the back, so that the posterior fibres are longer. The heart lies immediately above the central tendon, and the pericardium, the membrane round the heart, is attached to it.

- *LOOK at an umbrella (with a very curved shape if possible). The ribs of the umbrella are in the direction of the muscles fibres of the dome of the diaphragm. Imagine the point of the umbrella compressed into a flat trefoil shape to understand the position of the central tendon.*

Figure 10.10 is a view of the diaphragm from below (i.e. in the abdomen looking up to the under surface of the muscle). The diaphragm originates all around the lower margin of the thorax.

Beginning anteriorly, fibres originate from the xiphoid process of the sternum. Next, ribs 7 to 12 and their costal cartilages form the largest surface for the attachment of fibres. Posteriorly, the origin from the twelfth rib is interrupted by the muscles of the posterior abdominal wall, quadratus lumborum and psoas. These two muscles are bridged by fibrous bands, known as the lateral and medial arcuate ligaments, which provide a base for the attachment of the diaphragm. The most posterior fibres originate from the sides of the lumbar vertebrae by two bands, the right crus (from L1, L2, and L3) and the left crus (from L1 and L2), which arch over the aorta in the midline. The right crus is longer to overcome the resistance of the larger liver lying below the diaphragm on the right side.

Figure 10.10 follows the complete circle that forms the origin of the diaphragm, which can be summarised as follows. Sternal fibres: from the xiphoid process of the sternum. Costal fibres: from the inner surfaces of the 7th to 12th ribs. Lumbar fibres: from the arcuate ligaments over the muscles of the posterior abdominal wall, and from the lumbar vertebrae by two crura.

Figure 10.11 shows how the sternal origin is higher than the lumbar origin. The inferior vena cava passes through the central tendon, and the oesophagus passes through the muscular part just towards the left of the midline. The aorta lies posteriorly against the vertebral column.

Action of the diaphragm. When the diaphragm is *active*, the contractile muscle fibres pull the central tendon *downwards* and the dome becomes flatter.

When the diaphragm *relaxes*, the muscle fibres return to their resting length and the central tendon moves *upwards*.

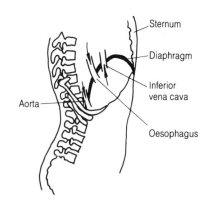

Fig. 10.11. Diaphragm viewed from the side.

10.4.4 Abdominal muscles in breathing

The muscles of the anterior abdominal wall can actively participate in breathing out. Contraction of the abdominal muscles raises the pressure inside the abdomen and the diaphragm is pushed *up*. The vertical diameter of the thorax is decreased and air is expelled from the lungs in expiration. The diaphragm and abdominal muscles cooperate in breathing movements in the following way. Inspiration: diaphragm descends, abdominals relax. Expiration: abdominals contract, diaphragm moves upwards.

- *PLACE YOUR HANDS on the anterior abdominal wall.*
  Breathe in deeply, lifting the ribs and feel the abdominals relax as the diaphragm moves down. Breathe out deeply, contracting the abdominals to expel more air.

During quiet breathing, the contribution of the abdominal muscles to the ventilation of the lungs varies in different individuals. In deep breathing, the contraction of the abdominal muscles increases the depth of expiration. The control of the muscle work of the abdominals is important in singing and in some relaxation techniques.

10.5 Movements of the pelvis

The bony pelvis is formed by the two hip bones and the sacrum (see Appendix 1). The two hip bones articulate together anteriorly by a cartilaginous joint (the pubic symphysis), and each articulates posteriorly with the sacrum at the sacroiliac joints. The weight of the trunk above tends to tilt the upper end of the sacrum forwards and the lower end backwards. This tendency for rotation of the sacrum is prevented by the sacrospinous and sacrotuberous ligaments, two strong bands which bind the sacrum to the hip bone (Fig. 10.12). The pelvis is a staging post for muscles passing upwards to the trunk or downwards to the lower limbs.

The muscles attached to the pelvis that act on the trunk are the rectus abdominis, the oblique abdominals, the erector spinae and the quadratus lumborum.

The muscles attached to the pelvis that act on the lower limbs are the gluteus maximus, medius and minimus, the hamstrings, the hip adductors, the rectus femoris, the tensor fascia lata and the sartorius (see Chapter 8).

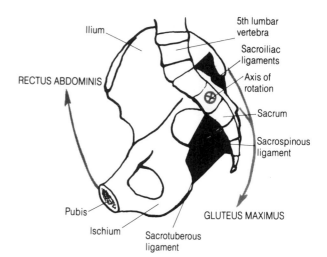

Fig. 10.12. Medial aspect of the right pelvis. Arrows indicate the direction of pull of the rectus abdominis and gluteus maximus in controlling pelvis tilt.

The tilt of the pelvis in relaxed standing largely depends on the opposing tension in the rectus abdominis pulling the pubis up towards the ribs, and the gluteus maximus pulling on the posterior surface of the sacrum in the opposite direction (Fig. 10.12). Lateral tilting of the pelvis when one leg is lifted off the ground is counteracted by contraction of the gluteus medius and minimus on the supported side (see Chapter 7). When the glutei and the knee flexors are weak, the tilting of the pelvis to the unsupported side can be counteracted by the contraction of the quadratus lumborum and the latissimus dorsi on that side; this is known as 'hip hitching'.

The iliopsoas (Fig. 8.9) links the lumbar spine and pelvis with the femur and is used to raise the legs when lying supine. If the knees are extended, iliopsoas has to develop a very large force to lift the weight of the leg acting on a long lever arm, and may pull on the lumbar spine causing back strain. Therefore, double leg raising, often used to exercise the abdominals, should be avoided.

The pelvic floor

The muscles of the floor of the pelvis are suspended from the bony walls of the pelvis, and from a fibrous arch, a thickened band in the pelvic fascia. This fibrous arch extends from the pubis anteriorly to the spine of the ischium posteriorly, and the main muscle of the pelvic floor, the *levator ani*, is attached to it. The fibres of the levator ani descend and then turn inwards to meet those from the opposite side in the midline (Fig. 10.13).

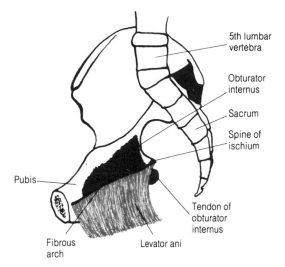

5th lumbar
vertebra

Obturator
internus

Sacrum

Spine of
ischium

Pubis

Tendon of
obturator
internus

Fibrous
arch

Levator ani

Fig. 10.13. Medial aspect of the right pelvis to show obturator internus and levator ani (cut).

Posteriorly to the levator ani, the pelvic floor is completed by the *coccygeus* which extends from the spine of the ischium to the lower part of the sacrum and the coccyx.

The functions of the pelvic floor are to support the pelvic organs, and to withstand any increase in pressure in the abdomen and pelvis, for example in lifting, coughing and sneezing. In women, the levator ani surrounds the vagina and supports the uterus.

Clinical note-pad 10D: Stress incontinence

Stretching of the muscle in childbirth may affect the action of the levator ani on the control of the bladder and the rectum. This leads to incontinence, particularly at times when there is a sharp rise in intra-abdominal pressure such as coughing, sneezing and laughing.

10.6 Nerve supply of the muscles of the trunk

The **posterior primary rami** of the spinal nerves supply all the deep muscles of the back, including the erector spinae, and in the cervical region supply the splenius capitis and cervicis (see Chapter 4, Section 4.2.1).

All the other muscles of the trunk are supplied by branches of the **anterior primary rami** of the spinal nerves. The spinal accessory (cranial) nerve, together with branches of C2 and C3, supplies the sternomastoid. Branches of C6, C7 and C8 supply

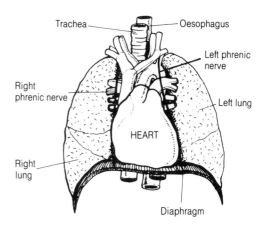

Fig. 10.14. Position and relations of the phrenic nerves in the thorax.

the scalene muscles, and S3 and S4 supply the muscles of the pelvic floor.

10.6.1 Phrenic nerves

The phrenic nerves are formed from branches of the third, fourth and fifth cervical nerves in the neck, and supply the diaphragm. Each nerve passes down the neck deep to the sternomastoid and enters the thorax. The right phrenic nerve lies on the pericardium covering the right atrium and pierces the central tendon of the diaphragm with the inferior vena cava. The left phrenic nerve lies on the pericardium over the left ventricle and pierces the diaphragm in front of the central tendon (Fig. 10.14).

Each phrenic nerve is the motor and sensory supply to the corresponding side of the diaphragm.

> ### Clinical note-pad 10E: Cervical spine injuries
>
> Injuries to the neck occur by falls from a height, a blow on the head, or violent free movements of the neck. If there is damage to the roots of the phrenic nerves (C3, C4 and C5), a loss of the action of the diaphragm in breathing occurs and a ventilator must be used.

10.6.2 Intercostal nerves

The muscles of the thoracic and abdominal walls are supplied by the intercostal nerves, T1–T12.

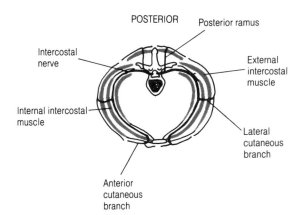

Fig. 10.15. Transverse section of an intercostal space with one pair of intercostal nerves.

Thoracic nerves 1–6 run parallel to the corresponding rib and deep to the internal intercostal muscles (Fig. 10.15).

Thoracic nerves 7–12 also supply the corresponding intercostal muscles, and continue forwards from the intercostal spaces to the muscles of the anterior abdominal wall. Each layer of the abdominal wall (the rectus abdominis, the external oblique, the internal oblique and the transversus) receives branches of thoracic nerves 7–12 from above downwards.

Thoracic nerve 12 is known as the subcostal nerve and branches to supply the quadratus lumborum.

10.7 Summary of the muscles of the trunk

(1) *Muscles moving the head and neck.* Sternocleidomastoid; scalenus anterior, medius and posterior; splenius capitis and cervicis.

(2) *Muscles moving the thorax in the ventilation of the lungs.* External and internal intercostals; diaphragm.

(3) *Deep posterior muscles of the back.* Erector spinae (sacrospinalis).

(4) *Abdominal muscles.* Anterior abdominal wall: rectus abdominis, external oblique, internal oblique, transversus. Posterior abdominal wall: quadratus lumborum.

(5) *Pelvic floor.* Levator ani and coccygeus.

At the end of this chapter, you should be able to:

(1) Summarise the functions of the trunk.

(2) Explain how the vertebral column is arranged to combine support and resilience in the upright posture.

(3) Demonstrate the movements of the trunk and list the muscles producing them. Explain how the starting position for lifting a load affects the stress on the back.

(4) Outline the position and actions of the muscles of the anterior abdominal wall, and list their collective functions.

(5) Describe the muscle action involved in ventilation of the lungs in quiet and deep breathing.

(6) List the muscles acting on the pelvis, and the function of the muscular floor of the pelvis.

(7) Outline the role of the phrenic and intercostal nerves in breathing.

Further Reading for Section 2

Akesson E.J., Loeb J.A. & Wilson-Pauwels L. (1990) *Thompson's Core Textbook of Anatomy*. JB Lippincott Co., Philadelphia.

Apley A.G. & Solomon L. (1994) *Concise System of Orthopaedics and Fractures*. Butterworth-Heinemann Ltd., Oxford.

Basmajian J.V. (1989) *Grant's Method of Anatomy*. 11th edn., Williams & Wilkins, London.

Caillet R. (1994) *Hand Pain and Impairment*. 4th edn., FA Davis Co., Philadelphia.

Kapandji J.I. (1982) *The Physiology of the Joints*, Vols. 1, 2 and 3. E & S Livingstone, Edinburgh.

Lehmkulh L.D. & Smith L.K. (1983) *Brunstrom's Clinical Kinesiology*. FA Davis Co., Philadelphia.

Moffat D.B. & Mottram R.F. (1987) *Anatomy and Physiology for Physiotherapists*. 2nd edn., Blackwell Science, Oxford.

Palastanga N., Field D. & Soames R. (1989) *Anatomy and Human Movement, Structure and Function*. Heinemann, Oxford.

Rasche P.J. & Burke R.K. (1989) *Kinesiology and Applied Anatomy, The Science of Human Movement*. 7th edn., Lea & Febinger, Philadelphia.

Stone R.J. & Stone J.A. (1990) *Atlas of Skeletal Muscles*. Wm.C Brown Publishers, USA.

Thompson C.W. & Ford R.T. (1993) *Manual of Structural Kinesiology*. 12th edn., CV Mosby Co., St. Louis.

Section 3 Integration of Movement
SENSATION, ACTION AND PERFORMANCE

11 / Sensory Background to Movement

All movement starts with a background of sensory information about the space around us, and about the position of the body, entering the central nervous system. As movement proceeds, this sensory activity changes from moment to moment.

- *THINK about the variety of incoming signals as you walk along a rough path towards a gate. From the eyes scanning the visual field ahead, sensing the movement of objects on either side of the path, and anticipating obstructions that must be avoided. From the skin of the feet detecting the roughness of the path. From the attitude and movement of the head in relation to the body to keep the balance. From the joints and muscles in the moving body parts.*

We are aware of some of the changes, but many of the responses to the changing input are entirely automatic. We do not fall over, we do recognise obstacles in our path and avoid them by changing direction. In the absence of information from the eyes, we rely more heavily on information from the other sources of input including sound and smell. Some of the automatic responses to the changing input are basic protective reflexes, and we may find ourselves doing them even when there is no threat. For example, we may blink and 'duck' the head when a bird flies towards the windscreen as we drive in a car along the road. If there is a deficit in the processing of sensory information due to neural damage or disease, the motor performance dependent on it cannot proceed normally.

11.1 Sensory subsystems in movement

The sensory system can be divided into subsystems, each providing specific information to the central nervous system. Three of these subsystems will be considered, with emphasis on their role in movement. The familiar description of 'five senses' (vision, hearing, taste, smell and touch) is incomplete with the omission of proprioception, the information about the position and the movement of body parts. The three main subsystems which provide the monitoring of changes during movement are the *somatosensory system*, the *vestibular system* and the *visual system*.

The **somatosensory** (or somaesthetic) **system** is our body sensation. It monitors a wide variety of stimuli from all over the body. From this system we know where the arms are in space, the pressure of a pencil held in the fingers, and how cold the wind is on our face.

The skin is part of this subsystem. The skin is not only a

simple sense organ for touch, but responds to the particular pressure and temperature of surfaces. In gripping, the feedback from all the receptors of the skin in contact with the object guides the muscle force that is required. Pressure receptors in the skin of the soles of the feet monitor the distribution of body weight over the feet, and therefore assist balance reactions.

Proprioceptors, which report the position and the movement of body parts from the muscles and joints are also part of the somatosensory system. The response of muscle spindles in the elbow flexors to an object held in the hand allows us to judge its weight. If you hold someone's hand, you are feeling touch, also the temperature and weight of the hand, and you may sense whether the person is tense or relaxed.

All these cues are possible due to the large variety of receptors in the skin, the joints and the muscles, which collectively respond to many types of stimulation.

The **vestibular system** detects movement of the head. It has been considered part of proprioception since it monitors the position and movement of the head, but the vestibule also functions with the visual system for the control of eye movements.

The receptors for this subsystem are found in the vestibule and semicircular canals of the ear, lying in the cavity of the temporal bone of the skull, behind the organ for sound (the cochlea). We are largely unaware of activity in this system, except when we are in a jerky lift or at the fairground. The vestibular system gives us our sense of stability, and it plays a vital role in keeping the body in balance during movement.

The **visual system** contributes to our sense of balance by providing visual information about the orientation of objects in the space around us. We use vertical and horizontal structures, such as walls, doors and furniture, to align the position of the body. Information from the eyes about the movement of objects held in the hand allows corrections to be made to make accurate and precise movements. When the eyes are closed, all movement becomes more difficult, and highly skilled movements become almost impossible.

11.2 Input from the skin, joints and muscles (somatosensory system)

The two main ascending pathways in the somatosensory system are: (a) the *medial lemniscus pathway* – posterior (dorsal) column; and (b) the *anterolateral pathway* – spinothalamic tracts. Both the systems link the receptors on one side of the body with the somatosensory area in the opposite parietal lobe. The antero-lateral pathway crosses at the spinal level, while the medial lemniscus crosses in the sensory decussation in the medulla of the brain. The pathways converge in the brain stem, and both synapse in the thalamus. All the fibres from *both* the anterolateral and medial lemniscus pathways pass through the internal capsule to end in the somatosensory area of the parietal lobe where the body parts are represented in a particular topographical arrangement (see Chapter 3, Section 3.4.2).

- *REVISE the composition of a spinal nerve from Chapter 4, and the position of ascending tracts of the spinal cord described in Chapter 3.*
- *LOOK at Figure 11.1 to follow the general plan of these two pathways.*

The function of each of the two sensory pathways is different, even though some of the sensation transmitted appears to be the same. The medial lemniscus pathway is concerned with fast acting information that has a high degree of discrimination. For example, changes in joint position occur rapidly during movement. The changing activity in the joint proprioceptors is conducted via this route. The anterolateral pathway on the other hand conducts the reponses from stimuli, such as temperature, that are neither urgent nor require precise location.

11.2.1 Medial lemniscus pathway (posterior/dorsal column)

The medial lemniscus pathway provides the route for several different modalities of sensation: touch, vibration, joint position and joint movement. This ascending route also plays a part in the interpretation of pain (see Section 11.2.3). The important role of the medial lemniscus pathway is in the combination of input from more than one modality to interpret complex sensations. For example, both two-point discrimination of touch and proprioception are involved in the ability to distinguish a particular texture. The size and shape of an object is judged by touch and by the movements of the hand required to hold it.

The activity in the medial lemniscus route is initiated by receptors that are fast adapting with large diameter axons. These receptors are found in the skin and also lying in muscles, tendons and joints (proprioceptors). The sensory neurones enter the posterior horn of the spinal cord, and then pass into the posterior (dorsal) column of white matter of the same side. (Many of the first order neurones branch to synapse in the posterior horn at the spinal level of entry.) The posterior column of white matter,

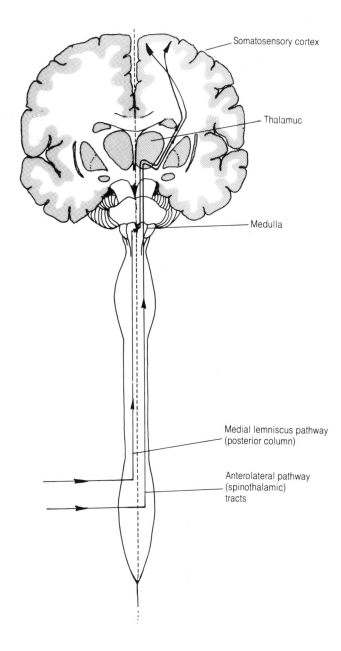

Somatosensory cortex

Thalamus

Medulla

Medial lemniscus pathway
(posterior column)

Anterolateral pathway
(spinothalamic)
tracts

Fig. 11.1. Frontal section of the brain
with spinal cord; ascending pathways
to the sensory cortex – general plan.

lying underneath the lamina of each vertebra, becomes larger as
it ascends the spinal cord collecting sensory fibres from each
spinal nerve. In the medulla of the brain, the neurones end in
the gracile and cuneate nuclei. At this level, the second order
neurones cross to the opposite side and pass through the brain
stem in the medial lemniscus to the thalamus. The third order
neurones project to the somatosensory cortex.

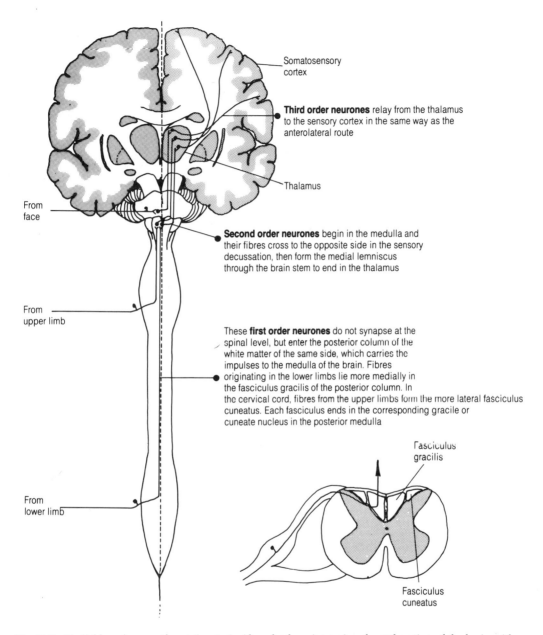

Somatosensory cortex

Third order neurones relay from the thalamus to the sensory cortex in the same way as the anterolateral route

Thalamus

From face

Second order neurones begin in the medulla and their fibres cross to the opposite side in the sensory decussation, then form the medial lemniscus through the brain stem to end in the thalamus

From upper limb

These **first order neurones** do not synapse at the spinal level, but enter the posterior column of the white matter of the same side, which carries the impulses to the medulla of the brain. Fibres originating in the lower limbs lie more medially in the fasciculus gracilis of the posterior column. In the cervical cord, fibres from the upper limbs form the more lateral fasciculus cuneatus. Each fasciculus ends in the corresponding gracile or cuneate nucleus in the posterior medulla

Fasciculus gracilis

From lower limb

Fasciculus cuneatus

Fig. 11.2. Medial lemniscus pathway (posterior/dorsal column) seen in a frontal section of the brain with spinal cord, and its position in the TS of the spinal cord (fasciculus cuneatus and fasciculus gracilis).

- *LOOK at Figure 11.2 to trace the route followed by the medial lemniscus pathway in the central nervous system. Identify the three orders of neurone.*

11.2.2 Anterolateral pathway (spinothalamic tracts)

This pathway is primarily concerned with the sensations of temperature and pain. The spinothalamic tracts play a supplementary role for touch sensation, but probably only become important when the medial lemniscus pathway is damaged.

Activity in the anterolateral pathway originates in sensory neurones with slowly adapting receptors in the skin. The sensory neurones have small diameter axons with slow conduction velocity. These sensory neurones enter the spinal cord and synapse in the posterior horn before crossing to the opposite side to enter the spinothalamic tract. The fibres of the spinothalamic tract lie in the anterolateral white matter of the spinal cord. This route has been divided into anterior and lateral spinothalamic tracts, but more recent work has shown no difference in the spread of fibre types across the spinothalamic tract. There is a topographical arrangement of the spinothalamic fibres in the white matter, with those from distal body segments more lateral, and proximal areas more medial.

The spinothalamic tract continues in the brain stem, to end in the thalamus. The third order neurones project from the thalamus to the somatosensory area in the parietal lobe.

- *LOOK at Figure 11.3 to trace the route followed by the anterolateral pathway in the central nervous system. Identify the three orders of neurone in the pathway.*

    Return to Figure 11.1 to find the fibres in the brain stem lying alongside those from the medial lemniscus pathway.

Some of the first order neurones in this **anterolateral pathway** synapse with interneurones in the spinal cord before synapsing with the second order neurones, i.e. before entering the ascending tract on the opposite side (see Section 11.2.3). In the brain stem, some of the second order neurones branch to link with the reticular formation.

The **posterior columns** are ipsilateral, i.e. they contain fibres carrying sensation from the same side of the body. Fibres from the lower limbs are mostly medial and form the fasciculus gracilis. As more fibres enter the spinal cord (travelling from sacral to cervical segments) they are added laterally. In this way, the fibres from the upper limb form the fasciculus cuneatus. Some of the fibres from proprioceptors in the *lower limb* leave the posterior column and form the ascending *posterior spinocerebellar tract* in the lateral white matter. These fibres rejoin the second order neurones of the posterior column as they cross in the medulla of

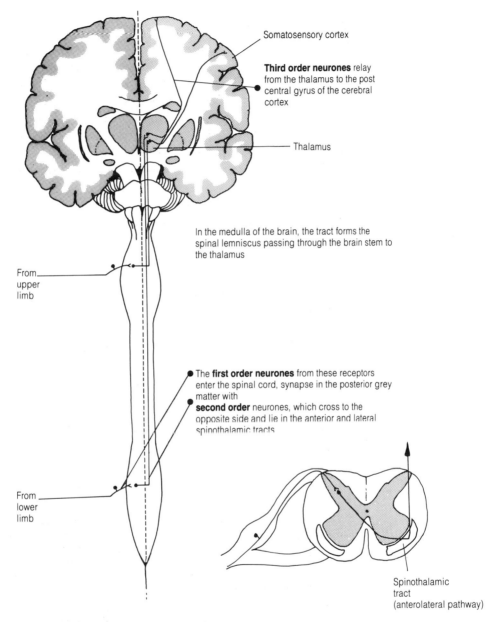

Somatosensory cortex

Third order neurones relay from the thalamus to the post central gyrus of the cerebral cortex

Thalamus

In the medulla of the brain, the tract forms the spinal lemniscus passing through the brain stem to the thalamus

From upper limb

The **first order neurones** from these receptors enter the spinal cord, synapse in the posterior grey matter with **second order** neurones, which cross to the opposite side and lie in the anterior and lateral spinothalamic tracts

From lower limb

Spinothalamic tract (anterolateral pathway)

Fig. 11.3. Anterolateral pathway (spinothalamic) seen in a frontal section of the brain with spinal cord and its position in the TS of the spinal cord.

the brain. In the medial lemniscus all the fibres carrying proprioception information are lying together. Figure 11.4 shows the position of the main ascending tracts in position in the spinal cord at the level of the cervical segments. A similar section at the level of the lumbar segments would have a smaller posterior column with no fasciculus cuneatus.

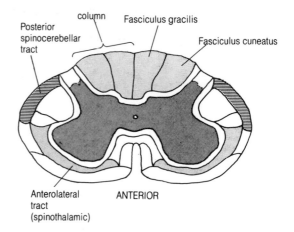

Fig. 11.4. TS spinal cord . Position of the ascending tracts at the level of the cervical segments.

Sensory information from the face

Receptors in the skin and the muscles of the face and mouth enter the brain stem mainly in the *trigeminal* (fifth cranial) nerve and synapse in the sensory nuclei of this nerve. Second order neurones cross to the opposite side and lie alongside the medial lemniscus to reach the thalamus. Third order fibres end in the region representing the face in the somatosensory cortex in the parietal lobe. Input from this trigeminal system is important for the sensory background to the movements of facial expression, swallowing and speaking.

Clinical note-pad 11A: Sensory loss in spinal cord damage

Sensory loss occurs when the posterior roots of the spinal nerves and/or the posterior column of white matter are damaged in the following ways:

(1) degeneration of myelin in the spinal cord in multiple sclerosis;

(2) infection, e.g. AIDS; or

(3) diseases involving the vertebral column and/or intervertebral discs, e.g. ankylosing spondylitis and prolapsed discs.

The outcome depends on the segmental level and the extent of the spinal cord damage. Sensory loss occurs on the same side of the body below the spinal level affected, so that cervical damage affects upper and lower limb function. Loss of position and movement sense in the lower limbs gives a poor prospect for walking. The overall sensory loss is severe in bilateral lesion of the posterior columns.

11.2.3 The interpretation of pain

Pain is a subjective sensation and many aspects of the experience of pain cannot be explained by activity in one specific route from pain receptors to the somatosensory cortex. The gate theory of pain attempts to explain how a painful stimulus may be interpreted in different ways at different times and by different individuals. There are interneurones in the substantia gelatinosa of the posterior horn of the spinal cord that act as a spinal cord mechanism for the transmission of pain into the two ascending pathways to the brain. Figure 11.5a shows how some large diameter fibres of the medial lemniscus route, and some small diameter fibres of the anterolateral route, synapse with cells in the substantia gelatinosa (SG). These in turn synapse with larger transmission cells (T cells), whose axons cross the spinal cord to lie in the anterolateral pathway of the opposite side. The interneurones in the substantia gelatinosa form what is known as the *pain gate*.

Activity in the small diameter fibres stimulates the T cells and impulses enter the anterolateral system so that pain is felt. The pain gate is *open* (Fig. 11.5b).

If there is activity in the large diameter fibres which form the posterior column of white matter, the SG cells are stimulated and these in turn *inhibit* the transmission cells. This prevents activity entering the anterolateral pathway and no pain is felt. The gate is *closed* (Fig. 11.5c).

In this way, the transmission of pain impulses depends on the balance of activity in the first order neurones of the medial lemniscus and the anterolateral routes.

The pain gate theory explains how stimulation of the skin over a painful area by rubbing often reduces pain; the tactile stimuli increase the activity in large diameter fibres and close the gate. The effectiveness of acupuncture in the relief of pain may be partly explained by the stimulation of large diameter fibres. Electrical devices applied to the skin, or implanted in the posterior column of the spinal cord, can be used to relieve severe intractable pain. Patients can then control the stimulation of large diameter fibres and close the gate.

Descending pathways in the spinal cord from the *reticular formation* of the brain stem also synapse with interneurones in the fasciculus proprius (see Fig. 3.27b) at the spinal level and in turn *inhibit* the transmission cells (Fig. 11.5a). This suggests how brain centres can influence whether or not pain is felt. The pain from an injury may not be felt by a footballer or athlete while

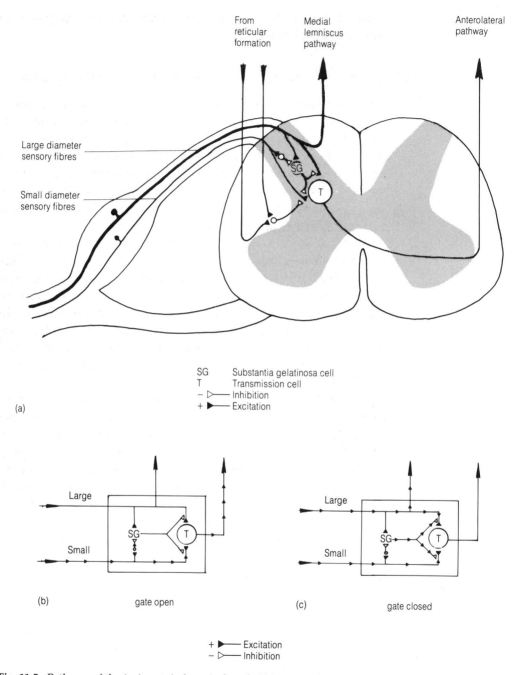

Fig. 11.5. Pathway of the 'pain gate', the spinal cord: (a) input and output to the SG and T cells in the posterior horn of the spinal cord; (b) pain gate open, less inhibition of T cells by SG cells; (c) pain gate closed, more inhibition of T cells by SG cells. SG = cells in substantia gelatinosa; T = transmission cells.

there is a high level of activity in the descending pathways during the match or race.

11.3 Input from the position of the head (vestibular system)

The vestibular system monitors the position of the head in relation to the body and the movement of the head in relation to the space around the body. The brain processes this information to control the muscles of the trunk (axial muscles) and keep the body in balance. The vestibular system also links with the nerves supplying the eye muscles, via the brain stem, so that the eyes can be kept 'on target'. This will be discussed in more detail in Section 11.4, the visual system.

The receptors which activate the vestibular pathway are in the *vestibule* and *semicircular canals* of the inner ear which consist of five fluid filled sacs communicating with each other, arranged in the form of: (a) two oval bulbs, about 5 mm in diameter, known as the utricle and saccule, that together form the **vestibule**; and (b) three **semicircular canals**, about 1 mm in diameter, lying above and behind the utricle and saccule. One canal lies in each of the three planes of the head – superior, posterior and lateral (Fig. 11.6).

The proprioceptors found in the walls of these sacs respond to movement of the fluid in the sacs as the head moves in space and in relation to gravity. Each receptor responds to a particular direction and velocity of head movement. Together, the receptors are important for maintaining the balance of the body, and for monitoring the movement of the head. We are not generally aware of vestibular activity, so that it may be difficult at first to appreciate its importance in everyday movement.

In the **vestibule**, the receptor areas which lie in the walls of

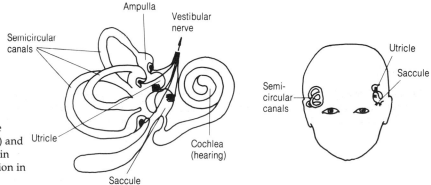

Fig. 11.6. Vestibule (utricle and saccule) and semicircular canals in the inner ear. Position in the head.

the utricle and saccule are called otoliths or maculae. The receptor cells have projecting cilia embedded in a jelly like mass, which contains particles of calcium called otoconia (Fig. 11.7a). If the head tilts, the fluid in the sacs lags behind the movement of the walls of the utricle and saccule, the cilia are bent and the sensory cells are stimulated (Fig. 11.7b). Sideways tilting of the head results in increased firing of impulses from one saccule and less from the opposite saccule. The otoliths on the base of the utricle signal when the head is bent forwards and backwards. In horizontal movement of the head and body, for example when sitting in a car or a train moving forwards, the otoconia lag behind the movement of the wall of the sac, the cilia are again bent and the sensory cells stimulated (Fig. 11.7c).

A simple way to try to understand the mechanism of the utricle or saccule is to imagine a football filled with fluid. If the football is tilted or moved steadily in a horizontal direction, there is always a delay in the movement of the fluid inside the football. This moment of delay would be signalled by flexible pins projecting from the inner side.

The **semicircular canals** are thin tubes with relatively less fluid than the utricle and saccule. Receptor areas in the semicircular canals are found in the ampulla, a swelling at the base of each canal. Sensory cells in the ampulla also have cilia embedded in a jelly like structure called the cupula, but there are no calcium particles (Fig. 11.8a). The cupula forms a flap like a swing door, moving backwards and forwards in response to movement of the fluid along the canal as the head moves. As the cupula bends, the cilia move and the hair cells are stimulated. Rotation of the head affects the canal lying in the same plane of movement. Figure 11.8 shows the direction of head movement that stimulates each of the canals on the left side of the head.

The five fluid filled sacs of the vestibule and semicircular canals form the anatomical structure known as the membranous

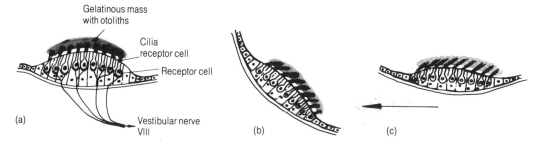

Fig. 11.7. Otolith receptors in the utricle and saccule: (a) head upright; (b) head tilted; (c) head movement.

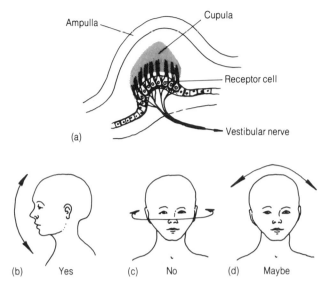

Ampulla

Cupula

Receptor cell

Vestibular nerve

(a)

Fig. 11.8. (a) Cupula in the ampulla of a semicircular canal. (b), (c) and (d) Directions of head movement for stimulation of each canal on the left side of the head: (b) 'yes'; (c) 'no'; (d) 'maybe'.

(b)   Yes

(c)   No

(d)   Maybe

labyrinth. Although individual receptors may respond to a greater extent in particular movements of the head, it is the combined effect of movement of the fluid in all the cavities that is integrated in the vestibular nucleus. The automatic responses to stimulation of these receptors are known as *vestibular* or *labyrinthine reflexes*.

Return to Chapter 4, Section 4.4.2 and Figure 4.10 to revise the pathways in and out of the vestibular nucleus. The vestibulo-ocular reflex, which maintains a constant image on the retina as the head moves, has already been described. The vestibulospinal reflex keeps the body in balance if you start to fall to one side. The vestibule signals the change in head position, and the extensor muscles on the same side of the body increase their activity via the vestibulospinal tracts. The neck muscles on the opposite side also contract to keep the head upright.

Clinical note-pad 11B: Vertigo

Vertigo is a sense of rotation together with a sense of imbalance of the head, which occurs in many disorders of the vestibule. Menière's disease (unknown cause and occurs mainly in men over 40 years), motion sickness and viral infection all produce vertigo. Nausea and dizziness accompany the instability.

11.4 Input from the eyes

Light entering the eyes passes through several transparent layers of cells and blood vessels to reach the rods and cones, the primary receptor cells. The retina itself is like a 'mini brain' and some processing occurs in its layers of cells before transmission along the fibres of the optic nerve to the brain.

One function of the retina is to act as a system for signalling movement in the environment around the body. When we move in a particular direction, the eyes are fixed on the centre of the visual field ahead. Images of objects moving on either side of us are signalled by the receptors in the periphery of the retina. When the eyes follow a moving object, such as a tool held in the hand, images from the tool remain stationary on the retina and those from the background sweep across the retina. In both cases, the retina is transmitting information about the changes in the visual environment during movement.

The visual pathway, from the eyes to the striate cortex in the occipital lobes of the cerebral hemispheres (Fig. 11.9), branches in the midbrain just before the lateral geniculate nucleus. These fibres, which synapse in the superior colliculus of the midbrain, allow the visual system to cooperate with the vestibular system in keeping the body balanced during movement.

The contribution of the eyes to our sense of balance can be demonstrated as follows.

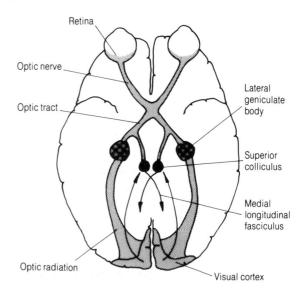

Fig. 11.9. The visual system.

- *STAND on one leg with the eyes open, and then with the eyes closed. Notice how much you sway, and may fall over when the eyes are closed.*
- *TRY running over rough ground at night. The fine adjustments needed to place the feet accurately and with the correct force are more difficult without the visual input.*

The visual input becomes more important during movement as a target is approached. In reaching out to grasp a glass of water, or running to jump on a bus, visual information is crucial in the final stage of gripping the glass or negotiating the step.

Clinical note-pad 11C: Visual impairment

The visually impaired person has to rely on alternative input for detecting the presence of obstacles, the nature of supporting surfaces and the form of objects to be manipulated. Touch, pressure, sound and proprioception all help to compensate for loss of vision. Perceptual and cognitive functions such as spatial awareness, recognition from sound and smell, and semantic memory are also important.

In this chapter we have outlined a variety of sensory information entering the central nervous system during movement. Within the central nervous system the overall patterns of signals at any one moment are integrated and processed at different levels. Like a radio receiver with an infinite number of channels, the sensory input is tuned to 'listen' to particular combinations of signals so that they can be recognised and acted on.

Vision probably plays the major role in the overall sensory information involved in movement. The visual system is not only a monitor of visual changes in the external environment, but it also reinforces proprioceptive information about the movement of body parts, and cooperates with the vestibular system in maintaining the balance of the body.

The sensory system has a remarkable capacity to adapt to loss, particularly in the young. The reorganisation of neurones to compensate for the loss may involve axons growing new branches to make new connections, and the diversion of activity along previously unused routes.

At the end of this chapter, you should be able to:

(1) Distinguish the functions of the three main parts of the sensory system: somatosensory, vestibular and visual.

(2) Describe in outline the two main ascending pathways of the somatosensory system in the central nervous system: medial lemniscus (posterior column) and anterolateral (spinothalamic). Appreciate the difference between the fast discriminating function of the medial lemniscus route, compared with the slower, more diffuse function of the anterolateral tracts.

(3) Summarise the interpretation of pain based on the pain gate theory.

(4) Give a brief summary of the role of the vestibular system in the maintenance of balance during movement, including the names and position of the receptors which respond to changes in the position of the head.

(5) Appreciate the importance of vision in movement.

12 / Motor Control

All the movements we make in daily activities, such as dressing, speaking, eating, writing and walking, are controlled by motor centres in the brain. Activity passes down from these motor centres in descending pathways to the motor neurones of the cranial nerves in the movements of speaking, eating and facial expressions, and to the motor neurones of spinal nerves in the movements of the limbs and trunk. The motor system moves the arms in skillful activity, the legs in walking, and controls the background posture of the whole body. The same system is involved in movements of the tongue, lips and larynx needed for speech.

In the brain, the motor areas of the cerebral cortex interact with the basal ganglia and the cerebellum to form the highest level of motor control. Motor nuclei in the brain stem are particularly concerned with the control of the posture and the balance of the body as the movement proceeds. Motor control in the spinal level is the result of a variety of influences from the descending pathways from the brain, and from the proprioceptors in the muscles and tendons themselves.

The activity of the spinal motor neurones will be considered first, and then the influence from descending pathways from the brain.

12.1 Lower motor neurones: motor activity at the spinal level

The lower motor neurones form the final route to the muscles in all movement, both voluntary and reflex. The cell bodies of the lower motor neurones lie in the anterior horn of the spinal cord and in the nuclei of the cranial nerves. The axons of the lower motor neurones lie in the peripheral nerves supplying the muscles (see Fig. 1.15).

Lower motor neurones are stimulated by activity in: (a) the descending pathways which terminate in the anterior horn of the spinal cord at all levels (see Section 12.2); and (b) local spinal reflexes. Two of the local spinal reflexes are the *myotatic (stretch) reflex* and the *Golgi tendon reflex*.

12.1.1 The myotatic reflex: static and dynamic activity

Activity in the myotatic unit, which maintains a muscle at constant length to hold a position, has been described in Chapter 1 (Section 1.6). During movement, muscles **do change in length**, and the level of reflex activity is modified by changing the 'setting' of the spindles. The intrafusal fibres of the muscle spindles are supplied by the smaller fusimotor (gamma) neurones.

If these neurones are excited by impulses from descending pathways in the spinal cord, the intrafusal fibres of the spindle contract. The spindle then becomes taut and more sensitive to length changes in the muscle (Fig. 12.1a). On the other hand, if the impulses from the descending tracts inhibit fusimotor neurones, the spindle becomes slack and only responds to marked changes in the length of the muscle (Fig. 12.1b). In this way, the higher levels of the central nervous system modify spinal stretch reflex activity during movement.

Consider the hand performing fine manipulative movements, such as doing up buttons and tieing shoe laces. Stretch reflex activity must be damped in the muscles of the hand to allow rapid length changes to occur. At the same time, muscles of the

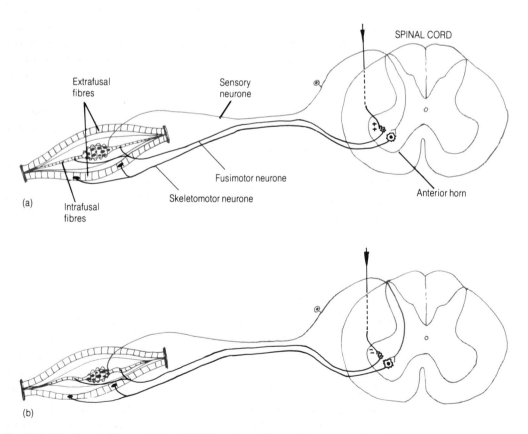

Fig. 12.1. Muscle spindle sensitivity: (a) high – descending pathways stimulate fusimotor neurones, the intrafusal fibres contract and the muscle spindle is very sensitive to distortion; (b) low – descending pathways inhibit fusimotor neurones, intrafusal fibres are slack and the muscle spindle is less sensitive to distortion.

shoulder and arm perform background activity to hold the
postion of the limb and allow the fingers to move accurately.
The spindles in the supporting muscles are set at a high level, so
that any change in length is resisted. During movements of the
whole limb, the setting of the spindles in all the active muscle
groups is continually monitored by the cerebellum as the
movement proceeds.

Static and dynamic intrafusal fibres

If we look in more detail at the structure of the muscle spindle
shown in Figure 1.19, two different types of intrafusal fibres can
be identified. Both types have a primary sensory ending wound
round the central area (the annulospiral endings described in
Chapter 1). In addition, some of the intrafusal fibres have
secondary sensory endings towards the periphery of the fibre,
known as flower spray endings, which respond to the rate of
change in length of the muscle during movement. The two types
of intrafusal fibre are: (a) *nuclear bag fibres* with a bulge in the
middle where the nuclei are found and secondary sensory
endings are present; and (b) *nuclear chain fibres* which are thinner
and have nuclei which are lined up in a row.

The **nuclear bag** (dynamic) **fibres** respond to rapid changes
in length of the muscle, while the **nuclear chain** (static) **fibres**
respond to prolonged slow stretch. The muscle spindles, therefore, relay detailed information about both the length, and the
rate of change in length, of a muscle during movement to
the spinal cord. Stretch reflex activity can then be adjusted to the
appropriate level during the progress of a movement.

12.1.2 Golgi tendon reflex

Receptors are also found in the tendons of muscles. They lie
embedded in the collagen fibres of the tendon and in series with
the muscle fibres. Remember that the muscle spindles lie in
parallel with the muscle fibres. The Golgi tendon organs are not
activated by the tension present in muscles at rest, since they
have a higher threshold of stimulation than muscle spindles.
When the tension in a muscle rises rapidly, the muscle pulls on
the tendon and the Golgi tendon organs are stimulated. Figure
12.2 shows the Golgi tendon reflex pathway. The sensory
neurones synapse with small interneurones which are inhibitory
to the lower motor neurones. The result is that *less* activity
reaches the muscle, and the tension is reduced by *relaxation* of

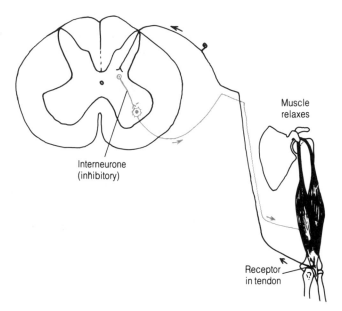

Muscle
relaxes

Interneurone
(inhibitory)

Receptor
in tendon

Fig. 12.2. Golgi tendon reflex.

the muscle. The tendon organs therefore act as a protective mechanism to prevent sudden rise in tension which might tear a muscle or tendon, and also cooperate with the muscle spindles by providing a control system for muscle tension.

Clinical note-pad 12A: Lower motor neurone lesion

Interruption of lower motor neurones may be due to damage of the cells in the anterior horn of the spinal cord (for example in polio-myelitis), or to the motor axons in peripheral nerves (for example in peripheral nerve injury). The result is loss of tendon reflexes, and of muscle tone in the absence of stretch reflex activity. The muscles usually feel limp and have no 'life' (hypotonia). Muscle wasting occurs with time and there is risk of contractures (see clinical note-pad 1A). Note: hypertonia can occur in a limb in lower motor neurone lesion when there is overactivity in the unaffected muscles.

12.2 Upper motor neurones: brain stem and cortical levels

The neurones which link motor areas in the brain with the spinal cord and with the cranial nerve nuclei are know as *upper motor neurones*. They lie in descending tracts in the brain stem and the spinal cord. The collective output from these upper motor neurones influences the level of activity in the lower motor neurones of the spinal cord, which in turn controls the active muscles during movement.

Upper motor neurones synapse at all levels in the spinal cord with alpha motor neurones supplying Type I and Type II muscle fibres (see Section 1.4.1), and also with gamma motor neurones innervating the intrafusal fibres of muscle spindles. In this way, the upper motor neurones affect both the recruitment of motor units, and the level of stretch reflex activity in the muscles.

12.2.1 Motor centres in the brain stem and descending pathways

The upper motor neurones that originate in subcortical motor areas of the brain relay in various motor nuclei in the brain and form polysynaptic routes to the lower motor neurones.

Figure 12.3 shows the **input** to the motor centres in the brain stem.

The **tectum** of the midbrain contains two pairs of nuclei, the superior and inferior colliculli. Visual and auditory information is processed in these nuclei. The output to the muscles of the neck initiates changes in the position of the head in response to the sound or to the changes in the visual field. Examples of this response can be observed in driving a car, standing on an unstable surface, and in group activities, such as team games.

The **red nucleus** in the midbrain (sometimes included with the basal ganglia) is a motor nucleus that provides a link between the cerebellum and the lower motor neurones of the spinal cord on the opposite side. There is no direct descending pathway from the cerebellum to the lower motor neurones.

The **vestibular nucleus** in the medulla receives input from the vestibule of the ear (see Chapter 4, Fig. 4.12, and Chapter 11, Section 11.3). The descending tract from the vestibular nucleus links to the lower motor neurones of the extensor muscles which provide support for the body as the head turns during movement.

The **reticular formation** which extends along the core of the brain stem is a collection of nuclei that are loosely connected. The reticular formation receives ascending somatosensory information from the spinal cord, and also descending fibres from the cerebral cortex which terminate bilaterally. There are two areas of the reticular formation which probably play a role in the support and balance of the body during movement. The medial group of neurones originates in the pons, and the lateral group originates in the medulla.

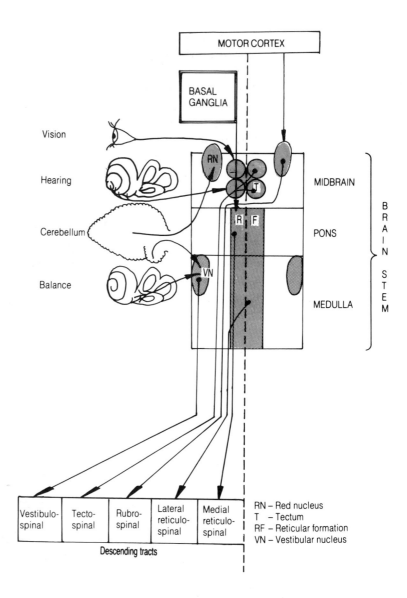

Fig. 12.3. Motor centres in the brain stem (diagrammatic). Origin of the descending tracts from the brain stem centres is shown.

Descending pathways from the brain stem motor centres

The axons of upper motor neurones originating in the motor areas of the brain stem are:

(1) the tectospinal tract from the tectum of the midbrain;

(2) the rubrospinal tract from the red nucleus of the midbrain;

(3) the vestibulospinal tract from the vestibular nucleus in the medulla; and

(4) the reticulospinal tracts (medial and lateral) from the reticular formation in the pons and medulla respectively.

The tectospinal tract, concerned with the control of head movements, is only present in the cervical segments.

The descending tracts synapse with skeletomotor (alpha) and fusimotor (gamma) motor neurones at the spinal level (Fig. 12.4). Some fibres are excitatory and others are inhibitory. The overall action of these pathways on the fusimotor neurones is inhibitory, to eliminate unwanted tone, so allowing skillful movement to take place.

The main function of the rubrospinal and lateral reticulospinal tracts is in positioning and support by the proximal muscles of the limbs during movement. For example, the muscles around the shoulder region, the elbow and the wrist, which support the upper limb during fine manipulation movements of the hand, are mainly activated via these routes. The vestibulospinal and medial reticulospinal tracts are more concerned with the activation of the muscles of the neck and trunk to counteract the

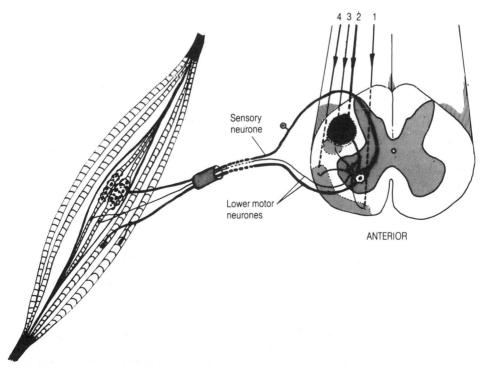

Fig. 12.4. Position of the descending tracts in the spinal cord and their termination on the skeletomotor and fusimotor neurones in the spinal cord: 1 = vestibulospinal tract; 2 = lateral corticospinal tract; 3 = rubrospinal tract; 4 = tectospinal tract.

effects of gravity, and to maintain the posture and balance of the whole body.

12.2.2 Motor areas of the cerebral cortex and descending pathways

Upper motor neurones originating in the *primary motor area* (described in Chapter 3, Section 3.4.1) form a fast direct route via the brain stem and the spinal cord to the lower motor neurones. The neurones in the primary motor cortex are large pyramidal cells with large diameter fast conducting axons. The descending tracts from this area are:

(1) the lateral and anterior *corticospinal* tracts; and

(2) the *corticobulbar* (or corticonuclear) tracts.

The **corticospinal tracts** descend from the primary motor area through the brain stem to the spinal cord. Neurones of the premotor cortex and the primary somatosensory area also contribute some fibres to the corticospinal tracts.

The corticospinal fibres converge as they enter the posterior limb of the internal capsule (see Chapter 3, Fig. 3.15). Passing into the brain stem, the fibres lie anteriorly in the cerebral peduncles of the midbrain, and continue down through the pons. At the level of the medulla, 85% of the fibres cross to the opposite side and enter the lateral white matter of the spinal cord to become the *lateral corticospinal tract*. The other fibres continue anteriorly in the white matter of the spinal cord as the *anterior corticospinal tract*. The area where the fibres cross in the medulla is known as the decussation of the pyramids (see Fig. 3.17c). Fibres of both tracts terminate in the spinal cord, where they synapse with lower motor neurones. The anterior corticospinal fibres cross at the level of the segment they supply. Some corticospinal fibres relay via interneurones at the spinal level.

The **corticobulbar tract** fibres originate in the same cortical areas. In the midbrain, pons and medulla of the brain stem, the fibres terminate in the motor nuclei of cranial nerves III–XII.

Movement of the muscles on one side of the body is initiated by the motor areas of the opposite cerebral cortex. The corticobulbar fibres link via cranial nerves with the muscles of the face, and the corticospinal fibres link via spinal nerves with the muscles of the limbs and trunk. The most important function of the corticospinal tract is the voluntary control of skilled precision

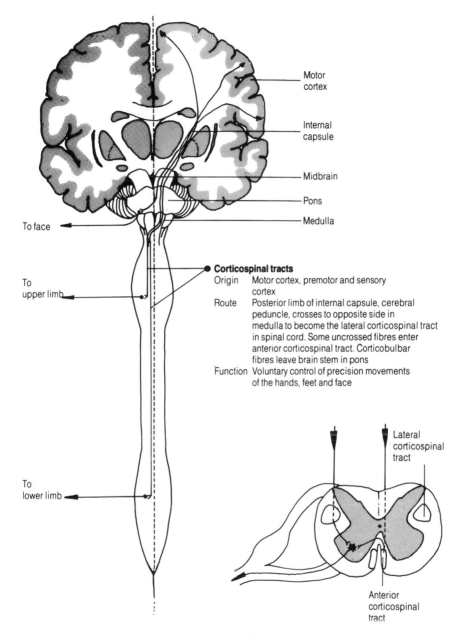

Motor cortex

Internal capsule

Midbrain

Pons

Medulla

To face

To upper limb

Corticospinal tracts
Origin   Motor cortex, premotor and sensory
            cortex
Route   Posterior limb of internal capsule, cerebral
            peduncle, crosses to opposite side in
            medulla to become the lateral corticospinal tract
            in spinal cord. Some uncrossed fibres enter
            anterior corticospinal tract. Corticobulbar
            fibres leave brain stem in pons
Function   Voluntary control of precision movements
            of the hands, feet and face

Lateral corticospinal tract

To lower limb

Anterior corticospinal tract

Fig. 12.5. Frontal section of the brain with the spinal cord. Pathway of the corticospinal and corticobulbar tracts. Transverse section of the spinal cord shows the position of the corticospinal tracts.

movements of the distal muscle groups of the limbs. The muscles involved in speech, facial expression and eye movements are controlled via the corticobulbar tracts.

Figure 12.5 shows the route followed by the corticospinal and corticobulbar tracts.

Summary of upper motor neurones

The upper motor neurones have been divided into the following.

(1) The *pyramidal system* for the direct descending pathway from the cortical motor areas to the lower motor neurones.

(2) The *extrapyramidal system* for all the other descending pathways from the brain to the lower motor neurones. These routes are largely polysynaptic.

The division into pyramidal and extrapyramidal was originally based on the assumption that the motor cortex, activating the pyramidal system, is concerned with voluntary movement, while the extrapyramidal system is involved in background postural activity during movement. Recent evidence suggests that the only special function of the pyramidal system is in the control of precision movements of the hands and feet. The extrapyramidal system is involved in all movements, both voluntary and reflex.

Clinical note-pad 12B: Upper motor neurone lesion

Interruption of upper motor neurones may be due to a cerebral vascular accident, brain injury or cerebral tumour. The outcome is variable. Lesions can cause increased tendon reflexes and spasticity due to loss of higher centre control of the stretch reflex. Movement is often most affected in the fine coordinated movements of the fingers and hands. Abnormal movement patterns may appear. The upper limb may show flexor synergy, and the lower limb may demonstrate an extensor synergy, so that normal movements are difficult to perform. There is a risk of muscle contracture.

- Hemiplegia is an upper motor neurone lesion affecting motor and/or sensory loss on one side of the body. It is usually due to damage to the contralateral cerebral hemisphere, or to the brain stem above the level of crossing of the corticospinal tracts in the medulla.

12.3 Basal ganglia and cerebellum

The highest level of control of motor activity is composed of the cortical motor areas together with the basal ganglia and cerebellum. The cortical motor areas include the primary motor area, the premotor area and the supplementary motor area. Both the basal ganglia and the cerebellum interact with them.

12.3.1 Basal ganglia

The individual nuclei of the basal ganglia link together to form a functional unit (see Chapter 3, Section 3.5). Most of the input to the basal ganglia is from the cerebral cortex, and the system of basal ganglia projects back to the cortex of the same side via the thalamus. Two control loops are formed in this way: (a) cortex, caudate and putamen (striatum), globus pallidus, thalamus, cortex; and (b) cortex, caudate and putamen (striatum), globus pallidus, substantia nigra, thalamus, cortex (Fig. 12.6). This interaction between the motor cortex and the basal ganglia forms a high level motor control system for the forward planning and execution of voluntary movement.

The basal ganglia have no direct link with the spinal cord. Their influence on the lower motor neurones is via descending pyramidal and extrapyramidal pathways from the cortical motor areas.

12.3.2 Cerebellum

The cerebellum links with the motor cortex of the opposite side by a loop which crosses the midline (Fig. 12.7). Corticospinal

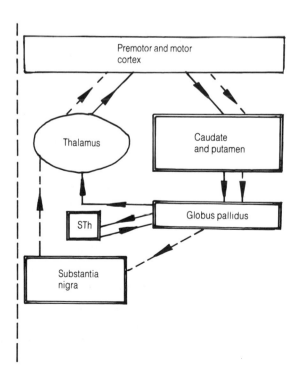

Fig. 12.6. Motor control loops between the basal ganglia and the motor cortex. STh = subthalamic nucleus.

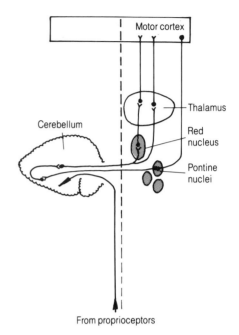

Fig. 12.7. Motor control loop between the cerebellum and the motor cortex crossing the midline.

fibres originating in the motor cortex branch in the brain stem to synapse in the *pontine nuclei* and then link with the opposite cerebellar cortex. In this way, there is a fast input from the motor cortex to the cerebellum which crosses the midline. A return pathway links the cerebellum across the midline back to the motor cortex via the thalamus.

The cortical control loop with the cerebellum allows for comparison of the intended movement with the sensory information reaching the cerebellum from the proprioceptors in the muscles and joints of the body. The cerebellum then modifies the activity of the motor cortex via the return loop, to correct the progress and timing during the muscle activity, and also to bring the movement to a halt at the right moment.

The cerebellum has no direct descending tracts to the spinal cord, but exerts an influence on the lower motor neurones via the brain stem nuclei (red nucleus, vestibular nucleus and reticular formation) and their descending pathways (see Section 12.2.1).

12.4 Summary of the three levels of motor control

The motor system functions at three levels of control.

The **spinal level** executes movement patterns based on spinal reflexes and on the activity received from higher levels of the nervous system. The muscle spindles play a major part in the spinal control of muscles during movement by their effect on the activity in the lower motor neurones.

The **brain stem** contains the nuclei with the cells of origin of many of the descending extrapyramidal tracts, which modify activity at the spinal level to maintain the posture and balance of the body. Input to the brain stem nuclei is mainly from the eyes, the vestibule of the ear, and from proprioceptors via the cerebellum.

The **higher centres** (cortical motor areas, basal ganglia and cerebellum) plan and execute movement with constant reference to the changing sensory information from the external environment and from the active muscles. Movement can be modified during its progress and the end goal achieved. Fine coordinated movements of the hands and fingers require the highest level of motor control.

In the motor system as a whole, it is the lower motor neurones in the spinal cord that form the final common pathway to the muscles. Movements are controlled by the influence of the motor centres in the brain, with their descending pathways of upper motor neurones, on the lower motor neurones. The primary motor cortex and the motor centres in the brain stem have direct links to the spinal cord, while the basal ganglia and the cerebellum exert their control mainly via their connections with the motor cortex.

At the end of this chapter, you should be able to:

(1) Define a lower motor neurone and an upper motor neurone and distinguish between them in relation to effects of lesion.

(2) Augment the understanding of the myotatic unit (stretch reflex) from Chapter 3 to include: (a) changes in the sensitivity of the muscle spindles; and (b) modification of stretch reflex activity via descending pathways during movement.

(3) Name the motor centres in the brain stem and their descending pathways in the spinal cord. Outline their role in the control of background posture during movement.

(4) Describe the descending pathways from the primary motor cortex: corticobulbar and corticospinal. Distinguish the function of the corticobulbar and corticospinal tracts in the control of

skilled precision movements of the eyes, the face, and the distal musculature of the limbs.

(5) Augment the knowledge of the basal ganglia and the cerebellum from Chapter 3 to include the control loops between each of these two brain areas and the motor cortex. Distinguish the function of the basal ganglia and the cerebellum in the planning and the modification of movement respectively.

(6) Summarise the three levels of control in the motor system: spinal, brain stem and higher centres.

13 / Integration and Performance

The integration of input from the sensory system with activity in the motor system is an essential part of movement performance to reach a particular goal. The simple movement of pouring water from a kettle into a cup involves integration of the input from visual, tactile and proprioceptive pathways with activity in the motor centres controlling the muscles of the upper limb.

In the execution of movement we can consider that motor commands are generated in the central nervous system, which sets up the particular pattern and timing of nerve impulses to the muscles to perform the movement. The muscle groups are activated in a specific sequence, with each group producing the correct force, direction and timing of action. The motor commands for a particular movement have been called a *motor programme* or *engram*. The early stages of the development of a motor programme involve the integration of sensory input with the motor commands. With practice, learned movements can be performed without relying so heavily on feedback from the sensory system. Stored motor programmes can then be activated, and the movement can proceed without moment to moment reference to sensory input. This has been compared with the activation of a computer programme, for example a programme to draw a coloured shape on the screen. The analogy is, however, too simplistic, and more recently the motor programme has been redefined. Motor commands for a sequence of movements may have motor programmes for each component of the activity with sensory feedback included in the programme.

The integration of sensory and motor information occurs at all levels in the central nervous system. In this chapter, some of the mechanisms for the local integration of activity in networks of neurones will be considered, followed by integration at the spinal and brain stem levels. Finally, the performance of skilled movement is outlined with special reference to the role of the cerebellum and the basal ganglia.

13.1 Integration in neurone pools

We have described how impulses pass from one neurone to another at a synapse in Chapter 1, Section 1.5.1. Collections of neurones in the central nervous system that have a particular function are called neurone pools (see Chapter 1, Fig. 1.14). The motor neurones in the anterior horn of the spinal cord which supply a group of muscles form a neurone pool. The nuclei of cranial nerves are other examples of neurone pools. We will now consider some of the ways in which groups of neurones can regulate their own input and output.

Within a network of neurones, the axons of each neurone branch to synapse with many other neurones (divergence), and each cell body receives branches from many other neurones (convergence) (Fig. 13.1). An example of convergence is in the motor neurone pools of the spinal cord where neurones receive input from all the descending pathways (see Chapter 12, Fig. 12.4). Divergence allows the input from one source to be relayed in different directions at the same time. It has been estimated that each of the neurones in the brain has 100 inputs converging on to it, and each neurone diverges to 100 other neurones. The number of possibilities for the route of impulses through a neurone network in the brain is therefore enormous.

The balance of excitatory and inhibitory influences within a group of neurones affects its output. There are several ways in which this balance may be changed.

Neurotransmitters

The most common neurotransmitter substance in the nervous system is acetylcholine. In the brain, several other substances have been identified such as dopamine, GABA, serotonin and enkephalin. Dopamine is an inhibitory transmitter released by neurones in the substantia nigra (one of the basal ganglia). In addition, the sensitivity of neurones to transmitter substances can be changed by the presence of other chemicals known as

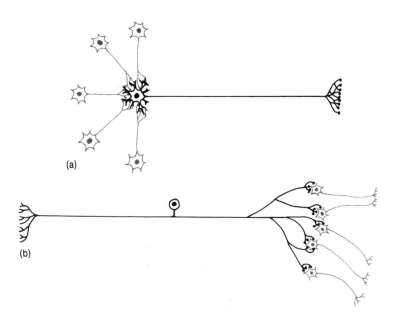

Fig. 13.1. Neurone circuits: (a) convergence – several presynaptic neurones synapse with one postsynaptic neurone; (b) divergence – one presynaptic neurone synapses with several postsynaptic neurones.

neuropeptides. The effect of a change in sensitivity is to regulate the amount of information entering or leaving a particular group of neurones. In diseases of the central nervous system, it may be the balance of excitatory and inhibitory transmitter substances produced by groups of neurones that is disturbed with the result that abnormal movements are produced. Parkinson's disease is an example of this.

Presynaptic inhibition

Inhibition of neurones also occurs in the central nervous system by a 'blocking' mechanism, whereby the excitatory transmitter substance is inhibited before it can be released. This is known as presynaptic inhibition. A presynaptic neurone releases the inhibitory transmitter on to the synaptic knobs of the excitatory neurone as shown in Figure 13.2. An example of presynaptic inhibition is the activity of the cells of the substantia gelatinosa in the 'pain gate' mechanism which regulates the activity of the pain transmission cells (see Fig. 11.6). Another example is the suppression of stretch reflex activity by descending tracts from the medulla of the brain. Descending fibres from the medulla exert presynaptic inhibition on the sensory neurones entering the spinal cord from muscle spindles. This provides a mechanism for changing the level of stretch reflex activity.

Feedback inhibition

Activity in a neurone may be fed back to the same neurone by a collateral or branch which synapses with a small inhibitory interneurone (formerly known as a Renshaw cell) (Fig. 13.3). The effect of activity in these interneurones is inhibition. In this way, lower motor neurone activity can be modified at the spinal level by a local feedback circuit. Similar recurrent branches of

Fig. 13.2. Presynaptic inhibition. An inhibitory synapse is formed by one presynaptic neurone on the synaptic knobs of a second presynaptic neurone, preventing the release of its transmitter substance.

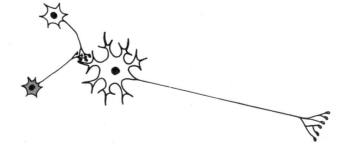

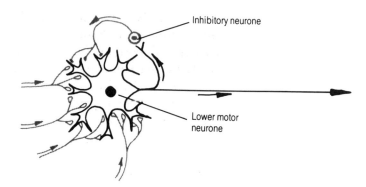

Fig. 13.3. Feedback inhibition of a lower motor neurone via a collateral which synapses with an inhibitory interneurone.

axons are found in neurones in the cerebral cortex and the limbic system.

Feedback also occurs between groups of neurones. The output from one group of neurones is fed back to either inhibit or to excite a preceding group of neurones. The effect is to either limit or extend the activity after the input to the original group has stopped. The feedback may be inhibitory (negative feedback), or alternatively the effect may be excitatory (positive feedback).

Synergy

The performance of a particular pattern of movement, or synergy, is the combined result of different levels of activity in all the active muscle groups. For example, the leg swing in walking involves the hip flexors and lateral rotators, the knee extensors and the ankle dorsiflexors. Synergy is achieved by the correct modulation of activity in all the motor neurone pools in the spinal cord which execute this particular movement pattern.

13.2 Spinal integration

13.2.1 Interneurones

The integration of spinal reflex activity is the function of the large number of interneurones which connect both sides, and different levels, of the spinal cord. The interneurones that spread activity up and down the cord lie in the intersegmental tract (fasciculus proprius) (see Chapter 3, Fig. 3.25c).

The flexor and crossed extensor reflexes have already been described in Chapter 3, Section 3.14.3. The spread of activity across the spinal cord and to the other pair of limbs via interneurones is an example of integration at the spinal level. The pattern of movement performed in the flexor and crossed extensor reflexes is basic to many natural movements, such as walking. Consequently, if we try to oppose this pattern by swinging the same arm forwards as the swinging leg, it feels unnatural and awkward.

The spread of activity across the spinal cord by interneurones is also the basis of *associated reactions*.

- *ASK a partner to remove an elastic band placed round the fingers and thumb of one hand without using the other hand. Watch how the complex movements attempting to release the fingers from the band are mirrored in the untied hand.*

The associated reaction movements may become exaggerated when the interruption of descending pathways releases spinal reflexes from the control by higher centres.

13.2.2 Reciprocal innervation

All movements require the integration of activity in opposing muscle groups, which is the result of reciprocal innervation of the lower motor neurones of the particular muscle groups involved. Opposing muscle groups, for example flexors and extensors, abductors and adductors, acting round a joint cooperate during movement. Excitation of one group is accompanied by inhibition of the antagonist group which then relaxes and allows the agonist to contract. In spinal reflex movements, the sensory neurones entering the spinal cord branch in the posterior horn of the grey matter. A branch of each neurone excites the alpha motor neurones of one group of muscles, while the other branch relays to interneurones that form an inhibitory synapse with the motor neurones supplying the opposing muscle group (Fig. 13.4). This is known as reciprocal innervation or reciprocal inhibition, whereby the activity in opposing muscle groups is balanced and graded during movement.

The *development* of integrative activity in opposing muscle groups is seen in young babies. The dominance of flexor activity is evident at birth when the baby lies with bent arms and legs, and curled fingers (Fig. 13.5a). By 4 months, the extensors of the arm can be used to lift the head and chest from the floor in prone lying (Fig. 13.5b). By 6 months, the legs extend to take the body weight if the baby is held upright. The arms also reach out in extension to grasp objects in the hand. The early movements are flexor/extensor patterns. Later the ability to integrate activity

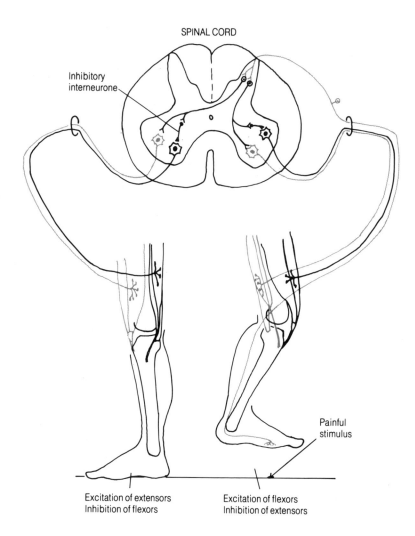

Fig. 13.4. Reciprocal innervation. Excitation of the agonist and inhibition of the antagonist groups of muscles in flexion of one limb and extension of the other.

SPINAL CORD

Inhibitory interneurone

Painful stimulus

Excitation of extensors
Inhibition of flexors

Excitation of flexors
Inhibition of extensors

in muscles acting as synergists and fixators allows more complex movement patterns to develop.

13.3 Integration in the brain stem

The brain stem is largely concerned with the integration of activity related to postural support during movement.

The development of brain stem reflexes can be seen in the young child. The first stage in control of posture is head control. At birth, there is no head control, but by 1 to 2 months, the *tonic labyrinthine reflex* develops and the vestibular nucleus in the brain stem can integrate the position of the head with the body, so that the head moves with the body (Fig. 13.6a).

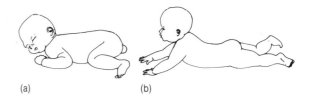

Fig. 13.5. Early development of extensor activity: (a) flexed position of the newborn in prone lying; (b) by 3 months the neck extends to lift the head, the arms and the legs are extended.

(a)   (b)

Movements of the head stimulate the *tonic neck reflexes* in the young baby. Turning the head to one side results in extension of the limbs on the same side, and flexion of the opposite limb (Fig. 13.6b). Turning the head upwards increases activity in the flexors of the lower limbs; turning the head downwards increases flexion in the upper limbs. (These are known as *symmetrical tonic neck reflexes*.)

By 7 months, the baby has voluntary control of the head and eye movements, and the righting reflexes are established. The neck and body *righting reflexes* allow the baby to rotate about the vertical axis and roll over from prone to supine, and supine to prone lying. The rotation of the head stimulates stretch receptors in the neck muscles, and the response is contraction of the rotators of the trunk so that the body starts to turn. Pressure on the side of the body then stimulates the body righting reflex which rotates the pelvis to complete the turn.

The final stage is the development of the more complex *equilibrium reactions* which occurs between 1 and 2 years of age. These automatic adjustments of the position of the head and body allow the body segments to align over the feet in standing and walking. The tonic neck and righting reflexes become modified with the development of the equilibrium reactions, but they remain as basic movement patterns. For example, the position of the head and arms in the asymmetrical tonic neck reflex is often adopted in dance movements.

The equilibrium reactions remain as an essential background to the highly skilled movement patterns acquired in the adult. In neurological deficits that involve movement, equilibrium reactions must be re-educated before normal voluntary movements can occur.

Fig. 13.6. Development of brain stem reflexes: (a) labyrinthine reflex – newborn to 6 months when the head is held upright on the trunk; (b) asymmetric tonic neck reflex.

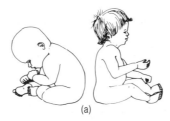

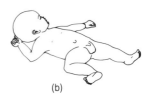

(a)   (b)

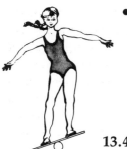

- *OBSERVE the equilibrium reactions in the adult by asking a partner to try to balance on a board resting on a cylinder or pipe as shown in Figure 13.7. As each foot moves, the body is thrown off balance. Notice the simultaneous changes in the hips, the trunk and the head as the body tries to maintain balance over the feet. Also notice how the eyes remain looking ahead.*

Fig. 13.7. Equilibrium reactions. As the body is thrown off balance, the body segments realign and the eyes look straight ahead.

13.4 Performance

13.4.1 Open and closed loop movements

Voluntary movement can be divided into two types: (a) *open loop* or *ballistic* movement, which once initiated must follow its course; and (b) *closed loop*, which is guided movement, always variable and subject to fine adjustment.

Open loop movements are performed in response to the activation of a motor programme, and proceed without change. The accuracy of these movements depends on the ability to assemble the correct motor commands before the movement begins. Once the movement has been initiated, no modification can be made.

An example of this type of movement is throwing a ball. Once the ball has been released, control over its flight has ended. Other everyday examples of this type of movement are brushing the hair, chopping vegetables, and pressing a key of a typewriter or piano.

Closed loop movements involve feedback of sensory information from the proprioceptors and from the exteroceptors (visual, auditory and tactile) as the movement proceeds. 'Error correction' is applied to the output in the motor system to achieve the desired performance. Examples of a closed loop type of movement are hand sewing, writing and drawing with care.

Most of our daily activities are a combination of **both** of these types of movement. For example, brushing the hair starts as a ballistic movement, but this becomes modified as the brush encounters different friction with each stroke, and as the hair is brushed into one's personal style.

13.4.2 Performance of skilled movements

A motor skill is a sequence of movements that are performed to achieve a particular goal with appropriate speed and accuracy. The acquisition of a motor skill involves a learning period when the correct motor programmes are developed in the central nervous system, and the activity in all the groups of muscles is gradually modified to produce the correct force and timimg. We learn to perform a complex motor skill, such as swinging a golf club, driving a car, or manipulating a paint brush on canvas; we make the movements slowly at first, then repeat them many times relying heavily on feedback from the eyes, the skin and the muscles. Eventually the motor programmes can be executed with accuracy, unless significant changes in the environment occur during the progress.

The **cerebellum** plays a major role in the performance of skilled movement by storing motor commands which have been developed with repetition. In this way, the cerebellum acts as a *'skills bank'*. If there is any change in the pattern of input to the cerebellum (for example a driver may change to a new car), then the stored motor pattern can be updated, and after a short period of practice, the movements become automatic again. Various theories have been developed to explain the role of the cerebellum in the acquisition of motor skills. The theories are based on detailed knowledge of the cellular structure of the cerebellar cortex and on the results of damage to the cerebellum.

Cellular structure of the cerebellum

The **cerebellar cortex** has three layers which are distributed uniformly over all the surface of the cerebellum (Fig. 13.8). This is different from the cerebral cortex where the arrangement and type of neurones varies in different areas.

The middle layer of the cerebellar cortex has a layer of large **Purkinje cells**, which have extensive and complex systems of dendrites reaching to the superficial (molecular) layer. The axons of the Purkinje cells form the only *output* from the cerebellar cortex. These axons end in the deep nuclei of the cerebellum and then relay to the brain stem.

The *input* is made up of two systems of incoming fibres that affect the activity of the Purkinje cells.

(1) **Climbing fibres** which originate only in the inferior nucleus of the olive in the medulla. Each fibre winds round the dendrites of one Purkinje cell. This forms a fast route for the excitation of the Purkinje cells.

(2) **Mossy fibres** which originate in all the other areas of input to the cerebellum. The mossy fibres synapse with granule cells in the deeper cell layer before sending ascending axons to the

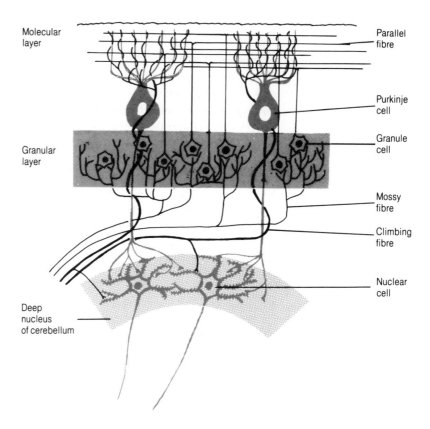

Molecular layer

Parallel fibre

Purkinje cell

Granule cell

Granular layer

Mossy fibre

Climbing fibre

Nuclear cell

Deep nucleus of cerebellum

Fig. 13.8. Cellular structure of the cerebellar cortex (simplified), showing Purkinje cells, granule cells and deep nuclear cells.

molecular layer. Each axon divides into two to form the *parallel fibres* which traverse the molecular layer of the cortex like telephone wires, and each branches to make contact with a large number of Purkinje cells. The activity in the mossy fibres provides input from a large number of sources in the body. The activity is then spread by the parallel fibres to the output from a large number of Purkinje cells.

During the early stages of motor learning, the Purkinje cells are excited by the climbing fibres, which are stimulated by the motor cortex via the olivary nucleus in the brain stem (Fig. 13.7b). The performance of each movement produces a particular pattern of sensory feedback from the muscles, skin, eyes and ears, which is carried via the mossy fibres and the parallel fibres to the Purkinje cells. After many repetitions of the same sequence, motor programmes of successful movements are stored by the Purkinje cells, and excitation by the climbing fibres from the cortex is no longer required. If any updating of the sequence is required, the olivary route via the climbing fibres is involved again until a new motor programme is generated.

Input and output connections with the cerebellum

There are three main functions of the cerebellum.

(1) The planning and initiation of movement, together with the storage of plans as a 'skills bank'. The anatomical pathway for this function is mainly the motor control loop with the motor cortex described in Chapter 12, Section 12.3.2, Figure 12.7.

(2) The coordination of brain stem reflexes for the maintenance of posture and equilibrium during movement (see Section 13.3). The input to the cerebellum from the vestibule of the ear is an important part of this function. The vestibule signals the position of the head in space, and also integrates with visual input via the vestibulo-ocular reflex (Chapter 4, Section 4.4.2, Fig. 4.10). The output for this pathway is via the vestibulospinal tracts to the axial muscles of the head, neck and trunk (Chapter 12, Fig. 12.3).

(3) The cerebellum monitors and modifies the progress of goal directed movements, acting as a correction device. The modification of muscle activity required to correct any error is partly based on *input* from the ascending tracts of the somatosensory system, which includes proprioceptive information about body position and movement. This can be compared with the *input* from the motor cortex about intended movement. The *output* pathway is to the brain stem nuclei and via their descending tracts to the motor neurones of the spinal cord. The cerebellum has been compared with the control system of a guided missile which ensures its arrival on target.

Basal ganglia

The **basal ganglia** function at a high level in movement performance. The movements influenced by the basal ganglia include background posture, basic movement patterns such as standing and walking, and skilled motor actions. The basal ganglia have output links with the premotor and supplementary motor areas which suggest a role in the *planning* of movement as well as its execution.

Also at the cortical level, the basal ganglia receive input from many sensory areas and therefore may play a role in the integration of *sensory information related to action*. All movements are associated with particular sensory parameters which are task related. The value of cueing for some patients with Parkinson's disease provides evidence of this role of the basal ganglia.

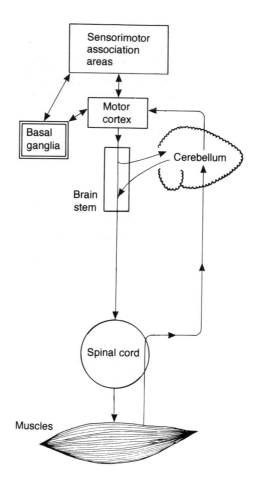

Fig. 13.9. Interaction of the basal ganglia and the cerebellum with cortical areas, the brain stem and the spinal cord.

- *LOOK at Figure 13.9 to follow a summary of how the cerebellum and the basal ganglia interact in different ways with cortical areas, the motor nuclei in the brain stem, and the spinal cord.*

13.5 Behavioural aspects of movement

The way we perform daily tasks such as dressing and cooking depends on our mood and on how alert we feel at the time. In this section, a brief outline of the brain areas concerned with behavioural aspects of movement will be given.

Reticular formation

By its position in the central core of the brain stem, and its numerous links with the sensory and motor systems, the reticular formation has an effect on the way we perform movement. If there is a high level of activity in the reticular formation, the level of arousal is high, and the muscles seem to 'spring into action'. A low arousal state, that we may feel on waking from a night's sleep, reduces our capacity to move with speed and accuracy. This reflects the absence of overall stimulation of the cerebral cortex from the reticular activating system (ARAS) seen in Figure 3.18. The addition of an extra stimulus, such as an alarm clock or door bell ringing, increases the input to the system and we feel more able to move quickly.

Neurones in the reticular formation are non-specific, they are stimulated by different types of sensation. Collaterals from the anterolateral ascending tracts are given off to the reticular formation as they pass through the brain stem. Reticular neurones project to most areas of the cerebral cortex either directly, or indirectly via the thalamus (Fig. 13.10). Activity in these ascending fibres makes the cerebral cortex more receptive to stimulation, and general alertness is increased.

The reticular formation receives information from the various motor centres in the brain, particularly the basal ganglia and the vestibular nuclei, and relays into the reticulospinal tracts to both the alpha and gamma motor neurones in the spinal cord. In this way, the integration of activity in the reticular neurones exerts an influence on the performance of movement, especially the postural adjustments involved.

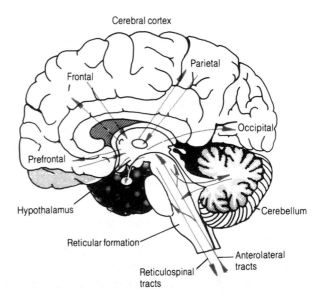

Fig. 13.10. Sagittal section of the brain to show reticular formation. Collaterals of the anterolateral system, the link with the cerebellum, and the arousal system to the cerebral cortex are shown.

Affect

The brain areas concerned with our emotional feelings are the *limbic system*, the *prefrontal cortex* and the *hypothalamus* (see Chapter 3, Section 3.8). Some of the connections between these brain areas are shown in Figure 13.11.

The structures which form the **limbic system** can be divided into those which connect with the forebrain, and those linking to the midbrain: these two areas are linked by the fornix, which is a large tract of white matter. The hypothalamus lies in between the limbic forebrain and midbrain.

The limbic forebrain links with the **prefrontal cortex** which is concerned with subjective feelings of emotion. Sensory information filters back down from the cerebral cortex to the limbic forebrain and affects its overall activity. The limbic midbrain links with the reticular formation. Pathways from the hippocampus to the basal ganglia suggest that the limbic system plays a role in the long-term memory of motor skills.

The **hypothalamus** is the area of the brain that responds to stress in the body. The stress stimulus or stressor may originate outside the body, such as pain to the skin, a loud noise, or an object rapidly approaching the eyes; or the stressor may be

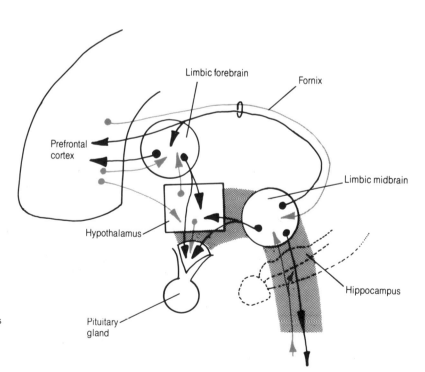

Fig. 13.11. Connections between the limbic system, hypothalamus and prefrontal cortex.

internal, such as feelings of anxiety or depression. The result of these stressors is activity in the sympathetic nervous system which prepares the body for action by speeding up the heart, opening up the airways of the lungs and so on. The same responses occur in the athlete preparing to start a race, so that the muscles spring into action when the starting pistol fires. A stress response of short duration is helpful in preparing the body for action, but if it is prolonged then stress diseases may develop.

13.6 Summary of the basic components in movement performance

Muscle components

The groups of muscles involved in a movement can be divided into three functional components.

(1) **Posture** and **balance** – the function of the muscles of the trunk controlled by the vestibular and medial reticulospinal tracts from the brain stem, and by spinal reflex activity.

(2) **Positioning** and **support** – the function of the proximal limb muscles (shoulder and elbow, hip and knee) controlled by the cerebellum and red nucleus, and the lateral reticulospinal tract from the midbrain.

(3) **Skilled** and **precision movement** – the function of the distal muscle groups of the limbs (the hand and foot), the muscles involved in speech, facial expression and eye movements, controlled by the primary motor and premotor cortex via the corticobulbar and corticospinal tracts.

The activity in each of the components is monitored and regulated throughout the progress of the movement.

Neural components

The **neural** components of a movement, shown diagrammatically in Figure 13.12, can be divided into the following.

(1) **Planning** – the function of the cerebral cortex (sensory and supplementary motor areas), the basal ganglia and the cerebellum. Movement of short duration depends particularly on planning by the basal ganglia, since no correction can be applied

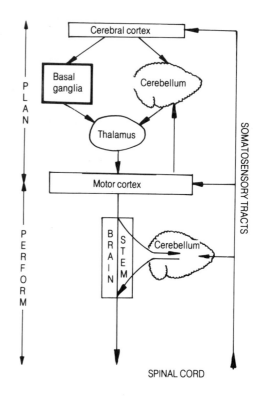

Fig. 13.12. Plan of the brain areas involved in planning and performance of movement.

once the movement has started. Prolonged movements are more dependent on the cerebellum which can modify programmes based on input from the muscles. Planning also involves the premotor areas receiving input from the sensory areas.

(2) **Performance** – the function of the cortical motor areas and the output to the spinal cord. The cerebellum provides an error correction to the movements, based on sensory feedback from the muscles as the movement proceeds.

The accuracy and precision of the performance of skilled movements depends on the accumulation of stored motor patterns in the cerebellum as the result of repetition of the same sequence of movements.

The acquisition of a complex motor skill, such as learning to ride a bicycle, is an event that most of us remember. The movements involved in propelling the bicycle require strength and bilateral coordination of the extensor muscles of the legs to overcome the resistance offered by the pedals. The leg movements must then be accompanied by appropriate movements of the head and trunk to balance over the seat of the bicycle. Repetition of the combined movements of the legs, the trunk and the head acting together eventually achieves the balance required. Next, the responses to various external changes, such as the surface of the road, turning corners and traffic, must be learnt, so adjusting the initial skill of riding. It is during the early stages of learning that conscious control of the individual movements is still necessary. Finally, the performance of all the movements becomes automatic. All our conscious effort can then be directed towards enjoying the scenery, and the pleasure that we gain from the exercise depends on our mood at the time.

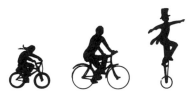

At the end of this chapter, you should be able to:

(1) Appreciate the importance of integration between the sensory and motor systems for the planning and performance of movement.

(2) Augment the knowledge of the properties of nervous tissue from Chapter 3 to include neurotransmitter substances, presynaptic and feedback inhibition.

(3) Appreciate the role of interneurones in the spinal cord for the integration of activity at the spinal level. Describe the mechanism of reciprocal innervation in the regulation of activity in opposing muscle groups.

(4) Describe the development of brain stem reflexes from birth to the equilibrium reactions of the adult for the maintenance of balance.

(5) Define a motor programme, and distinguish between open loop and closed loop movements.

(6) Augment the knowledge of the cerebellum in Chapter 12 to include (a) cellular structure and (b) input and output connections with the motor cortex, the vestibule and the spinal cord.

(7) Augment the knowledge of the basal ganglia from Chapter 12 to include the connections with the premotor, supplementary

motor, and the somatosensory areas for the planning and execution of movement.

(8) Outline the behavioural aspects of movement performance including arousal and affect.

(9) Draw a chart to show the interaction of the main brain areas in the planning and performance of movement.

Further Reading for Section 3

Carpenter R.H.S. (1990) *Neurophysiology*. 2nd edn., Edward Arnold, London.

Coen C.W. (1987) *Functions of the Brain. Edited papers from lectures at Wolfson College*. Oxford Univeristy Press, Oxford.

Cohen H. (1993) edited by, *Neuroscience for Rehabilitation*. JP Lippincott Co., Philadelphia.

Ganong W.F. (1993) *Review of Medical Physiology*. A Lange Medical Book, Prentice-Hall, London.

Grieve J. (1993) *Neuropsychology for Occupational Therapists*. Blackwell Science, Oxford.

Guyton A.G. (1991) *Basic Neuroscience*. WB Saunders, New York.

Higgins J.R. (1977) *Human Movement: An Integrated Approach*. CV Mosby Co., St. Louis.

Illingworth R.S. (1987) *The Development of the Infant and Young Child*. 9th edn., Churchill Livingstone, Edinburgh.

Kidd G. (1986) The myotatic reflex. In *Cash's Textbook of Neurology for Physiotherapists*. (ed by P.A. Downie) Faber & Faber, London.

Kiernan J.A. (1987) *Introduction to human neuroscience*. JB Lippincott, Philadelphia.

Melzack R. & Wall P. (1989) *The Challenge of Pain*. Penguin, London.

Noback C.R. (1991) *The Nervous System*. 4th edn., Williams & Wilkins, London.

Schmidt R.F. (edited by) (1985) *Fundamentals of Neurophysiology*. 3rd edn., Springer Verlag, New York.

Sheridan M.D. (1990) *From Birth to Five Years*. Aust. Council Educ. Res. (AT) State Mutual Publishing Inc., New York.

Smyth M.M. & Wing A. (1984) *The Psychology of Human Movement*. Academic Press.

Appendix 1   Bones

Right clavicle – superior aspect

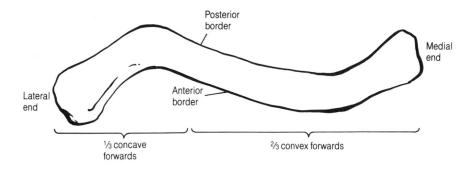

Posterior border
Medial end
Lateral end
Anterior border
⅓ concave forwards
⅔ convex forwards

Right scapula – anterior aspect

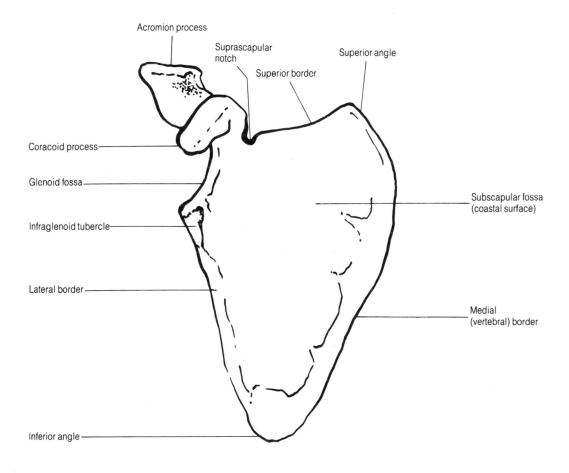

Acromion process
Suprascapular notch
Superior border
Superior angle
Coracoid process
Glenoid fossa
Subscapular fossa (coastal surface)
Infraglenoid tubercle
Lateral border
Medial (vertebral) border
Inferior angle

Right clavicle – inferior aspect

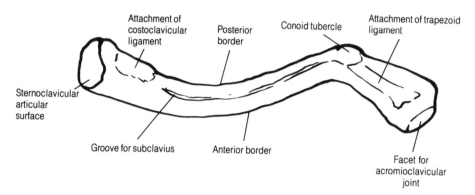

Attachment of costoclavicular ligament

Posterior border

Conoid tubercle

Attachment of trapezoid ligament

Sternoclavicular articular surface

Groove for subclavius

Anterior border

Facet for acromioclavicular joint

Right scapula – posterior aspect

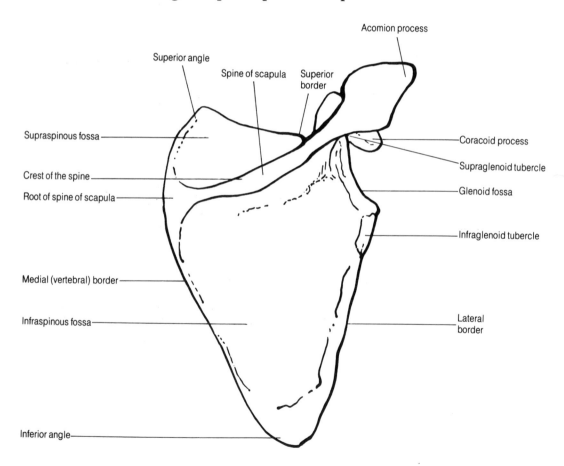

Acomion process

Superior angle

Spine of scapula

Superior border

Supraspinous fossa

Coracoid process

Supraglenoid tubercle

Crest of the spine

Glenoid fossa

Root of spine of scapula

Infraglenoid tubercle

Medial (vertebral) border

Infraspinous fossa

Lateral border

Inferior angle

Right humerus

Anterior aspect

Posterior aspect

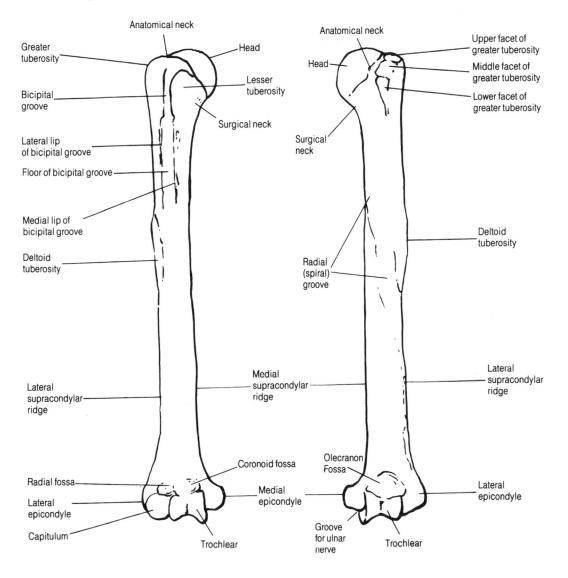

Right radius and ulna

Anterior aspect

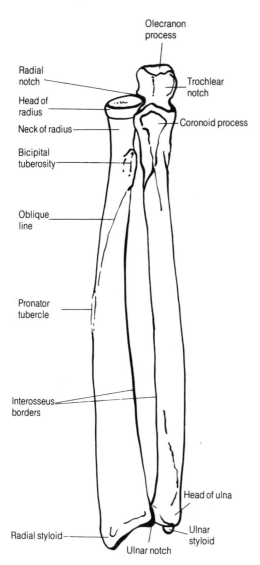

Olecranon process

Radial notch

Trochlear notch

Head of radius

Neck of radius

Coronoid process

Bicipital tuberosity

Oblique line

Pronator tubercle

Interosseus borders

Head of ulna

Radial styloid

Ulnar styloid

Ulnar notch

Posterior aspect

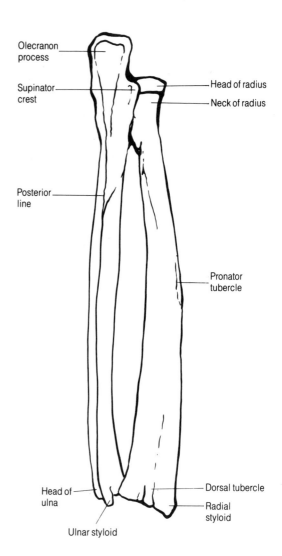

Olecranon process

Supinator crest

Head of radius

Neck of radius

Posterior line

Pronator tubercle

Head of ulna

Dorsal tubercle

Radial styloid

Ulnar styloid

Right hand – palmar aspect

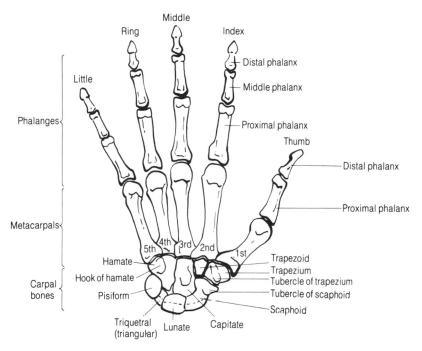

Right hand – dorsal aspect

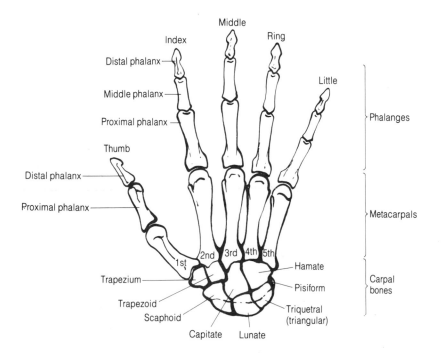

Pelvis – anterior aspect

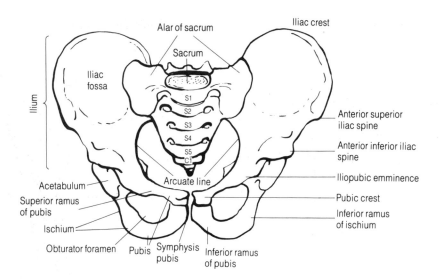

Pelvis – posterior aspect

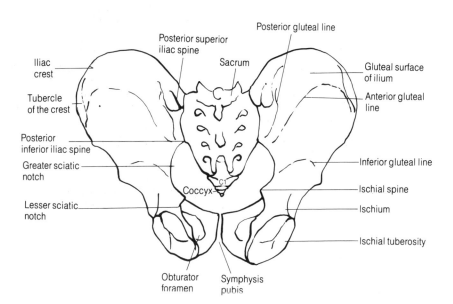

Right femur

Anterior aspect

Posterior aspect

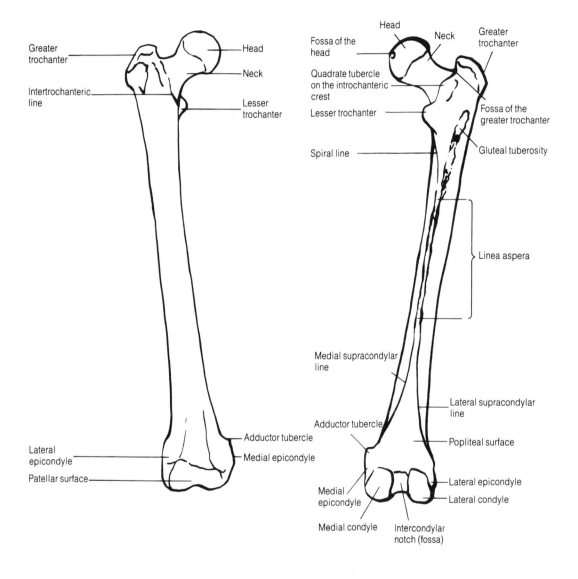

Right tibia and fibula

Anterior aspect

Posterior aspect

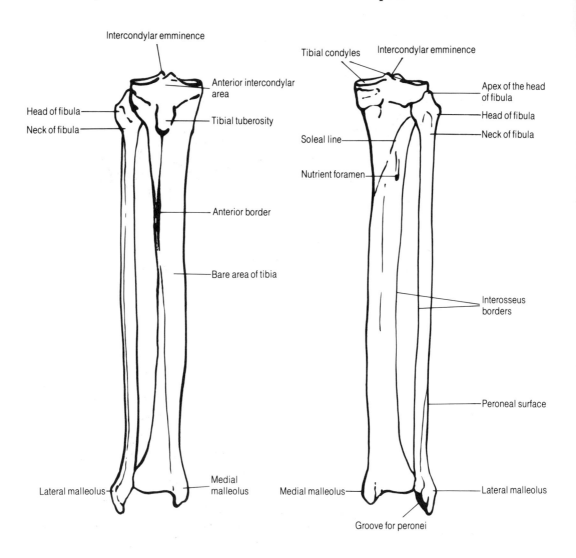

Right foot

Lateral aspect

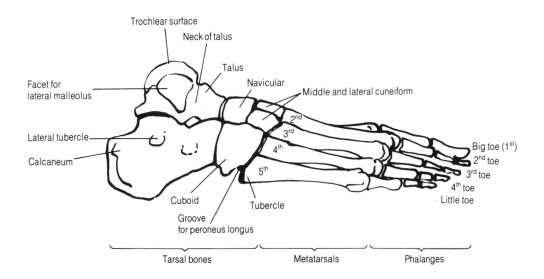

Trochlear surface
Neck of talus
Talus
Navicular
Facet for
lateral malleolus
Middle and lateral cuneiform
Lateral tubercle
Calcaneum
Cuboid
Tubercle
Groove
for peroneus longus
Big toe (1st)
2nd toe
3rd toe
4th toe
Little toe

Tarsal bones | Metatarsals | Phalanges

Medial aspect

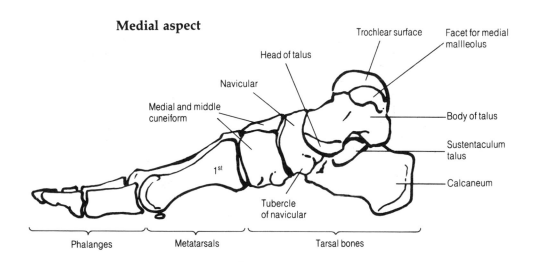

Trochlear surface
Facet for medial mallleolus
Head of talus
Navicular
Medial and middle cuneiform
Body of talus
Sustentaculum talus
Calcaneum
Tubercle of navicular

Phalanges | Metatarsals | Tarsal bones

A typical (thoracic) vertebra

Superior aspect

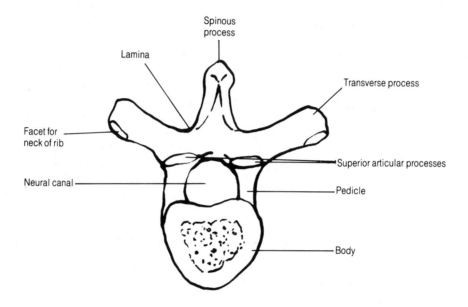

Spinous process

Lamina

Transverse process

Facet for neck of rib

Superior articular processes

Neural canal

Pedicle

Body

Lateral aspect

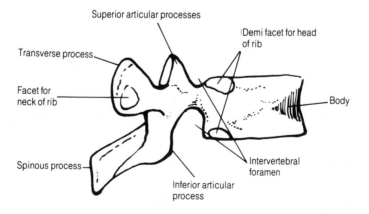

Superior articular processes

Demi facet for head of rib

Transverse process

Facet for neck of rib

Body

Spinous process

Intervertebral foramen

Inferior articular process

Appendix 2 Segmental Nerve Supply of Muscles

Table A2.1.
Cranial nerves

Note: Cranial nerves supplying muscles contain sensory proprioceptor fibres, except the facial nerve. Proprioception from facial muscles is carried in the trigeminal nerve.

I	Olfactory	Sensory from roof of the nose. Smell
II	Optic	Sensory from retina of the eye. Vision
III	Oculomotor	Motor to four of the muscles of the eye (superior, inferior and medial rectus, inferior oblique), motor to the sphincter muscle of the iris and the ciliary muscle of the lens
IV	Trochlear	Motor to the superior oblique eye muscle
V	Trigeminal	Sensory to skin of the face and anterior tongue Motor to salivary glands and muscles of mastication (temporalis and masseter)
VI	Abducens	Motor to the lateral rectus eye muscle
VII	Facial	Sensory to anterior tongue. Taste Motor to muscles of the face and salivary glands
VIII	Vestibulocochlear	Sensory from vestibule. Balance Sensory from cochlear of ear. Sound
IX	Glossopharyngeal	Sensory from posterior tongue. Taste Motor to salivary glands and pharynx
X	Vagus	Sensory and motor to pharynx, larynx, thoracic and abdominal organs
XI	Spinal Accessory Cranial root Spinal root (C1–C5)	Motor to the muscles of the pharynx and larynx Motor to sternomastoid and trapezius
XII	Hypoglossal	Motor to muscles of the tongue

Table A2.2.
Spinal nerves.

Segmental origin in the spinal cord of the nerves supplying the muscle groups moving the limbs

C5, C6	Shoulder	Abductors and lateral rotators
C5, C6, C7, C8		Flexors, extensors, adductors and medial rotators
C5, C6	Elbow	Flexors
C7, C8		Extensors
C5, C6	Forearm	Supinators
C6, C7, C8		Pronators
C6, C7, C8	Wrist	Flexors, extensors and deviators
C7, C8, T1	Digits	Long flexors and extensors
C8, T1	Hand	Intrinsic muscles
L2, L3	Hip	Flexors
L2, L3, L4		Adductors
L4, L5, S1		Extensors, medial and lateral rotators and abductors
L2, L3, L4	Knee	Extensors
L4, L5, S1, S2		Flexors
L4, L5, S1,	Ankle	Dorsiflexors
L4, L5, S1, S2		Plantarflexors
L4, L5, S1	Foot	Invertors
L5, S1		Evertors
L5, S1, S2		Intrinsic muscles

Table A2.3. Segmental innervation of the muscles of the upper limb (after Basmajian, J. (ed) (1980) Grant's Method of Anatomy, 10th edn, published by Williams & Wilkins)

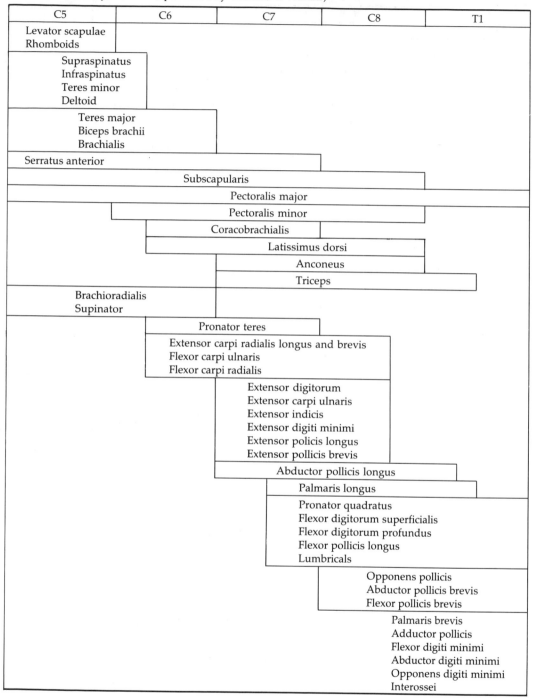

C5	C6	C7	C8	T1
Levator scapulae Rhomboids				
Supraspinatus Infraspinatus Teres minor Deltoid				
Teres major Biceps brachii Brachialis				
Serratus anterior				
Subscapularis				
Pectoralis major				
Pectoralis minor				
Coracobrachialis				
Latissimus dorsi				
Anconeus				
Triceps				
Brachioradialis Supinator				
Pronator teres				
Extensor carpi radialis longus and brevis Flexor carpi ulnaris Flexor carpi radialis				
Extensor digitorum Extensor carpi ulnaris Extensor indicis Extensor digiti minimi Extensor policis longus Extensor pollicis brevis				
Abductor pollicis longus				
Palmaris longus				
Pronator quadratus Flexor digitorum superficialis Flexor digitorum profundus Flexor pollicis longus Lumbricals				
Opponens pollicis Abductor pollicis brevis Flexor pollicis brevis				
Palmaris brevis Adductor pollicis Flexor digiti minimi Abductor digiti minimi Opponens digiti minimi Interossei				

Table A2.4. Segmental innervation of the muscles of the lower limb (after Basmajian, J. (ed) (1980) Grant's Method of Anatomy, 10th edn, published by Williams & Wilkins)

L2	L3	L4	L5	S1	S2
+ L1 Iliacus					
+ L1 Psoas					
		Tensor fascia lata			
		Gluteus medius			
		Gluteus minimus			
		Quadratus femoris			
		Inferior gemellus			
			Superior gemellus		
			Gluteus maximus		
			Obturator intermus		
			Piriformis		
Sartorius					
Pectineus					
Adductor longus					
	Quadriceps femoris				
Gracilis					
Adductor brevis					
	Obturator externus				
	Adductor magnus				
		Semitendinosus			
		Semimembranosus			
			Biceps femoris		
		Tibialis anterior			
		Extensor hallucis longus			
		Extensor digitorum longus			
		Popliteus			
		Plantaris			
			Gastrocnemius		
			Soleus		
			Peroneus longus		
			Peroneus brevis		
			Tibialis posterior		
			Flexor digitorum longus		
			Flexor hallucis longus		
		Extensor hallucis brevis			
		Extensor digitorum brevis			
			Flexor digitorum brevi		
			Abductor hallucis		
			Flexor hallucis brevis		
			Lumbricals		
				Adductor hallucis	
				Abductor digiti minimi	
				Flexor digiti minimi	
				Flexor accessorius	
				Interosseii	

Glossary

abduction   movement of a body segment that takes it away from the midline of the body in a coronal (frontal) plane.

acetyl choline   a neurotransmitter released at a synapse in many parts of the nervous system, e.g. a neuromuscular junction, and in the autonomic NS (except post ganglionic sympathetic).

action potential   reversal of the membrane potential in a localised area of a neurone or muscle fibre due to the movement of charged particles (ions) across the membrane.

adduction   movement of a body segment towards the midline of the body in a coronal (frontal) plane.

aerobic metabolism   chemical reactions in mitochondria which replenish ATP using oxygen and glucose.

affect   mood and emotion. Affective disorders include depression.

afferent   carrying impulses and information towards the central nervous system (sensory).

agonist   (prime mover) a muscle which contracts to perform a specific movement.

alpha motor neurone   *see* skeletomotor neurone.

ampulla   specialised receptor area in one of the semicircular canals of the inner ear.

anaerobic glycolysis   production of ATP from the breakdown of glycogen without oxygen.

antagonist   a muscle which opposes the action of the agonist (prime mover).

anterior root   of spinal nerve contains motor (efferent) axons.

aponeurosis   a broad sheet of dense fibrous tissue which: (i) attaches muscles to each other, e.g. abdominal muscles; or (ii) forms the attachment of a muscle to bone, e.g. tensor fascia lata; or (iii) forms a protective layer for tendons, e.g. plantar aponeurosis.

arthroplasty   replacement of a joint by an artificial one.

astereognosis   inability to identify an object by manipulation in the hand without vision.

ataxia   movement errors that include the inability to accurately place a body part, or to to perform smooth coordinated movement of the limbs.

ATP (adenosine triphosphate) major energy storing molecule in the cells of the body.

autonomic NS part of the peripheral nervous system which innervates cardiac and smooth muscle, and glands.

axon main process of the neurone which conducts impulses away from the cell body to another neurone or an effector (sometimes called nerve fibre).

basal ganglia (nuclei) an interconnected collection of masses of grey matter within each cerebral hemisphere (adjacent to the thalamus), and in the mid brain.

bouton enlarged bulbous end of a terminal branch of an axon or dendrite.

brachial related to the upper limb.

brain stem the part of the hind brain which connects to the spinal cord. 3 components – mid brain, pons and medulla.

bursa a closed sac of fibrous tissue, containing synovial fluid found associated with the large joints.

bursitis inflammation of a bursa.

capsule sleeve of dense fibrous tissue surrounding and uniting the ends of the bones in a synovial joint.

carpal one of eight bones of the wrist, which link the radius and the ulna of the forearm with the metacarpals in the hand.

carpal tunnel anatomical space on the palmar surface of the wrist for the long tendons passing from the forearm into the hand.

cartilage type of connective tissue: (a) hyaline – covering the articular surfaces of synovial joints; (b) fibro – found in discs between vertebra and inside the knee joint.

cauda equina the lower spinal nerves which lie in the spinal canal below the level of the first lumbar vertebra.

cerebrospinal fluid circulates in the cavities of the brain, the central canal of the spinal cord and in the sub arachnoid space of the meninges.

central nervous system division of the nervous system containing the brain and spinal cord.

centre of gravity   the point where the weight of an object, a body segment, or the whole body acts vertically downwards.

cerebrovascular accident (CVA)   a stroke – the term used to describe rapidly developing focal brain damage as a result of reduction of blood flow (ischaemia) or a haemorrhage in the brain.

circumduction   a circular (conical) movement made by a body segment (not to be confused with rotation movement at a joint).

closed loop   motor control that uses feed back to make corrections during the progress of a movement.

cognition   the mental processes involved in planning, monitoring and modifying actions and behaviour in response to changes in the environment.

collagen   fibrous protein found in connective tissue which has tensile strength.

concentric muscle work   active muscles shorten to produce a movement.

conduction velocity   the speed at which a neurone conducts impulses.

contracture   permanent shortening of a muscle or tendon producing a deformity and limiting movement.

contralateral   on the opposite side, e.g. a tract that crosses the mid line.

coronal   the top of the head. A coronal section separates the front from the back. Abduction and adduction occur in the coronal/frontal plane.

corpus callosum   a thick band of axons connecting the right and left hemispheres in the forebrain.

corpus striatum   collective term used for the caudate, putamen and globus pallidus, which form the main components of the basal ganglia.

cortex   outer layer of an organ, e.g. surface grey matter of cerebral hemispheres or cerebellum.

cranial nerve   one of 12 pairs of nerves leaving the brain. Some nerves contain sensory axons, others contain motor axons and some nerves are mixed.

CT scan   computerised axial tomography. A thin fan shaped X-ray beam views a 'slice' of the brain. The X-ray tube revolves round the patient so that the brain is viewed from all angles. A computer combines all the views, and the changes in soft tissue at the lesion site are revealed in a single image.

dendrite   short branching process projecting from the cell body of a neurone.

depolarisation   a change in the electrical potential across the membrane of a neurone, produced by the movement of charged particles (ions).

dermatome   sensory innervation of one spinal nerve.

diaphysis   shaft of long bone.

diencephalon   part of the forebrain found buried deep in the cerebral hemispheres which includes the thalamus and hypothalamus.

dorsiflexion   movement of the foot at the ankle joint which lifts the toes up towards the leg.

dura mater   strong fibrous membrane surrounding the central nervous system.

dysmetria   inability to make active placement of a body part, for example, touching the nose.

eccentric muscle work   active muscle that is lengthening to control the effects of external forces, such as gravity.

efferent   carrying information away from the central nervous system (motor).

encapsulated receptor   a sensory receptor inside a tissue capsule.

epiphysis   end of a long bone which develops from a secondary centre of ossification.

epiphyseal plate   cartilaginous layer between the epiphysis and diaphysis of long bone during growth in length.

eversion   movement in the joints of the foot which turns the sole of the foot outwards or laterally.

excitation   changes in the membrane of a neurone which allows impulses to be propagated.

extension   movement in the sagittal plane back to the anatomical position from flexion and beyond, e.g. the straightening of a flexed elbow, hip or knee.

extensors   muscles which increase the joint angle or straighten a limb when they contract.

exteroreceptor   sensory receptor in the skin which responds to changes in the external environment, for example temperature, pressure.

extrafusal   the main muscle fibres which form a skeletal muscle.

extrapyramidal system   polysynaptic descending pathways from brain areas (basal ganglia and brainstem) involved in motor control, balance and posture.

fascia lata   *see* iliotibial tract.

fasciculus   bundle of muscle fibres or axons surrounded by fibrous connective tissue.

fast muscle fibres (glycolytic, Type II)   generate energy from glycogen without oxygen. Specialised for short bursts of high level muscle activity.

first order neurone   the initial neurone in a sensory system that carries information from the receptor to the central nervous system.

flaccidity   state of hypotonia in muscles characteristic of lower motor neurone lesions.

flexion   movement in the sagittal plane that bends body segments towards each other, e.g. bending the elbow and the knee.

flexors   muscles which decrease a joint angle or bend a limb when they contract.

force (muscle)   is generated by the tension in a muscle acting at its point of attachment to a bone.

forearm   body segment between the elbow and the wrist containing the radius and the ulna.

fusimotor neurone   innervates the intrafusal muscle fibres found inside a muscle spindle.

gamma motor neurone   *see* fusimotor neurone.

ganglion   a collection of cell bodies of neurones located in the peripheral nervous system.

girdle   the bones which attach the limbs to the body; the pectoral girdle for the upper limb, and the pelvic girdle for the lower limb.

grey matter   collections of the cell bodies of neurones, their dendrites and the neuroglia cells that support them within the central nervous system.

gyrus   a raised area of cortex seen on the surface of the cerebral hemisphere or cerebellum.

hemianopia   'blindness' in part of the visual field of one or both eyes, originating in a lesion in the occipital lobe of the cerebral hemisphere.

hippocampus   is a curved area of gyrus which lies deep in the medial temporal lobe, adjacent to the temporal part of the lateral ventricle. It forms part of the limbic system.

homunculus   a representation of the parts of the body in the brain, usually drawn as a distorted image of a person.

hypertonia   muscle tone that is higher than normal, resulting in increased resistance to passive stretch of a limb.

hypothenar   muscles in the palm of the hand at the base of the little finger.

hypotonia   muscle tone that is lower than normal, resulting in decreased resistance to passive stretch of a limb.

iliotibial tract (fascia lata)   band of dense fibrous tissue on the lateral side of the thigh, extending from the iliac crest to below the posterior aspect of the lateral tibial condyle.

impulse (nerve)   localised change in the membrane potential of a neurone, which activates the adjacent area of membrane, and the impulse travels down the axon in one direction only.

inhibition   changes in the cell membrane of neurones which make it more difficult for them to respond to a stimulus from any other source.

inhibitory interneurone   type of neurone found in the spinal cord that inhibits the activity of other neurones.

innervation connection of a nerve to another nerve, to a muscle, or to an end organ/gland.

insertion more distal/lateral attachment of a muscle to a bone, and the attachment which usually moves when the muscle contracts.

interneurone a neurone, usually with a short axon, that connects other neurones.

interoceptors (enteroceptors) receptors that respond to sensation inside the body, not related to position or movement.

intrafusal specialised muscle fibres of the muscle spindle innervated by annulospiral (sensory) and fusimotor motor nerve endings.

inversion movement in the joints of the foot which turns the sole of the foot inwards or medially.

ipsilateral the same side of the body. A tract that does not cross the mid line.

isometric (static) muscle work active muscles remain the same length to hold a position.

kyphosis an increase in the primary thoracic curve of the spine, which may appear as rounded shoulders.

labyrinth (bony) system of tunnels within part of the temporal bone containing the utricle, saccule and semicircular canals.

lentiform nucleus the putamen and globus pallidus of the basal ganglia.

lesion focal damage of brain tissue, vascular in origin.

lever a rigid bar (or bone) which moves about a pivot (fulcrum).

ligament dense fibrous tissue which joins bone to bone around a joint in the form of a cord or band. The fibrous capsule which surrounds synovial joints is also known as a capsular ligament.

limbic system a complex system of interconnected structures in the cerebral hemispheres and the diencephalon. The main components are the cingulate gyrus of the medial cerebral cortex, and the hippocampus of the temporal lobe.

lobe   discrete rounded part of an organ, e.g. the brain.

lordosis   an increase in the secondary lumbar curve of the spine, often referred to as hollow back.

lower motor neurone   spinal motor neurones, originating in the anterior horn of the grey matter whose axons supply skeletal muscle (is also used to describe the neurones of cranial motor nerves).

lower motor neurone lesion   interruption of nerve impulses at any point in a lower motor neurone. The result is loss of muscle tone and of tendon reflexes.

membrane potential   the electrical potential due to the distribution of ions across a cell membrane.

meninges   the membranes that surround and protect the brain and spinal cord.

metacarpal   one of five bones found in the palm of the hand and the base of the thumb. The metacarpals join the distal row of carpals to the proximal phalanges of the fingers and the thumb.

metatarsal   one of five bones in the forefoot which link the distal row of tarsals with the proximal phalanges of the toes.

mitochondrion   sausage–shaped structure with a double membrane, found in the cytoplasm of cells, forming the site of production of ATP.

mixed nerve   contains both sensory and motor axons.

modality   a specific type of stimulus, e.g. tactile, visual, auditory.

moment of force   the product of the magnitude of a force and its distance from the fulcrum (centre of the joint).

motor (efferent) neurone   a neurone which innervates and activates muscular or other tissue.

motor program   a plan for action that includes force, timing and sequence of muscle activity.

motor unit   one motor neurone in the spinal cord and all the muscle fibres supplied by it.

MRI   magnetic resonance imaging. A strong magnetic field is produced by electromagnets distributed around the head. A radio pulse excites the hydrogen atoms in the water in the brain tissue. A computer translates the signals from the movement of the hydrogen atoms into an image, which identifies where lesions have occured.

muscle fibre   multi-nucleated unit of structure of skeletal muscle.

muscle spindle   complex receptor found lying in parallel with skeletal muscle fibres for sensing changes in muscle length.

muscle tone   constant tension in muscles resulting from background neural activity in the myotatic reflex. Clinically, the resistance that is felt by the therapist when passively manipulating the limb of a patient.

myelin sheath   a fatty layer surrounding the axon of some neurones which acts as an insulator and increases the rate of conduction of impulses.

myofibril   strand of protein along the whole length of a muscle fibre. There are several hundred myofibrils in each muscle fibre.

myofilaments   strands of actin and myosin, arranged in a particular way in a sarcomere.

myotatic reflex   monosynaptic reflex which is the basis of muscle tone.

myotome   all the muscles supplied by one spinal segment and its pair of spinal nerves.

nerve tract   bundle of parallel axons in the central nervous system carrying information towards (ascending) or away from (descending) centres in the brain.

neuroglia   support cells in the nervous system, other than neurones, which are not primarily involved in the propagation of nerve impulses.

neuromuscular junction   specialised synapse between a motor neurone and a muscle fibre.

neurone cell body   main cellular structure of a neurone containing the nucleus and organelles.

neuropathy   a pathology that affects the peripheral nervous system.

neurotransmitter a specific chemical released by a pre-synaptic neurone that crosses the synaptic cleft and stimulates or inhibits the postsynaptic neurone.

nociceptor a pain receptor.

nucleus pulposus semi-fluid central portion of the inter-vertebral disc.

nystagmus movement of the eyes from side to side with alternate slow and fast phases.

opposition movement which turns the pad or the tip of the thumb towards one or more fingers.

organelle specialised part of the cytoplasm of a cell, each type with a specific function, e.g. the mitochondrion is the site of production of ATP.

osteoblast bone forming cell.

osteoclast cell that absorbs bone in the remodelling during growth or repair.

pennate muscle fasciculi of muscle fibres arranged diagonally along a common tendon like a feather.

peripheral nervous system the division of the nervous system consisting of nerves and ganglia.

phalanx bone of a finger or toe (plural – phalanges).

pia mater innermost layer of the meninges covering the brain and spinal cord.

plane of movement a fixed line of reference passing through the body in a particular direction.

> **sagittal plane** passes through the body from front to back, dividing it into right and left halves.

> **coronal (frontal) plane** passes through the body from top to bottom, dividing it into anterior and posterior halves.

> **transverse (horizontal) plane** passes through the body horizontally, dividing it into upper and lower parts.

plantar flexion movement of the foot at the ankle joint which points the toes down; or in standing, lifts the body on to the toes.

plaque   an area of demyelination in the central nervous system.

plexus   network of nerves or blood vessels branching and joining, e.g. brachial plexus.

popliteal   posterior region of the knee.

power grip   holds an object with all the fingers flexed around it, and the thumb is opposed to them.

power (muscle)   the product of force times speed of movement. A high level of muscle power is required for fast dynamic movement such as jumping and throwing.

precision grip   holds an object between the pads or the tips of the thumb and one, two or three fingers.

preganglionic neurone   a neurone in the autonomic nervous system which innervates an autonomic ganglion, (**postganglionic neurone** innervates a tissue or an organ, e.g. the heart).

presynaptic   the side of a synapse that releases the neuro-transmitter, (**postsynaptic** neurone receives the neurotransmitter).

prime mover (agonist)   a muscle which contracts to perform a particular movement.

pronation   rotation movement of the forearm that turns the palm of the hand down or backwards.

pyramidal system   monosynaptic descending pathway from the motor cortex to the lower motor neurones.

receptor   specialised area of membrane at the distal end of a sensory neurone, that responds to a specific type of stimulus.

reciprocal innervation   the integration of spinal motor neurones to excite one muscle group and inhibit the opposing group.

red nucleus   an area of grey matter in the mid brain receiving fibres from the cerebellum and projecting fibres into the rubro-spinal tract for the positioning of proximal muscles of the limbs.

reticular formation   diffuse network of neurones in the brain stem.

retinaculum   band of dense fibrous tissue which binds the tendons of muscles and prevents bowstring.

rigidity   the resistance to passive movement over the whole range of a joint of a limb, due to presence of abnormal muscle tone.

sarcomere   unit of the myofibril between adjacent Z lines.

scoliosis   lateral curvature of the spine.

semicircular canals   thin tubes found in the inner ear with receptors responding to movements of the head in three planes.

sensory (afferent) neurone   carries nerve impulses from receptors in the body to the central nervous system.

sesamoid bone   found within a tendon, e.g. patella.

skeletomotor neurone   innervates skeletal muscle fibres.

slow muscle fibres   generate energy from ATP in the presence of oxygen. Specialised for long periods of muscle activity without fatigue.

somatosensory   part of the nervous system concerned with information from the body, including the skin, muscles and joints.

spasticity   a pathological state of hypertonia.

spinal nerve   one of 31 pairs of nerves leaving the spinal cord. Each nerve is formed by the joining of an anterior and a posterior root from the spinal cord.

spinal segment   portion of the spinal cord which gives origin to one pair of spinal nerves.

stereognosis   ability to identify an object by manipulation and without vision.

stretch reflex   see myotatic reflex.

striatum   caudate and putamen nuclei of the basal ganglia.

striate cortex   area of the cerebral cortex on the medial aspect of the occipital lobe where processing of visual information occurs.

subarachnoid space   the space between the arachnoid mater and the pia mater of the meninges.

substantia gelatinosa   a band of grey matter in the spinal cord round the apex of the posterior horn. The neurones form a spinal control mechanism in the transmission of pain to the brain.

sulcus (also know as a **fissure**)   a groove or furrow between adjacent gyri on the surface of the brain.

supination   rotation movement of the forearm which turns the palm of the hand up or forwards.

suture   fibrous joint between the bones of the skull.

symphysis   a secondary cartilaginous joint where the bones are joined by fibrocartilage.

synapse   a junction between a neurone with another neurone, a muscle fibre or a cell of a gland, where the transmission of nerve impulses occurs.

synaptic cleft   the microscopic space between the membranes of the presynaptic and postsynaptic neurones at a synapse.

syndesmosis   type of fibrous joint where the bones are a distance apart and they are connected by a sheet or band of fibrous tissue, e.g. middle radio-ulnar joint.

synergist   a muscle, other than the agonist or antagonist, whose activity assists in a movement.

synergy   coordinated activity in particular muscle groups to perform the movement of a limb.

synovial fluid   viscous fluid secreted by synovial membrane into the cavity of a joint or a tendon sheath.

synovial joint   the ends of two bones separated by a joint cavity and surrounded by a fibrous capsule lined with a synovial membrane.

tarsal   one of seven bones which link the tibia and fibula of the leg with the bones of the forefoot (metatarsals and phalanges).

tectum   roof of the mid brain.

tendon   cord or band of dense fibrous tissue which unites muscle to bone.

tendon organ reflex (Golgi)   inhibition (relaxation) of a muscle resulting from the stimulation of its tendon.

tension (muscle)   force generated by an active muscle to produce movement, or to resist movement.

thalamus   large oval mass of grey matter in the diencephalon on either side of the slit like third ventricle.

thenar   muscles in the palm of the hand at the base of the thumb.

tremor   involuntary rhythmic contractions of agonist and antagonist muscles, commonly in the distal segments of the limbs. May occur at rest, or on initiation of a movement (intention tremor).

tubercle   lump on a bone, created by muscle traction.

upper motor neurone   originates in a motor centre in the brain and affects the activity in lower motor neurones via descending pathways in the spinal cord.

upper motor neurone lesion   interruption of nerve impulses at any point in upper motor neurones, which results in exaggerated reflexes, abnormal movement patterns and changes in muscle tone.

ventricle   cavity inside the brain filled with cerebrospinal fluid.

vestibulo-ocular reflex   movement of the eyes in relation to the turning of the head which maintains a constant image on the retina.

vestibule   the middle part of the inner ear (utricle and saccule) with receptors responding to the position of the head with respect to gravity.

visual field   area of the visual world that is visible out of the eye in a given position.

white matter   parts of the nervous system which are mainly composed of bundles of axons, whose myelin sheaths give a white appearance.

Z line   the dark line seen by the electron microscope which marks the separation of adjacent sarcomeres in a myofibril.

Index

Index of clinical notepads